T0227021

Modern Management of High Grade Glioma, Part II

Guest Editors

ISAAC YANG, MD
SEUNGGU J. HAN, MD

NEUROSURGERY
CLINICS OF NORTH AMERICA

www.neurosurgery.theclinics.com

Consulting Editors
ANDREW T. PARSA, MD, PhD
PAUL C. McCORMICK, MD, MPH

July 2012 • Volume 23 • Number 3

SAUNDERS an imprint of ELSEVIER, Inc.

W.B. SAUNDERS COMPANY
A Division of Elsevier Inc.

1600 John F. Kennedy Blvd. • Suite 1800 • Philadelphia, PA 19103-2899

http://www.theclinics.com

NEUROSURGERY CLINICS OF NORTH AMERICA Volume 23, Number 3
July 2012 ISSN 1042-3680, ISBN-13: 978-1-4557-4945-4

Editor: Jessica McCool

Neurosurgery Clinics of North America (ISSN 1042-3680) is published quarterly by Elsevier Inc., 360 Park Avenue South, New York, NY 10010-1710. Months of issue are January, April, July, and October. Business and Editorial Offices: 1600 John F. Kennedy Blvd., Suite 1800, Philadelphia, PA 19103-2899. Customer Service Office: 11830 Westline Industrial Drive, St. Louis, MO 63146. Periodicals postage paid at New York, NY, and additional mailing offices. Subscription prices are $346.00 per year (US individuals), $531.00 per year (US institutions), $378.00 per year (Canadian individuals), $649.00 per year (Canadian institutions), $483.00 per year (international individuals), $649.00 per year (international institutions), $170.00 per year (US students), and $233.00 per year (international students). International air speed delivery is included in all *Clinics* subscription prices. All prices are subject to change without notice. **POSTMASTER:** Send address changes to *Neurosurgery Clinics of North America*, Elsevier Periodicals Customer Service, 11830 Westline Industrial Drive, St. Louis, MO 63146. **Customer Service: 1-800-654-2452 (US and Canada). From outside the US and Canada, call: 1-314-453-7041. Fax: 1-314-453-5170. E-mail: JournalsCustomerService-usa@elsevier.com (for print support) and journalsonlinesupport-usa@elsevier.com (for online support).**

Reprints. For copies of 100 or more, of articles in this publication, please contact the Commercial Reprints Department, Elsevier Inc., 360 Park Avenue South, New York, NY 10010-1710. Tel. (212) 633-3812; Fax: (212) 462-1935; E-mail: reprints@elsevier.com.

Neurosurgery Clinics of North America is covered in *MEDLINE/PubMed (Index Medicus), EMBASE/Excerpta Medica, and Current Contents/Clinical Medicine (CC/CM).*

Cover image from the American Association for Cancer Research: Vredenburgh JJ, Desjardins A, Herndon JE, et al. Bevacizumab plus irinotecan in recurrent glioblastoma multiforme. J Clin Oncol 2007;25(30):4722–9; with permission for print use only.

Printed and bound by CPI Group (UK) Ltd, Croydon, CR0 4YY

Transferred to Digital Print 2012

Contributors

CONSULTING EDITORS

ANDREW T. PARSA, MD, PhD
Associate Professor, Principal Investigator, Brain Tumor Research Center, Reza and Georgianna Khatib Endowed Chair in Skull Base Tumor Surgery, Department of Neurological Surgery, University of California, San Francisco, San Francisco, California

PAUL C. McCORMICK, MD, MPH, FACS
Herbert & Linda Gallen Professor of Neurological Surgery, Department of Neurological Surgery, Columbia University Medical Center, New York, New York

GUEST EDITORS

ISAAC YANG, MD
Assistant Professor, University of California, Los Angeles, David Geffen School of Medicine at UCLA, UCLA Department of Neurosurgery; UCLA Jonsson Comprehensive Cancer Center, UCLA Malignant Brain Tumor Program, Los Angeles, California

SEUNGGU J. HAN, MD
Department of Neurological Surgery, University of California, San Francisco, San Francisco, California

AUTHORS

ELIZABETH ALLCUT, MD
Wayne State University School of Medicine, Detroit, Michigan

ANUBHAV G. AMIN, BS
Departments of Neurosurgery and Oncology, The Johns Hopkins University School of Medicine, Baltimore, Maryland

MISHA AMOLIS, BS
Department of Neurological Surgery, University of California, Los Angeles, Los Angeles, California

ALEXANDROS BOURAS, MD
Brain Tumor Nanotechnology Laboratory, Department of Neurosurgery, Emory University School of Medicine, Winship Cancer Institute of Emory University, Atlanta, Georgia

TENE A. CAGE, MD
Department of Neurological Surgery, University of California, San Francisco, San Francisco, California

FRANCES CHOW, BA
Department of Neurosurgery, University of California, Los Angeles, David Geffen School of Medicine at UCLA, Los Angeles, California

WINWARD CHOY, BA
Department of Neurosurgery, David Geffen School of Medicine, University of California, Los Angeles, Los Angeles, California

CHAIM B. COLEN, MD, PhD
Director, Neurosurgical Oncology and Epilepsy Surgery, Assistant Professor, Department of Neurosurgery, Oakland Medical School, Beaumont Health System, Grosse Pointe, Detroit, Michigan

SAMUEL E. DAY, PhD
Medical Scientist Training Program, University of Colorado School of Medicine, Denver, Colorado

XIAOYAO FAN, BE
Norris Cotton Cancer Center, Lebanon; Thayer School of Engineering, Dartmouth College, Hanover, New Hampshire

CHRISTINA FONG, BS
Department of Neurosurgery, University of California, Los Angeles, Los Angeles, California

HEATHER M. GARCIA, BS
Department of Neurosurgery, University of California, Los Angeles, Los Angeles, California

MATTHEW C. GARRETT, MD
Resident, Department of Neurosurgery, David Geffen School of Medicine, University of California, Los Angeles, Los Angeles, California

NALIN GUPTA, MD, PhD
Departments of Neurological Surgery and Pediatrics, University of California, San Francisco, San Francisco, California

DAPHNE HAAS-KOGAN, MD
Departments of Pediatrics and Radiation Oncology, University of California, San Francisco, San Francisco, California

COSTAS G. HADJIPANAYIS, MD, PhD
Brain Tumor Nanotechnology Laboratory, Department of Neurosurgery, Emory University School of Medicine, Winship Cancer Institute of Emory University, Atlanta, Georgia

SEUNGGU J. HAN, MD
Department of Neurological Surgery, University of California, San Francisco, San Francisco, California

YASUAKI HARASAKI, MD
Department of Neurosurgery, University of Colorado School of Medicine, Denver, Colorado

BRENT T. HARRIS, MD, PhD
Department of Pathology and Neurology, Georgetown University Medical Center, Washington, DC

ALEXANDER HARTOV, PhD
Norris Cotton Cancer Center, Lebanon; Thayer School of Engineering, Dartmouth College, Hanover, New Hampshire

CHRISTOPHER JACKSON, BA
Departments of Neurological Surgery and Oncology, The Johns Hopkins University School of Medicine, Baltimore, Maryland

SONGBAI JI, DSc
Norris Cotton Cancer Center, Lebanon; Thayer School of Engineering, Dartmouth College, Hanover, New Hampshire

MILOTA KALUZOVA, PhD
Brain Tumor Nanotechnology Laboratory, Department of Neurosurgery, Emory University School of Medicine, Winship Cancer Institute of Emory University, Atlanta, Georgia

WON KIM, MD
Department of Neurosurgery, University of California, Los Angeles, Los Angeles, California

CAROL A. KRUSE, PhD
Professor, Department of Neurosurgery; Jonsson Comprehensive Cancer Center, University of California, Los Angeles, Los Angeles, California

FREDERIC LEBLOND, PhD
Norris Cotton Cancer Center, Lebanon; Thayer School of Engineering, Dartmouth College, Hanover, New Hampshire

LINDA M. LIAU, MD, PhD
Professor and Vice Chair of Neurosurgery, Director, UCLA Brain Tumor Program, Department of Neurosurgery, David Geffen School of Medicine, University of California, Los Angeles, Los Angeles, California

MICHAEL LIM, MD
Assistant Professor of Neurosurgery and Oncology, Departments of Neurological Surgery and Oncology, The Johns Hopkins Hospital, The Johns Hopkins University School of Medicine, Baltimore, Maryland

SABINE MUELLER, MD, PhD
Departments of Neurology and Pediatrics, University of California, San Francisco, San Francisco, California

DANIEL T. NAGASAWA, MD
Department of Neurosurgery, University of California, Los Angeles, David Geffen School of Medicine at UCLA, Los Angeles, California

EDJAH K. NDUOM, MD
Brain Tumor Nanotechnology Laboratory, Department of Neurosurgery, Emory University School of Medicine, Winship Cancer Institute of Emory University, Atlanta, Georgia

ANDREW T. PARSA, MD, PhD
Associate Professor, Principal Investigator, Brain Tumor Research Center, Reza and Georgianna Khatib Endowed Chair in Skull Base Tumor Surgery, Department of Neurological Surgery, University of California, San Francisco, San Francisco, California

KEITH D. PAULSEN, PhD
Norris Cotton Cancer Center, Lebanon; Thayer School of Engineering, Dartmouth College, Hanover; Dartmouth-Hitchcock Medical Center, Lebanon, New Hampshire

JILLIAN PHALLEN, BA
Department of Neurological Surgery, The Johns Hopkins University School of Medicine, Baltimore, Maryland

NADER POURATIAN, MD, PhD
Assistant Professor, Department of Neurosurgery, David Geffen School of Medicine, University of California, Los Angeles, Los Angeles, California

ROBERT M. PRINS, PhD
Department of Neurological Surgery; Jonsson Comprehensive Cancer Center, University of California, Los Angeles, Los Angeles, California

DAVID W. ROBERTS, MD
Dartmouth Medical School, Hanover; Section of Neurosurgery, Dartmouth-Hitchcock Medical Center; Norris Cotton Cancer Center, Lebanon, New Hampshire

JACOB RUZEVICK, BS
Department of Neurological Surgery and Oncology, The Johns Hopkins University School of Medicine, Baltimore, Maryland

MARKO SPASIC, BA
Department of Neurosurgery, David Geffen School of Medicine, University of California, Los Angeles, Los Angeles, California

KIMBERLY THILL, BS
Department of Neurosurgery, David Geffen School of Medicine, University of California, Los Angeles, Los Angeles, California

TOR D. TOSTESON, ScD
Dartmouth Medical School, Hanover; Norris Cotton Cancer Center, Lebanon, New Hampshire

ANDY TRANG, BS
Department of Neurosurgery, David Geffen School of Medicine, University of California, Los Angeles, Los Angeles, California

CLAIRE TU, BS
Department of Neurosurgery, University of California, Los Angeles, David Geffen School of Medicine at UCLA, Los Angeles, California

PABLO A. VALDÉS, BS
Dartmouth Medical School, Hanover; Section of Neurosurgery, Dartmouth-Hitchcock Medical Center, Lebanon; Thayer School of Engineering, Dartmouth College, Hanover, New Hampshire

ALLEN WAZIRI, MD
Assistant Professor, Department of Neurosurgery, University of Colorado School of Medicine, Denver, Colorado

BRIAN C. WILSON, PhD
Department of Medical Biophysics, Ontario Cancer Institute, University of Toronto, Toronto, Ontario, Canada

ISAAC YANG, MD
Assistant Professor, University of California, Los Angeles, David Geffen School of Medicine at UCLA, UCLA Department of Neurosurgery; UCLA Jonsson Comprehensive Cancer Center, UCLA Malignant Brain Tumor Program, Los Angeles, California

JIAN YANG, PhD
Department of Biological Chemistry, University of California, Los Angeles, Los Angeles, California

ANDREW YEW, MD
Department of Neurosurgery, University of California, Los Angeles, Los Angeles, California

CORINNA ZYGOURAKIS, MD
Resident, Department of Neurological Surgery, University of California, San Francisco, San Francisco, California

Contents

The CD133 epitope has been identified as a tumor marker for the purification of a subpopulation of glioblastoma multiforme (GBM) cells demonstrating cancer stem cell phenotypes. Isolated tumorsphere-forming CD133$^+$ GBM cells demonstrated heightened in vitro proliferation, self-renewal, and invasive capacity. Orthotopic transplantation of CD133$^+$ cells led to the formation of heterogeneous tumors that were phenocopies of the original patient tumor. In this article, the authors discuss the complex regulation of CD133 expression in gliomas, its role in tumorigenesis, and its potential as a marker for targeted and personalized therapeutic intervention.

High-grade gliomas are rapidly progressing and generally fatal neoplasms of the brain. Chemotherapy has continued to provide only limited benefit for patients harboring these tumors. The recurrence of common mutations, combined with the similarities of many of the acquired capabilities and characteristics of solid tumors, suggest many common therapeutic targets. During the past few decades, an increased understanding of many of the cellular regulatory mechanisms associated with carcinogenesis has provided an opportunity for the development of pathway-specific small molecule targeted inhibitors (SMIs). This article reviews the use of SMIs in the treatment of high-grade glioma.

This article provides historical background and current research involving the use of bevacizumab for the treatment of recurrent glioblastoma. Although bevacizumab, approved by the Food and Drug Administration, prolongs glioblastoma progression free survivial, decreases tumor vascularization, and reduces permeability of vessels, it does not seem to prolong overall survival. Despite slowed primary tumor progression, bevacizumab treatment may facilitate transformation to a more invasive phenotype. Adaptive responses, which make glioblastoma particularly resistant to various treatment modalities have been described. Conferred benefits, adverse effects, mechanisms of resistance, and potential areas for future research are discussed.

High-grade glioma continues to impart poor prognosis in spite of maximal treatment. Attempted gross total surgical resection followed by concurrent temozolomide and radiation therapy has become standard of care for glioblastoma. Ongoing clinical efforts have been directed at the further development of radiosensitizing agents that exploit tumor biology to maximize effects of concurrently administered radiation. The current article outlines the scientific rationale for the use of radiosensitizing agents and preliminary results from clinical trials using a variety of these approaches.

> Glioblastoma remains one of the most difficult cancers to treat and represents the most common primary malignancy of the brain. Although conventional treatments have found modest success in reducing the initial tumor burden, infiltrating cancer cells beyond the main mass are responsible for tumor recurrence and ultimate patient demise. Targeting residual infiltrating cancer cells requires the development of new treatment strategies. The emerging field of cancer nanotechnology holds promise in the use of multifunctional nanoparticles for imaging and targeted therapy of glioblastoma. This article examines the current state of nanotechnology in the treatment of glioblastoma and directions of further study.

> Endogenous vaults are ribonucleoproteins expressed throughout various cell types and across numerous species. Several central nervous system (CNS) tumors have been reported to exhibit high levels of major vault protein (MVP). The vault has been hypothesized to play a role in cellular transport. Although further studies are needed to elucidate the mechanisms of endogenous vault function, these advances may enable the development of targeted therapies to prevent cancer cells from acquiring MVP-related drug resistance. In addition, they seem suited for use as nanocapsules for delivering various therapeutic agents and immunogenic proteins, representing a promising prospect for CNS tumor immunotherapy.

> Immunotherapy is a potential new therapeutic option in patients with high-grade gliomas (HGGs). Phase I/II trials have assessed the efficacy of increasing immune activity using vaccines made from lymphokine-activated killer cells, cytotoxic T cells, autologous tumor cells, or dendritic cells. Studies to decrease tumor immunoresistance have focused on cytokine modulation of known immunosuppressive factors in the tumor microenvironment. Several early studies have reported a survival benefit using different forms of immunotherapy. This article discusses past clinical trials using immunotherapy in HGGs, their efficacy, limits, and biologic and clinical design challenges that must be overcome to advance immunotherapy for patients with HGGs.

> A novel mutation of isocitrate dehydrogenase-1 (IDH1) was recently found in a large percentage of secondary human gliomas. Unlike previously discovered prognostic molecular characteristics, IDH1 mutations were found across gliomas of many different grades and histologies. Further studies have illuminated its utility as a prognostic marker in low-grade and high-grade gliomas and its ability to aid the differentiation and diagnosis of various tumors with histologic ambiguity. As a metabolic enzyme, its inhibitory actions and neomorphic activity present a unique avenue in the understanding of these tumors and potentially a novel mechanism through which they may be treated.

NEUROSURGERY CLINICS OF NORTH AMERICA

DOWNLOAD Free App!

Review Articles
THE CLINICS

NOW AVAILABLE FOR YOUR iPhone and iPad

Preface

Modern Management of High Grade Glioma, Part II

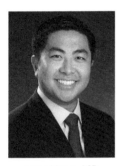 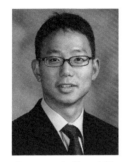

Isaac Yang, MD   Seunggu J. Han, MD
Guest Editors

Malignant glioblastoma is the most common primary brain tumor and has a poor prognosis. On average, overall survival is about one year and remains one of the most difficult challenges for the patients, families, treating clinicians, and scientific investigators in neuroscience, neurosurgery, radiation oncology, and neuro-oncology.

Despite the advances in research, knowledge, refinement of microsurgical neurosurgery, imaging, chemotherapy, and radiation, malignant glioma continues to pose a difficult challenge for those afflicted with this disease and those caregivers, family, and clinicians taking care of these patients. Recently, malignant glioma has gained an increase in public awareness as former Senator Ted Kennedy and late baseball great Gary Carter were stricken with this horrible disease. This year, over 13,000 Americans will also succumb to this affliction.

With this as the background, clinicians, investigators, and patients are courageously utilizing information, resources, and technology to improve the treatment and quality of life for patients with malignant glioma. The number of investigators and clinicians fighting brain cancer is increasing as evidenced by their growing numbers at the annual meetings for the Society of Neuro-Oncology and the AANS/CNS Section on Tumors. The work being done in clinical trials and research laboratories with novel therapies and the refinement of current strategies is moving us in the right direction.

This second half of a two-part issue of *Neurosurgery Clinics of North America* aims to provide a critical review of the modern management of malignant glioblastoma with contributions from leading researchers and world class clinicians in the field of neuro-oncology. We highlight the recent advances and evolving achievements in this rapidly developing field. There is a focus on increasingly targeted methods of immunotherapy and clinical trials, radiosensitizers, and small molecule chemotherapy for gliomas. Our issue also touches on improvements in surgical therapies with ALA, language mapping, and maximizing the quality of life in our glioma patients. Novel markers such as IDH1 and CD133 are also covered. Finally, on the cutting edge of nanotechnology, there is a focus on highlighting the potential implications of this technology for use in treating malignant glioma. These contributions are from some of the most cutting edge experts who are among the

Neurosurg Clin N Am 23 (2012) xiii–xiv
doi:10.1016/j.nec.2012.05.004

neurosurgery.theclinics.com

foremost brain tumor scientists investigating novel methods and improving our modern therapy against malignant glioblastoma.

As we improve our research, therapies, and understanding of malignant gliomas, we become better investigators and doctors trying to help our patients who are courageously fighting this formidable disease. Although we have made recent strides in our investigations, understanding, and clinical trials for this disease, there is still much research required and many advancements are yet to be made.

It is our sincere hope that our critical survey of the modern therapy for malignant glioma will spread knowledge in the field of neuro-oncology and inspire future research endeavors that will make a difference in the lives of our patients.

Isaac Yang, MD
UCLA Department of Neurosurgery
UCLA Jonsson Comprehensive Cancer Center
University of California, Los Angeles
David Geffen School of Medicine at UCLA
695 Charles East Young Drive South
UCLA Gonda 3357
Los Angeles, CA 90095-1761, USA

Seunggu J. Han, MD
Department of Neurological Surgery
University of California, San Francisco
505 Parnassus Avenue, M779
San Francisco, CA 94117, USA

E-mail addresses:
IYang@mednet.ucla.edu (I. Yang)
HanSJ@neurosurg.ucsf.edu (S.J. Han)

Immunotherapy for Glioma
Promises and Challenges

Seunggu J. Han, MD[a], Corinna Zygourakis, MD[a],
Michael Lim, MD[b], Andrew T. Parsa, MD, PhD[a],*

KEYWORDS

- Glioma • Glioblastoma multiforme • Brain tumors • Central nervous system • Immunotherapy
- Cytokines • B cells • T cells

KEY POINTS

- High-grade gliomas (glioblastoma multiforme) are the most common primary intracranial neoplasms and are associated with a poor prognosis, despite the current standard of care treatment (surgical resection, followed by radiation and temozolomide chemotherapy).
- There is active research investigating novel immunotherapies in the treatment of high-grade gliomas.
- Gliomas suppress immune function in the brain by limiting effective communication with immune cells, secreting immune-inhibitory cytokines and molecules, and expressing molecules that induce apoptosis of immune cells.
- To combat tumor-associated immunosuppression, there are 3 categories of immunotherapeutic approaches: cytokine immunotherapy, passive immunotherapy (including serotherapy and adoptive immunotherapy), and active immunotherapy.
- Although immunotherapeutic approaches have met with mixed success so far, immunotherapy continues to be actively pursued because of its potential to harness the potency, specificity, and memory of the immune system to attack infiltrating high-grade gliomas.

INTRODUCTION

The most common primary brain neoplasm, glioblastoma multiforme (GBM), is associated with a dismal prognosis. With the standard of care treatment regimen of aggressive surgical resection, radiation, and chemotherapy, the median survival remains only 14 months.[1] However, advances in conventional treatments (ie, radiation and chemotherapy) have brought only modest improvements in patient survival. As a result, new treatment modalities, such as immunotherapy, are being pursued.[2] This article describes the current strategies and results of immunotherapy for high-grade gliomas.

The central nervous system (CNS) has historically been considered an immune-privileged organ in which immune activity is significantly decreased.[3] Several unique anatomic and physiologic characteristics limit immune surveillance and response in the brain.[4] First, the CNS lacks a lymphatic system. Second, the brain is shielded from the peripheral circulatory system by the blood-brain barrier (BBB), and is therefore isolated from most peripheral immune cells, soluble factors, and plasma proteins. Third, the brain has high levels of immunoregulatory cells and factors that decrease immune function. Fourth, CNS cells express low baseline levels of major histocompatibility complex (MHC) molecules

Disclosures: The authors have no conflicts of interest to disclose.
[a] Department of Neurological Surgery, University of California at San Francisco, San Francisco, CA, USA;
[b] Department of Neurosurgery, The Johns Hopkins Hospital, Johns Hopkins University School of Medicine, Phipps Building, Room 123, 600 North Wolfe Street, Baltimore, MD 21287, USA
* Corresponding author. Department of Neurological Surgery, University of California at San Francisco, 505 Parnassus Avenue, Room M779, San Francisco, CA 94143.
E-mail address: parsaa@neurosurg.ucsf.edu

Neurosurg Clin N Am 23 (2012) 357–370
doi:10.1016/j.nec.2012.05.001
1042-3680/12/$ – see front matter © 2012 Published by Elsevier Inc.

responsible for antigen presentation to immune effector cells.[5]

Despite these factors, effective immune responses are performed in the CNS. Both the complement system[6] and the antigen-antibody system, including functional B cells,[7,8] are active in the CNS. In response to insults, CNS antigen-presenting cells (APCs), microglia, are activated, upregulate MHC and costimulatory molecules, and stimulate CD4-specific and CD8-specific T cell responses.[9–11] A small number of lymphocytes are found in normal, healthy brain,[12] and both naive lymphocytes[13] and activated T cells can cross the BBB.[12,14,15] Many different types of lymphocytes also infiltrate the CNS in the presence of disease, such as gliomas.[16–19] However, the magnitude and potency of these immune response in the CNS remain to be elucidated.[15]

TUMOR-ASSOCIATED IMMUNOSUPPRESSION

In addition to the classic hallmarks of cancer, gliomas display an additional unique feature: the ability to evade and suppress the immune system in various ways.[20] First, by limiting effective signaling between glioma and immune cells (by either expressing low levels or defective human leukocyte antigen [HLA]), glioma cells evade immune detection. A recent study by Facoetti and colleagues[21] found that approximately 50% of 47 glioma samples displayed loss of the HLA type I antigen, and a high proportion of these showed selective loss of HLA-A2 antigen as well. Loss of HLA type I antigen was more common among higher-grade tumors, suggesting a role of deficient antigen presentation in glioma progression.

Inhibition of antigen presentation by microglia and macrophages in the tumor microenvironment also contributes to the tumors' ability to escape immune detection. In vitro, the presence of glioma cells induces monocytes to reduce their phagocytic activity.[22] In addition, microglia within glioma tissue are deficient in proper antigen presentation for cytotoxic and helper T cell activation,[23] with, for example, significantly less MHC-II induction by microglia and macrophages from gliomas compared with normal brain tissue.[24] Stimulation of microglia in the presence of tumor cells also reduces the secretion of proinflammatory cytokines, such as tumor necrosis factor (TNF)-α, but increases the secretion of the inhibitory cytokine interleukin (IL)-10.[25]

The lymphocytic population is also altered in the presence of gliomas. CD4+ helper T cells have depressed function in both the peripheral blood and tumor microenvironment,[26,27] display weak proliferative responses, and produce lowered amounts of the T_H1 cytokine IL-2.[28] Most CD8+ T cells are not activated.[29] In patients with malignant gliomas, a subpopulation of T lymphocytes termed T regulatory cells (T_{reg}; eg, CD4+CD25+ cells) that suppresses activity of effector T cells is increased.[21,24,30–32] By downregulating the production of key cytokines, such as IL-2[33] and interferon (IFN)-γ[34,35] from target lymphocytes, these T_{regs} potently inhibit T cell activation, proliferation, and differentiation.[33] In vivo experiments have shown significantly improved survival after depleting T_{regs} in a murine model of glioma (GL261) by injecting an anti-T_{reg} antibody (anti-CD25+ monoclonal antibody [mAb]).[36,37]

Gliomas secrete various immune-inhibitory cytokines, such as IL-10,[38] and other immunomodulating molecules that play an important role in glioma-associated immunosuppression. Malignant glioma cells produce large amounts of prostaglandin E2,[39,40] which, in turn, inhibits IL-2 activation of lymphocytes.[41,42] They also express high levels of TGF-β2,[41,43] which is also known as glioblastoma cell–derived T cell suppressor factor (G-TsF) because of its potent inhibition of cytotoxic T cells.[44–46] Inhibition of signaling through the TGF-β2 pathway by antisense RNA in the C6 rat glioma model significantly prolonged survival[47] and, at times, eradicated the tumor.[48] These experiments strongly support the key role that TGF-β2 plays in the immunosuppression that seems essential for the survival of glioblastoma cells.

In addition to secreting immunosuppressive factors, glioma cells also express molecules that induce apoptosis of immune effectors, such as Fas ligand (FasL), galectin-1, and B7-H1, further contributing to their immunosuppressive properties.[49,50] FasL and its receptor Fas are important mediators of apoptosis in the immune system, particularly of CD8+ cytotoxic lymphocytes. High expression of FasL by human glioma cells is associated with low levels of T cell infiltration,[51] suggesting that FasL expression by tumor cells may contribute to T cell depletion in tumors by increased T cell apoptosis. However, the clinical significance of FasL expression levels remains to be determined. Like Fas/FasL, galectin-1 induces apoptosis in a variety of immune cell types through an alternate signaling pathway.[52] Overexpression of galectin-1 by gliomas[53] likely also contributes to increased apoptosis of T cells by gliomas, serving as another method of evasion from the antitumor activity of T lymphocytes. B7-H1 is a potent immunosuppressive surface molecule that induces T cell apoptosis via the PD-1 signaling pathway and is overexpressed in a subset of gliomas with particularly strong immunoresistant phenotypes.[50] Not only the glioma cells but also microglia in the presence of gliomas have increased levels of 2 of these proapoptotic factors, FasL and B7-H1.[54-56]

In addition, iatrogenic factors may cause systemic immunosuppression in patients with gliomas. Corticosteroids prescribed for tumor-associated edema may inhibit cytokine production and sequestration of CD4+ T cells.[57] However, recent evidence suggests that, at therapeutic doses, corticosteroids do not interfere with immunotherapy.[58] In addition, chemotherapeutic agents, such as temozolomide, can cause lymphopenia, particularly of the CD4+ population,[59] which may weaken the effect of immunotherapeutic modalities that depend on the CD4+ T cell response. Other chemotherapeutic agents, such as rapamycin, inhibit production of the proliferative cytokine IL-2[57] and may therefore exacerbate the immunosuppressive state in patients with high-grade gliomas.

IMMUNOTHERAPY

The major challenge in the management of malignant gliomas has been the inevitable recurrence of the tumor despite aggressive therapy. This problem highlights the infiltrative nature of high-grade gliomas, which have often already spread with evidence of diffuse microscopic disease beyond the tumor mass at the time of clinical presentation. The development of a successful mode of therapy requires systemic efficacy throughout the brain, with the ability to target tumor cells left behind after surgical resection and conventional adjuvant therapies. Such systemic therapy must also be highly specific for infiltrating tumor cells. Immunotherapy represents a promising modality, with the potential to harness the potency, specificity, and memory of the immune system to attack infiltrating glioma cells.

The main strategies in anti-glioma immunotherapy include cytokine therapy, passive immunotherapy, and active immunotherapy. Cytokine therapy is based on the concept that administration of immunomodulatory cytokines activates the immune system. Passive immunotherapy includes serotherapy, in which monoclonal antibodies are given to aid in immune recognition of tumor and to deliver toxins to tumor cells, and adoptive therapy, which involves tumor-specific immune cells that are expanded ex vivo and reintroduced to the patient. Active immunotherapy involves generating or augmenting the patient's own immune response to tumor antigens, typically by administrating tumor antigens or professional APCs.

Cytokine Therapy

Cytokines are potent immunomodulators, and immunotherapy with cytokines has been applied in oncology against a variety of tumors with variable success. To deliver cytokines to the CNS, different strategies have been explored, including injection/infusion of recombinant cytokines, vectors containing cytokine-encoding genes, cells that secrete cytokines, or cytokines linked to toxins.

The first clinical trial using cytokine immunotherapy showed promising results using intratumoral IFN-α in addition to surgery and radiotherapy,[60] but the study was limited by design flaws.[20] In contrast, Farkkila and colleagues[61] found that their IFN-γ neoadjuvant and adjuvant to radiotherapy regimen was well tolerated but did not offer a statistically significant survival benefit. Follow-up studies using systemic or intrathecal administration of IFN-α, IFN-γ, and/or IL-2 continued to find no significant improvement in survival, and patients in the treatment arm encountered considerable toxicities.[62-64] Current research is addressing improved targeting of cytokine delivery to reduce systemic toxicity and increase the effective cytokine concentrations within the tumor.

Viral vectors for local delivery of cytokines to glioma cells met with only limited success.[65-67] However, strategies using intratumoral implantation of various cell types genetically modified to produce cytokines produced more encouraging results. Injection of IL-2–secreting allogeneic fibroblasts into GL261 tumors in mice significantly delayed tumor development when injected before the tumor cells and prolonged survival in mice with established tumors.[68-70] Injection of neural stem/progenitor cells (which are attractive carrier cells because they can self-replicate, have prolonged survival, and migrate long distances) transfected to produce IL-2,[71] IL-4,[72] IL-12,[73] and IL-23,[74] improved survival in animals with established gliomas.

Alternate vehicles for intratumoral cytokine delivery include liposomes and biopolymer microspheres. Injection of liposomes containing a plasmid with the IFN-β gene into GL261 gliomas in mice induced a robust activation of natural killer cells,[75] IFN-β expression by tumor cells, significant infiltration of cytotoxic T cells, a 16-fold reduction in mean tumor volume, and a complete response in 40% of animals.[76] Biopolymer microspheres containing IL-2 were also effective in generating a specific response when injected into mice and rat gliomas.[77-79]

Cytokines have also been used to deliver toxins, such as *Pseudomonas* exotoxin, to attack glioma cells. Cytotoxic effects of *Pseudomonas* exotoxin conjugated to IL-4 (whose receptor is highly expressed on glioma but not normal brain cells[80,81]) against glioma cells have been shown in vitro.[81,82]

In the clinical trial of intratumoral injection of IL-4-*Pseudomonas* exotoxin for patients with high-grade glioma, 6 out of 9 patients showed evidence of tumor necrosis, with no significant toxicity found in any patient.[83] Clinical trials are currently underway to evaluate this modality's efficacy and maximum tolerated dose.[84,85]

Intratumoral injections of *Pseudomonas* exotoxin conjugated to IL-13R (which is similarly overexpressed in malignant gliomas[86–88]) is well tolerated in patients with recurrent malignant glioma.[89–91] Recent efforts have focused on optimizing the specificity and strength of the interaction between IL-13 and IL-13R of glioma cells,[92] as well as developing new modes to deliver the IL-toxin.[93] *Pseudomonas* exotoxin conjugated to TGF-α has also shown improvement in survival of mice bearing tumor xenografts, with greater improvements seen in mice that express the epidermal growth factor receptor (EGFR).[94,95] In a phase I clinical trial, 2 patients received intratumoral infusions of TGF-α conjugated to the *Pseudomonas* exotoxin and showed radiographic response with relative safety.[96]

Overall, immunotherapy with cytokines has shown safety, with variable efficacy. Thus, given the relative nonspecificity of cytokine therapy, it may prove most useful as an adjunct to other types of therapies. The potential use of cytokines as an adjunct to chemotherapy, termed chemoimmunotherapy, is an active area of development.[79,97]

Passive Immunotherapy

Serotherapy

Passive immunotherapy includes serotherapy and adoptive immunotherapy. Serotherapy uses monoclonal antibodies to effect an antitumor response or to achieve specific delivery of toxins, chemotherapy, or radiotherapy to tumor cells. An important determinant of its success is the identification of glioma-specific antigens (ie, specific antigens that are expressed on glioma cell surfaces but not on normal brain parenchyma). Targeted glioma antigens have included tenascin, EGFR and its mutated form EGFRvIII, chondroitin sulfate, vascular endothelial growth factor (VEGF) receptor, neural cell adhesion molecule (NCAM),[98] and hepatocyte growth factor/scatter factor.[99]

An extracellular matrix protein strongly expressed in gliomas but not normal brain, tenascin, is readily identified immunohistochemically by mAb 81C6.[100] Systemic administration of ^{131}I-conjugated 81C6 mAb to mice with human glioblastoma xenografts prolonged survival,[101,102] with evidence of radioisotope localization to the tumor.[103] Clinical trials of ^{131}I-conjugated 81C6 mAb given intrathecally have shown safety at low radiation doses, with

neurotoxicity and hematologic toxicity at higher doses.[104–106] Several phase I and II trials studying ^{131}I-conjugated 81C6 mAb injected into the surgical resection cavity in humans with glioblastoma have shown improved survival.[104,107–112]

Similar to tenascin, EGFR is specifically overexpressed by glioma cells, and signaling through EGFR is thought to play a key role in survival, proliferation, and progression of gliomas. In a clinical trial by Kalofonos and colleagues,[113] patients with high-grade gliomas were treated with ^{131}I-conjugated mAb to EGFR injected intravenously or infused into the internal carotid artery, with 6 out of 10 patients showing clinical response lasting 6 months to 3 years and no major toxicity. In another trial, a single intravenous injection of murine anti-EGFR mAb, EMD55900 (mAb 425), was given to 30 patients with malignant gliomas, showing binding of EMD55900 to the tumor in 73% of patients.[114] In a phase I/II study in which patients were given repeated infusions of EMD55900, toxicity was minimal, but no significant therapeutic benefit was found, because 46% of patients had progressed at 3 months.[115] Another trial using EMD55900 was stopped because of high levels of toxicity of inflammatory reactions.[116]

Several other phase I, II, and III trials have been conducted using EMD55900 conjugated to [125]iodine,[117–120] showing that the conjugated mAb localizes to the glioma and is well tolerated. Two phase II trials in which patients received radiolabeled mAb following standard resection and radiation therapy showed a median survival of 15.6 months[119] and 13.5 months respectively.[120] Phase III trials are currently ongoing.[117] Another trial, which used a humanized anti-EGFR antibody, h-R3, designed to inhibit the kinase activity of the EGFR receptor, showed no high-grade toxicity and an overall 38% response rate, with stable disease in 41% patients at a median follow-up of 29 months.[121]

EGFRvIII is a constitutively active mutant form of EGFR and, as a tumor antigen that likely has a large role in tumorigenicity, is an attractive target for serotherapy.[122] Systemic injections of the anti-EGFRvIII mAb 806 into mice with U87 glioma xenografts significantly reduced tumor volume and increased survival.[123]

These EGFR and EGFRvIII antibodies can provide specific targeted delivery of chemotherapeutics or toxins to glioma cells as well. Mamot and colleagues[124] used fragments of mAbs binding EGFR and EGFRvIII conjugated to immunoliposomes containing the cytotoxic drugs doxorubicin, vinorelbine, and methotrexate and observed successful intracellar delivery of these drugs to glioblastoma cells in vitro. They then showed efficacy in slowing tumor growth of EGFR-targeted immunoliposomes containing cetuximab in mouse xenograft models.[125] Antibodies have also been conjugated to several different toxins, with varying results.[126] The specificity of delivery of therapeutic agents by monoclonal antibodies to tumor-specific antigens holds great potential for limiting therapeutic toxicity in immunotherapy against gliomas.

Adoptive immunotherapy

Adoptive immunotherapy augments the antitumor response with the reintroduction of immune effector cells that have been isolated from the patient and expanded ex vivo under controlled conditions. Most adoptive immunotherapeutic strategies have used harvested lymphocytes stimulated with IL-2 to produce lymphokine-activated killer cells (LAKs). Others have used tumor-infiltrating lymphocytes; neural stem cells (discussed earlier), tumor-draining lymph node T cells; and non–MHC-restricted, cytotoxic T cell leukemic cell lines.

Jacobs and colleagues[127] reported the first clinical trial studying immunotherapy with LAKs. LAKs and IL-2 were infused directly into the tumor bed of patients with malignant glioma, with minimal toxicity,[128] and mean progression-free survival in this small cohort was 25 weeks.[129] Other trials using this technique found a small benefit in patient survival, but showed dose-limiting neural toxicity related to IL-2-induced cerebral edema.[130–132] A recent study by Dillman and colleagues[133] reported a median survival of 17.5 months in patients with GBM who had LAKs placed in the resection cavity, compared with 13.6 months in controls. In mouse models, LAKs coated with bispecific anti-CD3 and anti-glioma antibodies increase the LAK activity of peripheral blood lymphocytes against the xenograft gliomas.[134] The tumor-bed infusion of these coated LAKs in clinical trials showed promising results, with either partial or complete radiographic glioma regression in 8 of 10 patients.[135] None of the 10 patients suffered tumor recurrence during follow-up of 10 to 18 months, and 9 of the 10 control patients given untreated LAK cells developed recurrent tumor within 1 year.[135]

Tumor-infiltrating lymphocytes (TILs) found within glioma tissue contain a higher proportion of cytotoxic CD8+ T cells compared with peripheral blood. Because they are readily expanded in culture, presumably recognize 1 or more tumor antigens, and are much more cytotoxic to glioma cells than LAKs,[136] TILs are promising candidates for adoptive immunotherapy. In the GL261 murine glioma model, TILs were incubated with enzymatically digested GL261 cells and IL-2 and then infused intraperitoneally into mice harboring gliomas in the liver or brain.[137] The infusion reduced the number of liver metastases but did not lengthen the survival of animals with GL261 tumors in the brain, leading the investigators to conclude that the inefficacy of TIL therapy in the brain reflects the unique challenges of the immunosuppressive tumor microenvironment and that more efficient delivery systems need to be developed.[137] However, subsequent studies have reported success with TILs in treatment of intracranial gliomas in vitro.[138,139] Several clinical pilot studies have described the feasibility of reinfusion of IL-2 and autologous TILs expanded in vitro to patients systemically and locally with little toxicity,[140,141] but evidence for the efficacy of such a technique is currently lacking. Despite the drawbacks of TILs (including altered cellular signaling, decreased proliferation, defective cytokine secretion, decreased cytotoxic capacity, and a predisposition toward apoptosis[40,142–145]), the superior specificity of TILs compared with LAKs and early clinical success with TIL strategies warrant further investigation.

The use of tumor-draining lymph node T cells and non–MHC-restricted, cytotoxic T cell leukemic cell lines has also been explored. In a phase I trial, 12 patients with astrocytoma, anaplastic glioma, or GBM were initially given injections of T lymphocytes from tumor site–draining lymph nodes after activation and expansion ex vivo.[146] Partial regression was observed in 4 patients, and no long-term toxicity was seen during the 2-year follow-up period.[146] In another study, transfer of TALL-104 cells (non–MHC-restricted cytotoxic T cells derived from a patient with acute T-lymphoblastic leukemia) into tumor sites of U87 xenografts in mice significantly reduced tumor growth[147] and prolonged survival[148] by both direct tumoricidal action and recruitment of endogenous antitumor activity.[149] Geoerger and colleagues[150] subsequently showed evidence of significant cytotoxic activity of TALL-104 cells against several human glioblastoma cell lines in rat models, and stressed the importance of local, as opposed to systemic, administration of TALL-104 cells. Preclinical studies have characterized the cytotoxic activity, trafficking patterns, viability of TALL-104 cells under different conditions, and specific activity against brain tumor cells, concluding that TALL-104 cells are appropriate for human clinical trials.[151,152] TALL-104 implantation therapy shows killing of glioma cells, but not of normal brain cells, through a mechanism mediated by specific cytokine release, and their activity is not altered by the presence of radiotherapy or corticosteroids.[151]

In summary, like cytokine therapy, adoptive immunotherapy (using LAKs, TILs, or the other cell types discussed earlier) is not fully effective by itself, but may become an important adjuvant to standard treatments and other immunotherapies for primary gliomas.

Active Immunotherapy

Active immunotherapy involves priming or augmenting patients' immunity in vivo by vaccinating against tumor antigen. Tumor vaccines for malignant glioma have been the focus of great interest in recent years. However, successful development of glioma vaccines requires proper presentation of tumor antigens and induction of an effective, durable, antigen-specific T cell immune response. Early efforts in active immunotherapy used vaccines containing autologous tumor cells as a source of glioma tumor antigens, given with various cytokines for immune stimulation.[153–156] Despite evidence for the safety and feasibility of such techniques, many challenges in glioma vaccine development remain because of the innately poor antigen-presenting capacity of glioma tumor cells, with low levels of expressed costimulatory molecules.

To augment antigen presentation, professional APCs have been used in glioma vaccines. Recent interest has turned to dendritic cells (DCs), which have an abundant expression of costimulatory molecules and a great capacity for activating T lymphocytes. DCs that are exposed to tumor antigens are then used to initiate an antitumor response in the patient's endogenous T cells,[157] inducing T cell proliferation and generating cytotoxic responses in vitro.[158,159]

In clinical trials, autologous DCs are obtained from peripheral blood mononuclear cells or bone marrow, primed to maturation, exposed to tumor antigen in a variety of ways (including whole tumor cells, isolated peptides, tumor lysates,[160,161] or tumor RNA[161]), and then reintroduced to the patient. An early phase I trial used peptide-pulsed DCs isolated from peripheral blood and showed the generation of robust T cell infiltration into the tumor.[162] Initial efforts by Kikuchi and colleagues[163] used DCs fused to glioma cells and injected intradermally into patients with malignant gliomas. There were no adverse reactions, but a partial response in only 2 out of 8 patients was observed.[163] In a subsequent study by the same investigators, IL-12 was added to the formulation, and a more robust 50% radiographic tumor reduction was seen in 4 of 15 patients, with similar safety profiles.[164] A complete regression of glioma was achieved in the murine GL261 model when a regimen of intrasplenic vaccination with DC/tumor fused cells, local cranial radiotherapy, and

anti-CD134 mAb 7 was given.[165] Liau and colleagues[166] proposed that the most promising patient subgroup for DC vaccine therapy may be patients with small, quiescent tumors with low expression of tumor TGF-β. The phase II randomized trial using tumor lysate–pulsed DC vaccine for high-grade gliomas is ongoing.

The use of unselected tumor extracts to prime DCs in such nonspecific ways risks inducing autoimmunity against antigens of normal brain.[167] In efforts to avoid this potential hazard, focus has turned to more specific approaches using tumor-specific antigens, such as EGFRvIII, as targets for glioma vaccines. Preliminary studies using EGFRvIII peptide–pulsed DCs showed generation of cytotoxic activity against the U87 human glioma cell line.[168] A phase I trial using an EGFRvIII peptide–based vaccine showed that the therapy was well tolerated, with treated patients with GBM having a progression-free survival of 6.8 months and a median overall survival of 18.7 months from vaccination.[169] The phase II/III randomized trial of the EGFRvIII peptide vaccine with radiation and temozolomide is ongoing.

Another peptide-based vaccine currently under study is based on heat shock protein gp96 and its associated peptides isolated from patient's autologous tumor acquired at the time of surgery.[170–172] Preliminary results of the ongoing phase I/II trial have shown the vaccine to be well tolerated, with evidence of induction of tumor-specific responses.

Infectious agents have also been used to induce an antigen-specific immune response to gliomas. These vaccines contain viral or bacterial vectors that carry tumor antigen genes, and are based on the premise that an immune response to the highly immunogenic infectious agent should augment the response to the tumor antigen as well. Such an approach using *Listeria monocytogenes* has shown efficacy against extracranial but not intracranial tumors in animal models, suggesting the potential for efficacy in gliomas with improved delivery systems to the CNS.[173,174]

MULTIMODALITY IMMUNOTHERAPY

To enhance the effects of immunotherapy in combating high-grade gliomas, combinations of the approaches discussed earlier (cytokine therapy, passive and active immunotherapy) have been attempted. Cytokine and active immunotherapy strategies have been combined by introducing tumor cells or fibroblasts transfected to produce cytokines, such as IL-2, IL-4, IL-12, IL-18, IFN-α, and GM-CSF, alone or in combination with DCs.[16,175–178] Several studies suggest the promise of this strategy. Intratumoral administration of IL-2–producing tumor cells along with recombinant IL-12 significantly prolonged survival in mice with gliomas.[179] Tumor cells producing GM-CSF and/or B7-2, a costimulatory molecule, also increased survival in mice when injected locally into GBM.[180] In rat models, when complementary DNA (cDNA) of IFN-γ,[181] TNF-α,[67] and IL-4[182] was delivered retrovirally to glioma cells in situ, a strong immune response was generated and the established tumors were eliminated.

SUMMARY

The continued poor prognosis of patients with high-grade gliomas with current treatment protocols warrants new therapeutic approaches. Advanced-stage clinical trials of several promising immunotherapies are currently underway, and their results will determine the clinical value of these modalities. However, the challenges to immunotherapy remain numerous. Although immunotherapy and chemotherapy can potentially serve as coadjuvants, the current practice of administering temozolomide during and 6 months after radiation therapy interferes with the clinical testing of immunotherapies, which may be compromised both by concurrent chemotherapy and by the immunosuppression that accrues with time.

Another impediment to developing effective immunotherapy is the immunosuppressive characteristics that are the hallmark of malignant gliomas. Effective therapeutic strategies require overcoming these mechanisms by augmenting tumor antigen presentation, perhaps in a setting isolated from the tumor microenvironment. The heterogeneity of potential glioma antigens warrants research and investigation of multiple tumor-specific antigen targets. The optimal immunotherapy will likely use several of the strategies reviewed earlier and become a standard component of a combined multi-modal approach to malignant gliomas.

REFERENCES

1. Stupp R, Mason WP, van den Bent MJ, et al. Radiotherapy plus concomitant and adjuvant temozolomide for glioblastoma. N Engl J Med 2005; 352(10):987–96.
2. Pardoll D, Allison J. Cancer immunotherapy: breaking the barriers to harvest the crop. Nat Med 2004;10:887–92.
3. Medawar P. Immunity to homologous grafted skin; the fate of skin homografts transplanted to the brain, to subcutaneous tissue, and to the anterior chamber of the eye. Br J Exp Pathol 1948;29(1): 58–69.
4. Cserr HF, Knopf PM. Cervical lymphatics, the blood-brain barrier, and the immunoreactivity of the brain. In: Keene RW, Hickey WF, editors. Immunology of the nervous system. New York: Oxford University Press; 1997. p. 134–52.
5. Lampson L, Hickey WF. Monoclonal antibody analysis of MHC expression in human brain biopsies. Tissue ranging from "histologically normal" to that showing different levels of glial tumor involvement. J Immunol 1986;136:4052–62.
6. Levi-Strauss M, Mallat M. Primary cultures of murine astrocytes produce C3 and factor B, two components of the alternative pathway of complement activation. J Immunol 1987;139:2361–6.
7. Bernheimer H, Lassmann H, Suchanek G. Dynamics of IgG+, IgA+, and IgM+ plasma cells in the central nervous system of guinea pigs with chronic relapsing experimental allergic encephalomyelitis. Neuropathol Appl Neurobiol 1988;14:157–67.
8. Sandberg-Wollheim M, Zweiman B, Levinson AI, et al. Humoral immune responses within the human central nervous system following systemic immunization. J Neuroimmunol 1986;11(3):205–14.
9. Aloisi F, Ria F, Columba-Cabezas S, et al. Relative efficiency of microglia, astrocytes, dendritic cells and B cells in naive CD4+ T cell priming and Th1/Th2 cell restimulation. Eur J Immunol 1999; 29(9):2705–14.
10. Aloisi F, Ria F, Penna G, et al. Microglia are more efficient than astrocytes in antigen processing and in Th1 but not Th2 cell activation. J Immunol 1998;160(10):4671–80.
11. Brannan CA, Roberts MR. Resident microglia from adult mice are refractory to nitric oxide-inducing stimuli due to impaired NOS2 gene expression. Glia 2004;48(2):120–31.
12. Hickey WF, Kimura H. Graft-vs.-host disease elicits expression of class I and class II histocompatibility antigens and the presence of scattered T lymphocytes in rat central nervous system. Proc Natl Acad Sci U S A 1987;84(7):2082–6.
13. Krakowski M, Owens T. Naive T lymphocytes traffic to inflamed central nervous system, but require antigen recognition for activation. Eur J Immunol 2000;60:5731–9.
14. Hickey WF, Hsu BL, Kimura H. T-lymphocyte entry into the central nervous system. J Neurosci Res 1991;28(2):254–60.
15. Hickey WF. Basic principles of immunological surveillance of the normal central nervous system. Glia 2001;36(2):118–24.
16. Sampson JH, Archer GE, Ashley DM, et al. Subcutaneous vaccination with irradiated, cytokine-producing tumor cells stimulates CD8+ cell-mediated immunity against tumors located in the "immunologically privileged" central nervous system. Proc Natl Acad Sci U S A 1996;93(19):10399–404.

17. Gordon LB, Nolan SC, Cserr HF, et al. Growth of P511 mastocytoma cells in BALB/c mouse brain elicits CTL response without tumor elimination: a new tumor model for regional central nervous system immunity. J Immunol 1997;159(5):2399–408.

18. Badie B, Schartner JM, Paul J, et al. Dexamethasone-induced abolition of the inflammatory response in an experimental glioma model: a flow cytometry study. J Neurosurg 2000;93(4):634–9.

19. Sawamura Y, Hosokawa M, Kuppner MC, et al. Antitumor activity and surface phenotypes of human glioma-infiltrating lymphocytes after in vitro expansion in the presence of interleukin 2. Cancer Res 1989;49(7):1843–9.

20. Das S, Raizer JJ, Muro K. Immunotherapeutic treatment strategies for primary brain tumors. Curr Treat Options Oncol 2008;9(1):32–40.

21. Facoetti A, Nano R, Zelini P, et al. Human leukocyte antigen and antigen processing machinery component defects in astrocytic tumors. Clin Cancer Res 2005;11(23):8304–11.

22. Parney IF, Waldron JS, Parsa AT. Flow cytometry and in vitro analysis of human glioma-associated macrophages. Laboratory investigation. J Neurosurg 2009;110(3):572–82.

23. Flugel A, Labeur MS, Grasbon-Frodl EM, et al. Microglia only weakly present glioma antigen to cytotoxic T cells. Int J Dev Neurosci 1999;17(5–6): 547–56.

24. Schartner JM, Hagar AR, Van Handel M, et al. Impaired capacity for upregulation of MHC class II in tumor-associated microglia. Glia 2005;51(4): 279–85.

25. Kostianovsky AM, Maier LM, Anderson RC, et al. Astrocytic regulation of human monocytic/microglial activation. J Immunol 2008;181(8):5425–32.

26. Roszman TL, Brooks WH. Neural modulation of immune function. J Neuroimmunol 1985;10(1):59–69.

27. Roszman TL, Brooks WH, Steele C, et al. Pokeweed mitogen-induced immunoglobulin secretion by peripheral blood lymphocytes from patients with primary intracranial tumors. Characterization of T helper and B cell function. J Immunol 1985; 134(3):1545–50.

28. Elliott LH, Brooks WH, Roszman TL. Cytokinetic basis for the impaired activation of lymphocytes from patients with primary intracranial tumors. J Immunol 1984;132(3):1208–15.

29. Hussain SF, Heimberger AB. Immunotherapy for human glioma: innovative approaches and recent results. Expert Rev Anticancer Ther 2005;5(5):777–90.

30. Gerosa MA, Olivi A, Rosenblum ML, et al. Impaired immunocompetence in patients with malignant gliomas: the possible role of Tg-lymphocyte subpopulations. Neurosurgery 1982;10(5):571–3.

31. El Andaloussi A, Lesniak MS. An increase in CD4+CD25+FOXP3+ regulatory T cells in tumor-infiltrating lymphocytes of human glioblastoma multiforme. Neuro Oncol 2006;8(3):234–43.

32. Fecci PE, Mitchell DA, Whitesides JF, et al. Increased regulatory T-cell fraction amidst a diminished CD4 compartment explains cellular immune defects in patients with malignant glioma. Cancer Res 2006;66(6):3294–302.

33. Thornton AM, Shevach EM. CD4+CD25+ immunoregulatory T cells suppress polyclonal T cell activation in vitro by inhibiting interleukin 2 production. J Exp Med 1998;188(2):287–96.

34. Camara NO, Sebille F, Lechler RI. Human CD4+CD25+ regulatory cells have marked and sustained effects on CD8+ T cell activation. Eur J Immunol 2003;33(12):3473–83.

35. Piccirillo CA, Shevach EM. Cutting edge: control of CD8+ T cell activation by CD4+CD25+ immunoregulatory cells. J Immunol 2001;167(3):1137–40.

36. Fecci PE, Sweeney AE, Grossi PM, et al. Systemic anti-CD25 monoclonal antibody administration safely enhances immunity in murine glioma without eliminating regulatory T cells. Clin Cancer Res 2006;12(14 Pt 1):4294–305.

37. El Andaloussi A, Han Y, Lesniak MS. Prolongation of survival following depletion of CD4+CD25+ regulatory T cells in mice with experimental brain tumors. J Neurosurg 2006;105(3):430–7.

38. Nitta T, Hishii M, Sato K, et al. Selective expression of interleukin-10 gene within glioblastoma multiforme. Brain Res 1994;649(1–2):122–8.

39. Fontana A, Kristensen F, Dubs R, et al. Production of prostaglandin E and an interleukin-1 like factor by cultured astrocytes and C6 glioma cells. J Immunol 1982;129(6):2413–9.

40. Sawamura Y, Diserens AC, de Tribolet N. In vitro prostaglandin E2 production by glioblastoma cells and its effect on interleukin-2 activation of oncolytic lymphocytes. J Neurooncol 1990;9(2):125–30.

41. Couldwell WT, Yong VW, Dore-Duffy P, et al. Production of soluble autocrine inhibitory factors by human glioma cell lines. J Neurol Sci 1992;110(1–2):178–85.

42. Dix A, Brooks WH, Roszman TL, et al. Immune defects observed in patients with primary malignant brain tumors. J Neuroimmunol 1999;100(1–2):216–32.

43. Bodmer S, Strommer K, Frei K, et al. Immunosuppression and transforming growth factor-beta in glioblastoma. Preferential production of transforming growth factor-beta 2. J Immunol 1989;143(10): 3222–9.

44. Fontana A, Frei K, Bodmer S, et al. Transforming growth factor-beta inhibits the generation of cytotoxic T cells in virus-infected mice. J Immunol 1989;143(10):3230–4.

45. Suzumura A, Sawada M, Yamamoto H, et al. Transforming growth factor-beta suppresses activation and proliferation of microglia in vitro. J Immunol 1993;151(4):2150–8.

46. Fontana A, Hengartner H, de Tribolet N, et al. Glioblastoma cells release interleukin 1 and factors inhibiting interleukin 2-mediated effects. J Immunol 1984;132(4):1837–44.
47. Liau L, Fakhrai H, Black K. Prolonged survival of rats with intracranial C6 gliomas by treatment with TGF-beta antisense gene. Neurol Res 1998;20(8):742–7.
48. Fakhrai H, Dorigo O, Shawler DL, et al. Eradication of established intracranial rat gliomas by transforming growth factor beta antisense gene therapy. Proc Natl Acad Sci U S A 1996;93(7):2909–14.
49. Yang BC, Lin HK, Hor WS, et al. Mediation of enhanced transcription of the IL-10 gene in T cells, upon contact with human glioma cells, by Fas signaling through a protein kinase A-independent pathway. J Immunol 2003;171(8):3947–54.
50. Parsa AT, Waldron JS, Panner A, et al. Loss of tumor suppressor PTEN function increases B7-H1 expression and immunoresistance in glioma. Nat Med 2007;13(1):84–8.
51. Ichinose M, Masuoka J, Shiraishi T, et al. Fas ligand expression and depletion of T-cell infiltration in astrocytic tumors. Brain Tumor Pathol 2001;18(1):37–42.
52. Hahn HP, Pang M, He J, et al. Galectin-1 induces nuclear translocation of endonuclease G in caspase- and cytochrome c-independent T cell death. Cell Death Differ 2004;11(12):1277–86.
53. Rorive S, Belot N, Decaestecker C, et al. Galectin-1 is highly expressed in human gliomas with relevance for modulation of invasion of tumor astrocytes into the brain parenchyma. Glia 2001;33(3):241–55.
54. Badie B, Schartner J, Prabakaran S, et al. Expression of Fas ligand by microglia: possible role in glioma immune evasion. J Neuroimmunol 2001;120(1–2):19–24.
55. Dong H, Strome SE, Salomao DR, et al. Tumor-associated B7-H1 promotes T-cell apoptosis: a potential mechanism of immune evasion. Nat Med 2002;8(8):793–800.
56. Magnus T, Schreiner B, Korn T, et al. Microglial expression of the B7 family member B7 homolog 1 confers strong immune inhibition: implications for immune responses and autoimmunity in the CNS. J Neurosci 2005;25(10):2537–46.
57. Barshes NR, Goodpastor SE, Goss JA. Pharmacologic immunosuppression. Front Biosci 2004;9:411–20.
58. Lesniak MS, Gabikian P, Tyler BM, et al. Dexamethasone mediated inhibition of local IL-2 immunotherapy is dose dependent in experimental brain tumors. J Neurooncol 2004;70(1):23–8.
59. Su YB, Sohn S, Krown SE, et al. Selective CD4+ lymphopenia in melanoma patients treated with temozolomide: a toxicity with therapeutic implications. J Clin Oncol 2004;22(4):610–6.
60. Jereb B, Petric J, Lamovec J, et al. Intratumor application of human leukocyte interferon-alpha in patients with malignant brain tumors. Am J Clin Oncol 1989;12(1):1–7.
61. Farkkila M, Jääskeläinen J, Kallio M, et al. Randomised, controlled study of intratumoral recombinant gamma-interferon treatment in newly diagnosed glioblastoma. Br J Cancer 1994;70(1):138–41.
62. Merchant RE, McVicar DW, Merchant LH, et al. Treatment of recurrent malignant glioma by repeated intracerebral injections of human recombinant interleukin-2 alone or in combination with systemic interferon-alpha. Results of a phase I clinical trial. J Neurooncol 1992;12(1):75–83.
63. Buckner JC, Schomberg PJ, McGinnis WL, et al. A phase III study of radiation therapy plus carmustine with or without recombinant interferon-alpha in the treatment of patients with newly diagnosed high-grade glioma. Cancer 2001;92(2):420–33.
64. Chamberlain MC. A phase II trial of intracerebrospinal fluid alpha interferon in the treatment of neoplastic meningitis. Cancer 2002;94(10):2675–80.
65. Liu Y, Ehtesham M, Samoto K, et al. In situ adenoviral interleukin 12 gene transfer confers potent and long-lasting cytotoxic immunity in glioma. Cancer Gene Ther 2002;9(1):9–15.
66. Ren H, Boulikas T, Lundstrom K, et al. Immunogene therapy of recurrent glioblastoma multiforme with a liposomally encapsulated replication-incompetent Semliki forest virus vector carrying the human interleukin-12 gene–a phase I/II clinical protocol. J Neurooncol 2003;64(1–2):147–54.
67. Ehtesham M, Samoto K, Kabos P, et al. Treatment of intracranial glioma with in situ interferon-gamma and tumor necrosis factor-alpha gene transfer. Cancer Gene Ther 2002;9(11):925–34.
68. Lichtor T, Glick RP, Kim TS, et al. Prolonged survival of mice with glioma injected intracerebrally with double cytokine-secreting cells. J Neurosurg 1995;83:1038–44.
69. Lichtor T, Glick RP, Tarlock K, et al. Application of interleukin-2-secreting syngeneic/allogeneic fibroblasts in the treatment of primary and metastatic brain tumors. Cancer Gene Ther 2002;9(5):464–9.
70. Glick RP, Lichtor T, Panchal R, et al. Treatment with allogeneic interleukin-2 secreting fibroblasts protects against the development of malignant brain tumors. J Neurooncol 2003;64(1–2):139–46.
71. Kikuchi T, Joki T, Saitoh S, et al. Anti-tumor activity of interleukin-2-producing tumor cells and recombinant interleukin 12 against mouse glioma cells located in the central nervous system. Int J Cancer 1999;80(3):425–30.
72. Benedetti S, Pirola B, Pollo B, et al. Gene therapy of experimental brain tumors using neural progenitor cells. Nat Med 2000;6(4):447–50.

73. Ehtesham M, Kabos P, Kabosova A, et al. The use of interleukin 12-secreting neural stem cells for the treatment of intracranial glioma. Cancer Res 2002; 62(20):5657–63.

74. Yuan X, Hu J, Belladonna ML, et al. Interleukin-23-expressing bone marrow-derived neural stem-like cells exhibit antitumor activity against intracranial glioma. Cancer Res 2006;66(5):2630–8.

75. Mizuno M, Yoshida J. Effect of human interferon beta gene transfer upon human glioma, transplanted into nude mouse brain, involves induced natural killer cells. Cancer Immunol Immunother 1998;47(4):227–32.

76. Natsume A, Mizuno M, Ryuke Y, et al. Antitumor effect and cellular immunity activation by murine interferon-beta gene transfer against intracerebral glioma in mouse. Gene Ther 1999;6(9):1626–33.

77. Rhines LD, Sampath P, DiMeco F, et al. Local immunotherapy with interleukin-2 delivered from biodegradable polymer microspheres combined with interstitial chemotherapy: a novel treatment for experimental malignant glioma. Neurosurgery 2003;52(4):872–9 [discussion: 879–80].

78. Hanes J, Sills A, Zhao Z, et al. Controlled local delivery of interleukin-2 by biodegradable polymers protects animals from experimental brain tumors and liver tumors. Pharm Res 2001;18(7): 899–906.

79. Hsu W, Lesniak MS, Tyler B, et al. Local delivery of interleukin-2 and adriamycin is synergistic in the treatment of experimental malignant glioma. J Neurooncol 2005;74(2):135–40.

80. Puri RK, Leland P, Kreitman RJ, et al. Human neurological cancer cells express interleukin-4 (IL-4) receptors which are targets for the toxic effects of IL4-Pseudomonas exotoxin chimeric protein. Int J Cancer 1994;58(4):574–81.

81. Joshi BH, Leland P, Asher A, et al. In situ expression of interleukin-4 (IL-4) receptors in human brain tumors and cytotoxicity of a recombinant IL-4 cytotoxin in primary glioblastoma cell cultures. Cancer Res 2001;61(22):8058–61.

82. Joshi BH, Leland P, Silber J, et al. IL-4 receptors on human medulloblastoma tumours serve as a sensitive target for a circular permuted IL-4-Pseudomonas exotoxin fusion protein. Br J Cancer 2002; 86(2):285–91.

83. Rand RW, Kreitman RJ, Patronas N, et al. Intratumoral administration of recombinant circularly permuted interleukin-4-Pseudomonas exotoxin in patients with high-grade glioma. Clin Cancer Res 2000;6(6):2157–65.

84. Weber FW, Floeth F, Asher A, et al. Local convection enhanced delivery of IL4-Pseudomonas exotoxin (NBI-3001) for treatment of patients with recurrent malignant glioma. Acta Neurochir Suppl 2003;88:93–103.

85. Weber F, Asher A, Bucholz R, et al. Safety, tolerability, and tumor response of IL4-Pseudomonas exotoxin (NBI-3001) in patients with recurrent malignant glioma. J Neurooncol 2003;64(1–2): 125–37.

86. Kioi M, Kawakami K, Puri RK. Analysis of antitumor activity of an interleukin-13 (IL-13) receptor-targeted cytotoxin composed of IL-13 antagonist and Pseudomonas exotoxin. Clin Cancer Res 2004;10(18 Pt 1):6231–8.

87. Joshi BH, Leland P, Puri RK. Identification and characterization of interleukin-13 receptor in human medulloblastoma and targeting these receptors with interleukin-13-Pseudomonas exotoxin fusion protein. Croat Med J 2003;44(4):455–62.

88. Husain SR, Joshi BH, Puri RK. Interleukin-13 receptor as a unique target for anti-glioblastoma therapy. Int J Cancer 2001;92(2):168–75.

89. Kunwar S. Convection enhanced delivery of IL13-PE38QQR for treatment of recurrent malignant glioma: presentation of interim findings from ongoing phase 1 studies. Acta Neurochir Suppl 2003;88:105–11.

90. Kunwar S, Prados MD, Chang SM, et al. Direct intracerebral delivery of cintredekin besudotox (IL13-PE38QQR) in recurrent malignant glioma: a report by the Cintredekin Besudotox Intraparenchymal Study Group. J Clin Oncol 2007;25(7): 837–44.

91. Parney IF, Kunwar S, McDermott M, et al. Neuroradiographic changes following convection-enhanced delivery of the recombinant cytotoxin interleukin 13-PE38QQR for recurrent malignant glioma. J Neurosurg 2005;102(2):267–75.

92. Kioi M, Seetharam S, Puri RK. Targeting IL-13Ralpha2-positive cancer with a novel recombinant immunotoxin composed of a single-chain antibody and mutated Pseudomonas exotoxin. Mol Cancer Ther 2008;7(6):1579–87.

93. Vogelbaum MA, Sampson JH, Kunwar S, et al. Convection-enhanced delivery of cintredekin besudotox (interleukin-13-PE38QQR) followed by radiation therapy with and without temozolomide in newly diagnosed malignant gliomas: phase 1 study of final safety results. Neurosurgery 2007;61(5): 1031–7 [discussion: 1037–8].

94. Heimbrook DC, Stirdivant SM, Ahern JD, et al. Transforming growth factor alpha-Pseudomonas exotoxin fusion protein prolongs survival of nude mice bearing tumor xenografts. Proc Natl Acad Sci U S A 1990;87(12):4697–701.

95. Phillips PC, Levow C, Catterall M, et al. Transforming growth factor-alpha-Pseudomonas exotoxin fusion protein (TGF-alpha-PE38) treatment of subcutaneous and intracranial human glioma and medulloblastoma xenografts in athymic mice. Cancer Res 1994;54(4):1008–15.

96. Sampson JH, Akabani G, Archer GE, et al. Progress report of a phase I study of the intracerebral microinfusion of a recombinant chimeric protein composed of transforming growth factor (TGF)-alpha and a mutated form of the *Pseudomonas* exotoxin termed PE-38 (TP-38) for the treatment of malignant brain tumors. J Neurooncol 2003; 65(1):27–35.

97. Sampath P, Hanes J, DiMeco F, et al. Paracrine immunotherapy with interleukin-2 and local chemotherapy is synergistic in the treatment of experimental brain tumors. Cancer Res 1999;59(9): 2107–14.

98. Hopkins K, Papanastassiou V, Kemshead JT. The treatment of patients with recurrent malignant gliomas with intratumoral radioimmunoconjugates. Recent Results Cancer Res 1996;141:159–75.

99. Prasad G, Wang H, Hill DL, et al. Recent advances in experimental molecular therapeutics for malignant gliomas. Curr Med Chem Anticancer Agents 2004;4(4):347–61.

100. Bourdon MA, Wikstrand CJ, Furthmayr H, et al. Human glioma-mesenchymal extracellular matrix antigen defined by monoclonal antibody. Cancer Res 1983;43(6):2796–805.

101. Lee Y, Bullard DE, Humphrey PA, et al. Treatment of intracranial human glioma xenografts with 131I-labeled anti-tenascin monoclonal antibody 81C6. Cancer Res 1988;48(10):2904–10.

102. Lee YS, Bullard DE, Zalutsky MR, et al. Therapeutic efficacy of antiglioma mesenchymal extracellular matrix 131I-radiolabeled murine monoclonal antibody in a human glioma xenograft model. Cancer Res 1988;48(3):559–66.

103. Zalutsky MR, Moseley RP, Coakham HB, et al. Pharmacokinetics and tumor localization of 131I-labeled anti-tenascin monoclonal antibody 81C6 in patients with gliomas and other intracranial malignancies. Cancer Res 1989;49(10):2807–13.

104. Bigner DD, Brown MT, Friedman AH, et al. Iodine-131-labeled antitenascin monoclonal antibody 81C6 treatment of patients with recurrent malignant gliomas: phase I trial results. J Clin Oncol 1998; 16(6):2202–12.

105. Brown M, Coleman RE, Friedman AH, et al. Intrathecal 131I-labeled antitenascin monoclonal antibody 81C6 treatment of patients with leptomeningeal neoplasms or primary brain tumor resection cavities with subarachnoid communication: phase I trial results. Clin Cancer Res 1996;2(6):963–72.

106. Riva P, Franceschi G, Arista A, et al. Local application of radiolabeled monoclonal antibodies in the treatment of high grade malignant gliomas: a six-year clinical experience. Cancer 1997;80(Suppl 12):2733–42.

107. Akabani G, Cokgor I, Coleman RE, et al. Dosimetry and dose-response relationships in newly diagnosed patients with malignant gliomas treated with iodine-131-labeled anti-tenascin monoclonal antibody 81C6 therapy. Int J Radiat Oncol Biol Phys 2000; 46(4):947–58.

108. Reardon DA, Akabani G, Coleman RE, et al. Salvage radioimmunotherapy with murine iodine-131-labeled antitenascin monoclonal antibody 81C6 for patients with recurrent primary and metastatic malignant brain tumors: phase II study results. J Clin Oncol 2006;24(1):115–22.

109. Akabani G, Reardon DA, Coleman RE, et al. Dosimetry and radiographic analysis of 131I-labeled antitenascin 81C6 murine monoclonal antibody in newly diagnosed patients with malignant gliomas: a phase II study. J Nucl Med 2005;46(6):1042–51.

110. Reardon DA, Akabani G, Coleman RE, et al. Phase II trial of murine (131)I-labeled antitenascin monoclonal antibody 81C6 administered into surgically created resection cavities of patients with newly diagnosed malignant gliomas. J Clin Oncol 2002; 20(5):1389–97.

111. Cokgor I, Akabani G, Kuan CT, et al. Phase I trial results of iodine-131-labeled antitenascin monoclonal antibody 81C6 treatment of patients with newly diagnosed malignant gliomas. J Clin Oncol 2000;18(22):3862–72.

112. Reardon DA, Quinn JA, Akabani G, et al. Novel human IgG2b/murine chimeric antitenascin monoclonal antibody construct radiolabeled with 131I and administered into the surgically created resection cavity of patients with malignant glioma: phase I trial results. J Nucl Med 2006;47(6):912–8.

113. Kalofonos HP, Pawlikowska TR, Hemingway A, et al. Antibody guided diagnosis and therapy of brain gliomas using radiolabeled monoclonal antibodies against epidermal growth factor receptor and placental alkaline phosphatase. J Nucl Med 1989;30(10):1636–45.

114. Faillot T, Magdelénat H, Mady E, et al. A phase I study of an anti-epidermal growth factor receptor monoclonal antibody for the treatment of malignant gliomas. Neurosurgery 1996;39(3):478–83.

115. Stragliotto G, Vega F, Stasiecki P, et al. Multiple infusions of anti-epidermal growth factor receptor (EGFR) monoclonal antibody (EMD 55,900) in patients with recurrent malignant gliomas. Eur J Cancer 1996;32A(4):636–40.

116. Wersall P, Ohlsson I, Biberfeld P, et al. Intratumoral infusion of the monoclonal antibody, mAb 425, against the epidermal-growth-factor receptor in patients with advanced malignant glioma. Cancer Immunol Immunother 1997;44(3):157–64.

117. Brady LW. A new treatment for high grade gliomas of the brain. Bull Mem Acad R Med Belg 1998; 153(5–6):255–61 [discussion: 261–2].

118. Brady LW, Markoe AM, Woo DV, et al. Iodine-125-labeled anti-epidermal growth factor receptor-425

in the treatment of glioblastoma multiforme. A pilot study. Front Radiat Ther Oncol 1990;24:151–60 [discussion: 161–5].

119. Brady LW, Miyamoto C, Woo DV, et al. Malignant astrocytomas treated with iodine-125 labeled monoclonal antibody 425 against epidermal growth factor receptor: a phase II trial. Int J Radiat Oncol Biol Phys 1992;22(1):225–30.

120. Snelling L, Miyamoto CT, Bender H, et al. Epidermal growth factor receptor 425 monoclonal antibodies radiolabeled with iodine-125 in the adjuvant treatment of high-grade astrocytomas. Hybridoma 1995;14(2):111–4.

121. Ramos TC, Figueredo J, Catala M, et al. Treatment of high-grade glioma patients with the humanized anti-epidermal growth factor receptor (EGFR) antibody h-R3: report from a phase I/II trial. Cancer Biol Ther 2006;5(4):375–9.

122. Jungbluth AA, Stockert E, Huang HJ, et al. A monoclonal antibody recognizing human cancers with amplification/overexpression of the human epidermal growth factor receptor. Proc Natl Acad Sci U S A 2003;100(2):639–44.

123. Mishima K, Johns TG, Luwor RB, et al. Growth suppression of intracranial xenografted glioblastomas overexpressing mutant epidermal growth factor receptors by systemic administration of monoclonal antibody (mAb) 806, a novel monoclonal antibody directed to the receptor. Cancer Res 2001;61(14):5349–54.

124. Mamot C, Drummond DC, Greiser U, et al. Epidermal growth factor receptor (EGFR)-targeted immunoliposomes mediate specific and efficient drug delivery to EGFR- and EGFRvIII-overexpressing tumor cells. Cancer Res 2003;63(12):3154–61.

125. Mamot C, Drummond DC, Noble CO, et al. Epidermal growth factor receptor-targeted immunoliposomes significantly enhance the efficacy of multiple anticancer drugs in vivo. Cancer Res 2005;65(24):11631–8.

126. Hall WA. Targeted toxin therapy for malignant astrocytoma. Neurosurgery 2000;46(3):544–51 [discussion: 552].

127. Jacobs SK, Wilson DJ, Kornblith PL, et al. Interleukin-2 and autologous lymphokine-activated killer cells in the treatment of malignant glioma. Preliminary report. J Neurosurg 1986;64(5):743–9.

128. Merchant RE, Grant AJ, Merchant LH, et al. Adoptive immunotherapy for recurrent glioblastoma multiforme using lymphokine activated killer cells and recombinant interleukin-2. Cancer 1988;62(4):665–71.

129. Merchant RE, Merchant LH, Cook SH, et al. Intralesional infusion of lymphokine-activated killer (LAK) cells and recombinant interleukin-2 (rIL-2) for the treatment of patients with malignant brain tumor. Neurosurgery 1988;23(6):725–32.

130. Barba D, Saris SC, Holder C, et al. Intratumoral LAK cell and interleukin-2 therapy of human gliomas. J Neurosurg 1989;70(2):175–82.

131. Lillehei KO, Mitchell DH, Johnson SD, et al. Long-term follow-up of patients with recurrent malignant gliomas treated with adjuvant adoptive immunotherapy. Neurosurgery 1991;28(1):16–23.

132. Hayes RL, Koslow M, Hiesiger EM, et al. Improved long term survival after intracavitary interleukin-2 and lymphokine-activated killer cells for adults with recurrent malignant glioma. Cancer 1995;76(5):840–52.

133. Dillman RO, Duma CM, Schiltz PM, et al. Intracavitary placement of autologous lymphokine-activated killer (LAK) cells after resection of recurrent glioblastoma. J Immunother 2004;27(5):398–404.

134. Nitta T, Sato K, Okumura K, et al. Induction of cytotoxicity in human T cells coated with anti-glioma x anti-CD3 bispecific antibody against human glioma cells. J Neurosurg 1990;72(3):476–81.

135. Nitta T, Sato K, Yagita H, et al. Preliminary trial of specific targeting therapy against malignant glioma. Lancet 1990;335(8686):368–71.

136. Tsurushima H, Liu SQ, Tsuboi K, et al. Induction of human autologous cytotoxic T lymphocytes against minced tissues of glioblastoma multiforme. J Neurosurg 1996;84(2):258–63.

137. Saris SC, Spiess P, Lieberman DM, et al. Treatment of murine primary brain tumors with systemic interleukin-2 and tumor-infiltrating lymphocytes. J Neurosurg 1992;76(3):513–9.

138. Holladay FP, Heitz T, Wood GW. Antitumor activity against established intracerebral gliomas exhibited by cytotoxic T lymphocytes, but not by lymphokine-activated killer cells. J Neurosurg 1992;77(5):757–62.

139. Holladay FP, Heitz T, Chen YL, et al. Successful treatment of a malignant rat glioma with cytotoxic T lymphocytes. Neurosurgery 1992;31(3):528–33.

140. Holladay F, Heitz-Turner T, Bayer WL, et al. Autologous tumor cell vaccination combined with adoptive cellular immunotherapy in patients with grade III/IV astrocytoma. J Neurooncol 1996;27(2):179–89.

141. Quattrocchi KB, Miller CH, Cush S, et al. Pilot study of local autologous tumor infiltrating lymphocytes for the treatment of recurrent malignant gliomas. J Neurooncol 1999;45(2):141–57.

142. Miescher S, Stoeck M, Whiteside TL, et al. Altered activation pathways in T lymphocytes infiltrating human solid tumors. Transplant Proc 1988;20(2):344–6.

143. Miescher S, Whiteside TL, de Tribolet N, et al. In situ characterization, clonogenic potential, and antitumor cytolytic activity of T lymphocytes infiltrating human brain cancers. J Neurosurg 1988;68(3):438–48.

144. Roszman T, Elliott L, Brooks W. Modulation of T-cell function by gliomas. Immunol Today 1991;12(10):370–4.

145. Prins RM, Graf MR, Merchant RE. Cytotoxic T cells infiltrating a glioma express an aberrant phenotype that is associated with decreased function and apoptosis. Cancer Immunol Immunother 2001; 50(6):285–92.

146. Plautz GE, Miller DW, Barnett GH, et al. T cell adoptive immunotherapy of newly diagnosed gliomas. Clin Cancer Res 2000;6(6):2209–18.

147. Cesano A, Visonneau S, Santoli D. Treatment of experimental glioblastoma with a human major histocompatibility complex nonrestricted cytotoxic T cell line. Cancer Res 1995;55(1):96–101.

148. Cesano A, Visonneau S, Santoli D. TALL-104 cell therapy of human solid tumors implanted in immuno-deficient (SCID) mice. Anticancer Res 1998;18(4A): 2289–95.

149. Cesano A, Visonneau S, Pasquini S, et al. Anti-tumor efficacy of a human major histocompatibility complex nonrestricted cytotoxic T-cell line (TALL-104) in immunocompetent mice bearing syngeneic leukemia. Cancer Res 1996;56(19):4444–52.

150. Geoerger B, Tang CB, Cesano A, et al. Antitumor activity of a human cytotoxic T-cell line (TALL-104) in brain tumor xenografts. Neuro Oncol 2000;2(2): 103–13.

151. Kruse CA, Visonneau S, Kleinschmidt-DeMasters BK, et al. The human leukemic T-cell line, TALL-104, is cytotoxic to human malignant brain tumors and traffics through brain tissue: implications for local adoptive immunotherapy. Cancer Res 2000;60(20): 5731–9.

152. Gomez GG, Read SB, Gerschenson LE, et al. Interactions of the allogeneic effector leukemic T cell line, TALL-104, with human malignant brain tumors. Neuro Oncol 2004;6(2):83–95.

153. Steiner HH, Bonsanto MM, Beckhove P, et al. Antitumor vaccination of patients with glioblastoma multiforme: a pilot study to assess feasibility, safety, and clinical benefit. J Clin Oncol 2004;22(21): 4272–81.

154. Sloan AE, Dansey R, Zamorano L, et al. Adoptive immunotherapy in patients with recurrent malignant glioma: preliminary results of using autologous whole-tumor vaccine plus granulocyte-macrophage colony-stimulating factor and adoptive transfer of anti-CD3-activated lymphocytes. Neurosurg Focus 2000;9(6):e9.

155. Ishikawa E, Tsuboi K, Yamamoto T, et al. Clinical trial of autologous formalin-fixed tumor vaccine for glioblastoma multiforme patients. Cancer Sci 2007;98(8): 1226–33.

156. Okada H, Lieberman FS, Walter KA, et al. Autologous glioma cell vaccine admixed with interleukin-4 gene transfected fibroblasts in the treatment of patients with malignant gliomas. J Transl Med 2007;5:67.

157. Thurner B, Röder C, Dieckmann D, et al. Generation of large numbers of fully mature and stable dendritic cells from leukapheresis products for clinical application. J Immunol Methods 1999;223(1): 1–15.

158. Siesjö P, Visse E, Sjögren H. Cure of established, intracerebral rat gliomas induced by therapeutic immunizations with tumor cells and purified APC or adjuvant IFN-gamma treatment. J Immunother Emphasis Tumor Immunol 1996;19(5):334–45.

159. Liau L, Black KL, Prins RM, et al. Treatment of intracranial gliomas with bone marrow-derived dendritic cells pulsed with tumor antigens. J Neurosurg 1999; 90(6):1115–24.

160. Yu JS, Liu G, Ying H, et al. Vaccination with tumor lysate-pulsed dendritic cells elicits antigen-specific, cytotoxic T-cells in patients with malignant glioma. Cancer Res 2004;64(14):4973–9.

161. Yamanaka R, Abe T, Yajima N, et al. Vaccination of recurrent glioma patients with tumour lysate-pulsed dendritic cells elicits immune responses: results of a clinical phase I/II trial. Br J Cancer 2003;89(7): 1172–9.

162. Yu JS, Wheeler CJ, Zeltzer PM, et al. Vaccination of malignant glioma patients with peptide-pulsed dendritic cells elicits systemic cytotoxicity and intracranial T-cell infiltration. Cancer Res 2001;61(3): 842–7.

163. Kikuchi T, Akasaki Y, Irie M, et al. Results of a phase I clinical trial of vaccination of glioma patients with fusions of dendritic and glioma cells. Cancer Immunol Immunother 2001;50(7):337–44.

164. Kikuchi T, Akasaki Y, Abe T, et al. Vaccination of glioma patients with fusions of dendritic and glioma cells and recombinant human interleukin 12. J Immunother 2004;27(6):452–9.

165. Kjaergaard J, Wang LX, Kuriyama H, et al. Active immunotherapy for advanced intracranial murine tumors by using dendritic cell-tumor cell fusion vaccines. J Neurosurg 2005;103(1):156–64.

166. Liau LM, Prins RM, Kiertscher SM, et al. Dendritic cell vaccination in glioblastoma patients induces systemic and intracranial T-cell responses modulated by the local central nervous system tumor microenvironment. Clin Cancer Res 2005;11(15):5515–25.

167. Ludewig B, Senbein AF, Odermatt B, et al. Immunotherapy with dendritic cells directed against tumor antigens shared with normal host cells results in severe autoimmune disease. J Exp Med 2000; 191(5):795–804.

168. Wu AH, Xiao J, Anker L, et al. Identification of EGFRvIII-derived CTL epitopes restricted by HLA A0201 for dendritic cell based immunotherapy of gliomas. J Neurooncol 2006;76(1):23–30.

169. Sampson JH, Archer GE, Mitchell DA, et al. An epidermal growth factor receptor variant III-targeted vaccine is safe and immunogenic in patients with glioblastoma multiforme. Mol Cancer Ther 2009; 8(10):2773–9.

170. Yang I, Han S, Parsa AT. Heat-shock protein vaccines as active immunotherapy against human gliomas. Expert Rev Anticancer Ther 2009;9(11):1577–82.

171. See AP, Pradilla G, Yang I, et al. Heat shock protein-peptide complex in the treatment of glioblastoma. Expert Rev Vaccines 2011;10(6):721–31.

172. Yang I, Fang S, Parsa AT. Heat shock proteins in glioblastomas. Neurosurg Clin N Am 2010;21(1):111–23.

173. Liau LM, Jensen ER, Kremen TJ, et al. Tumor immunity within the central nervous system stimulated by recombinant *Listeria monocytogenes* vaccination. Cancer Res 2002;62(8):2287–93.

174. Brockstedt DG, Giedlin MA, Leong ML, et al. *Listeria*-based cancer vaccines that segregate immunogenicity from toxicity. Proc Natl Acad Sci U S A 2004;101(38):13832–7.

175. Yang L, Ng KY, Lillehei KO. Cell-mediated immunotherapy: a new approach to the treatment of malignant glioma. Cancer Control 2003;10(2):138–47.

176. Kuwashima N, Nishimura F, Eguchi J, et al. Delivery of dendritic cells engineered to secrete IFN-alpha into central nervous system tumors enhances the efficacy of peripheral tumor cell vaccines: dependence on apoptotic pathways. J Immunol 2005;175(4):2730–40.

177. Okada H, Pollack IF, Lieberman F, et al. Gene therapy of malignant gliomas: a pilot study of vaccination with irradiated autologous glioma and dendritic cells admixed with IL-4 transduced fibroblasts to elicit an immune response. Hum Gene Ther 2001;12(5):575–95.

178. Yamanaka R, Honma J, Tsuchiya N, et al. Tumor lysate and IL-18 loaded dendritic cells elicits Th1 response, tumor-specific CD8+ cytotoxic T cells in patients with malignant glioma. J Neurooncol 2005;72(2):107–13.

179. Kikuchi T, Joki T, Akasaki Y, et al. Antitumor activity of interleukin 12 against interleukin 2-transduced mouse glioma cells. Cancer Lett 1999;135(1):47–51.

180. Parney IF, Petruk KC, Zhang C, et al. Granulocyte-macrophage colony-stimulating factor and B7-2 combination immunogene therapy in an allogeneic Hu-PBL-SCID/beige mouse-human glioblastoma multiforme model. Hum Gene Ther 1997;8(9):1073–85.

181. Saleh M, Jonas NK, Wiegmans A, et al. The treatment of established intracranial tumors by in situ retroviral IFN-gamma transfer. Gene Ther 2000;7(20):1715–24.

182. Benedetti S, Bruzzone MG, Pollo B, et al. Eradication of rat malignant gliomas by retroviral-mediated, in vivo delivery of the interleukin 4 gene. Cancer Res 1999;59(3):645–52.

Glioblastoma Multiforme Treatment with Clinical Trials for Surgical Resection (Aminolevulinic Acid)

David W. Roberts, MD[a,b,c,]*, Pablo A. Valdés, BS[a,b,d],
Brent T. Harris, MD, PhD[e], Alexander Hartov, PhD[c,d],
Xiaoyao Fan, BE[c,d], Songbai Ji, DSc[c,d],
Frederic Leblond, PhD[c,d], Tor D. Tosteson, ScD[a,c],
Brian C. Wilson, PhD[f], Keith D. Paulsen, PhD[c,d,g]

KEYWORDS

- 5-ALA • Fluorescence • Glioma • Surgery

KEY POINTS

- 5-aminolevulinic acid (5-ALA)-induced fluorescence is a user-friendly, technologically efficient, and clinically safe surgical adjunct for the identification of malignant glial tumor tissue.
- A multi-institutional clinical trial comparing fluorescence-guided versus white light tumor resection reported significant improvement in completeness of resection and 6-month progression-free survival; the trial was underpowered to show improvement in overall survival.
- The degree of 5-ALA-induced fluorescence correlates with histopathologic grade of tumor, degree of tumor cell infiltration, and proliferation indices.
- Quantitative methodologies for assessment of tissue fluorescence have significantly improved the ability to detect tumor tissue and intraoperative diagnostic performance, as assessed by receiver operating characteristic curve analysis.
- These developments extend the applicability of this technology to additional tumor histologies and provide the rationale for further instrumentation development.

Over the past 2 decades, increasing evidence has accumulated correlating more complete surgical resection of malignant glioma with improved survival. Numerous surgical technologies have been developed to facilitate optimal resection, many of which function to guide the surgeon during resection. This article focuses on the use of 5-aminolevulinic acid (5-ALA)-induced fluorescence and its present role in the surgical resection of high-grade gliomas.

Disclosure of funding: National Institutes of Health Grant Nos. R01NS052274-01A2 and K25CA138578. Carl Zeiss Surgical GmbH (Oberkochen, Germany) for operating microscope equipment. Medtronic Navigation (Louisville, CO) for the StealthStation Treon navigation system. DUSA Pharmaceuticals (Tarrytown, NY) for supplying the ALA.

[a] Dartmouth Medical School, Hanover, NH, USA; [b] Section of Neurosurgery, Dartmouth-Hitchcock Medical Center, Lebanon, NH, USA; [c] Norris Cotton Cancer Center, Lebanon, NH, USA; [d] Thayer School of Engineering, Dartmouth College, Hanover, NH, USA; [e] Department of Pathology and Neurology, Georgetown University Medical Center, Washington, DC, USA; [f] Department of Medical Biophysics, Ontario Cancer Institute, University of Toronto, Toronto, Ontario, Canada; [g] Dartmouth-Hitchcock Medical Center, Lebanon, NH, USA
* Corresponding author. Section of Neurosurgery, Dartmouth-Hitchcock Medical Center, Lebanon, NH 03756.
E-mail address: david.w.roberts@dartmouth.edu

5-ALA is a precursor in the hemoglobin synthesis pathway, and exogenous, oral administration of this molecule several hours before surgery leads to the preferential accumulation of the molecule protoporphyrin IX (PpIX) within tumor cells. Under blue-violet light conditions, the fluorophore PpIX emits light in the red region of the visible spectrum, enabling identification of tumor tissue that might otherwise be difficult to distinguish from normal brain. Several commercial operating microscope systems have been adapted to use this phenomenon, providing the illumination and optical apparatus for reliable and efficient fluorescence guidance during surgery.

The greatest impediment to wider clinical application of this technology has been the limited access to 5-ALA for use in intracranial tumor resection. Approved for intracranial use in Europe, Canada, and Japan, 5-ALA in the United States has not yet received such approval by the US Food and Drug Administration (FDA). Clinical investigation in the United States at the time of this writing requires an Investigational New Drug (IND) exemption, and all clinical studies in the United States have been performed under this exemption.

EARLY WORK

One of the earliest reports of the use of 5-ALA-induced fluorescence for tumor resection was that published by Stummer in 2000.[1] In this study, 52 patients with subsequently confirmed glioblastoma multiforme (GBM) underwent fluorescence-guided resection in which all fluorescent tissue considered safe to resect was removed. Absence of contrast-enhancing tumor on postoperative magnetic resonance imaging (MRI) was documented in 33 patients (63%), with 18 of the 19 patients with residual enhancement having had residual fluorescence intraoperatively, the location of which was considered to preclude safe resection. Intraoperatively, 2 types of fluorescence were noted: solid fluorescence, which corresponded with coalescent tumor on histology, and vague fluorescence, representing infiltrative tumor. Independent factors significantly associated with survival in multivariate analysis were patient age, residual intraoperative fluorescence, and residual contrast enhancement on postoperative MRI. There was no perioperative mortality, 1 case of new, permanent morbidity (severe hemiparesis), and 3 patients with transient worsening of preexisting symptoms. No serious adverse events related to the ingestion of 5-ALA were observed.[1] This positive and encouraging experience showed the safety and feasibility of using 5-ALA-induced fluorescence as a surgical guide.

THE GERMAN MULTI-INSTITUTIONAL TRIAL

The publication in 2006 of a randomized multi-institutional study comparing 5-ALA-induced fluorescence-guided surgery with conventional white light surgery for malignant glioma[2] represented the first randomized surgical study for malignant glioma and was a landmark in fluorescence-guided surgical resection. Seventeen centers enrolled 322 patients in this study, the primary end points of which were residual contrast-enhancing tumor on early postoperative MRI and 6-month progression-free survival assessed by MRI. The study was terminated at interim analysis, with 270 patients randomized between the 5-ALA (139 patients) and white-light (131 patients) groups.[2]

Complete resection of contrast-enhancing tumor on MRI was achieved in 90 (65%) of 5-ALA patients and in 47 (36%) of white-light patients, a difference significant to $P<.0001$. Six-month progression-free survival was observed in 41% versus 21.1% of patients in the respective treatment groups, a difference that again was highly significant ($P<.0003$). There was no difference in severe adverse events at 7 days. The study was not powered to show a difference in overall survival, although restratification based on early postoperative MRI showed that patients without residual contrast-enhancing tumor of postoperative MRI had a survival advantage. Subgroup analysis also showed a longer time to reintervention for older patients (age >55 years: 10.2 months [5-ALA group] versus 7.1 months [white-light group]).[2]

The large number of well-documented patients undergoing GBM resection in the German ALA Glioma Study Group afforded an opportunity to look at the effect of completeness of resection on postoperative MRI with overall survival in patients stratified with respect to the recursive partitioning analysis (RPA) of the Radiation Therapy Oncology Group (RTOG).[3] Historically, the confounding variable of patient selection bias has rendered difficult the interpretation of any intervention effect in malignant glioma, and this partitioning strategy recognizes the important prognostic variables of age, Karnofsky Performance Scale (KPS), neurologic condition, and mental status.

The 243 patients with newly diagnosed GBM in the multicenter German study, independent of their assignment to 5-ALA or white-light groups, were looked at with respect to their RTOG-RPA class. Median overall survival times for classes III, IV, and V were 17.8, 14.7, and 10.7 months, respectively; 2-year survival in these classes were 26%, 12%, and 7%. Stratification for completeness of resection within RPA class revealed clear differences: for class IV, survival with complete resection was 17.7 months versus 12.9 months with incomplete resection, and for class V, survival of 13.7 months versus 10.4 months. Two-year survival within class IV was 21.0% versus 4.4%, and within class V, 11.1% versus 2.6%. The number of patients within class III was too small to detect significant differences. Overall, the predictive capability of the RTOG-RPA classes was confirmed by the ALA Glioma Study Group, and differences in survival seen in class IV and class V support a relationship between maximum cytoreduction and survival.[4]

In the 2006 report of the ALA Glioma Study Group, only marginal differences were found between the 5-ALA and white-light groups. In a 2011 study, the investigators looked more closely at the issue of neurologic morbidity using the final intent-to-treat patient populations of their study (176 patients in the 5-ALA group and 173 in the white-light group). This analysis again confirmed the earlier findings of more complete tumor resection and improved progression-free survival. Using the National Institutes of Health Stroke Scale (NIH-SS) as a measure of neurologic status, the analysis also showed

a higher incidence of deterioration in the NIH-SS by 1 or more points at the 48-hour postoperative time point in the 5-ALA group (26.2% vs 14.5%; $P = .02$). This measure was no longer statistically significant at 7 days, and at 3 months, the percentages with neurologic deterioration of 1 point or greater were 19.6% versus 18.6%, respectively. KPS scores showed no statistically significant differences between the 2 groups (deterioration in the KPS score at 6 weeks postoperatively seen in 32.9% for the ALA group vs 28.8% for the white-light group, $P = 1.0$, and deterioration at 6 months seen in 35.7% and 49.1%, respectively, $P = .12$). Patients at risk of neurologic deterioration were those with preexisting neurologic deficits unresponsive to steroids, consistent with these deficits more likely related to tumor infiltration than surrounding edema.[5]

Further analysis in this same study attempted to assess the trade-off between a higher incidence of temporary and generally mild neurologic deterioration with 5-ALA-guided resection and improved likelihood of complete resection. In long-term

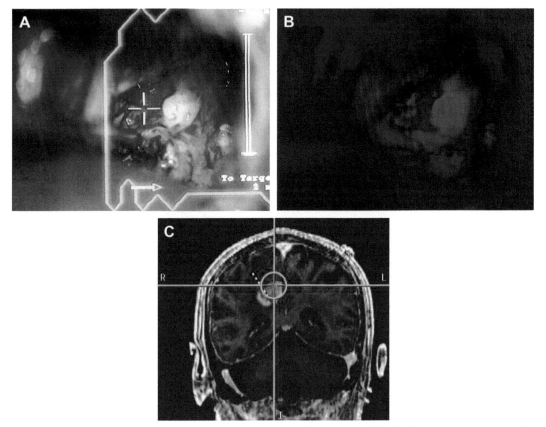

Fig. 1. (*A*) White-light operating microscope image at partial resection of this left parietal GBM tumor in a 79-year-old man. (*B*) Blue-violet light image of the same operative field. (*C*) Image guidance monitor image showing location of the focal point of the operating microscope at corresponding time during the procedure.

follow-up, a higher incidence of repeat surgery was found in the white-light group (39% vs 30%, $P = .0311$). Stratification by completeness of resection showed quicker time to progression and neurologic deterioration in those patients with incomplete resection ($P = .0036$).[5]

DARTMOUTH STUDIES

The aim of an initial investigative study at our institution using 5-ALA-induced fluorescence guidance in 11 patients with newly diagnosed GBM was to study the correlation between intraoperative visual fluorescence and preoperative MRI features as well as between fluorescence and histopathology (**Figs. 1** and **2**). Using a study design in which multiple locations of fluorescence assessment were spatially coregistered with preoperative MRI using image guidance, highly significant differences were found between fluorescent and nonfluorescent tissue in 2 measures of MRI contrast enhancement (gadolinium-enhanced signal intensity, $P = .018$; and normalized contrast ratio, $P<.001$).[6]

Biopsy specimens were obtained at each of 124 spatially coregistered sites in these 11 patients, 86 of which (69.4%) reported intraoperative fluorescence. Eighty-two of these 86 specimens (95.3%) were positive for tumor cells; 3 specimens (3.5%) showed either necrosis or abnormal, prominent vasculature, and 1 specimen (1.2%) showed no abnormality. Of the 38 nonfluorescent specimens, 28 (73.7%) were positive for tumor cells, 8 (21.1%) showed either necrosis or abnormal, prominent vasculature or reactive gliosis, and 2 (5.3%) showed no abnormalities. The sensitivity of visual fluorescence to identify tumor in this study was 0.75 (95% confidence interval [CI], 0.65–0.82); the specificity, 0.71 (0.42–0.90); the positive predictive value, 0.95 (0.88–0.98); and the negative predictive value, 0.26

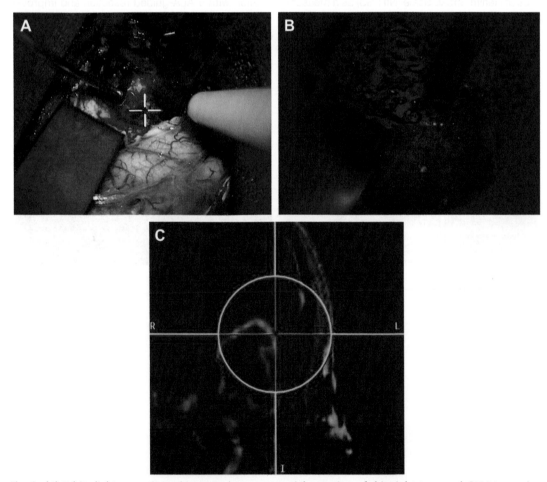

Fig. 2. (*A*) White-light operating microscope image at partial resection of this right temporal GBM tumor in a 68-year-old man. (*B*) Blue-violet light image of the same operative field. (*C*) Image guidance monitor image showing location of the focal point of the operating microscope at corresponding time during the procedure.

(0.14–0.43). As an indicator of abnormal tissue consistent with tumor, fluorescence had a positive predictive value of 0.99 (95% CI, 0.93–1.00). A low negative predictive value reflected the nonfluorescent property of fully necrotic tissue.[6]

Biopsy specimens in this study were also graded by World Health Organization (WHO) criteria for glial tumors (0–IV), independent of the overall WHO grade, which was IV for all patients. A Spearman rank correlation analysis was performed between this histologic grade and the level of visual fluorescence (0–3), yielding a correlation coefficient of 0.51 (P<.001). A similar analysis was performed between the degree of tumor infiltration in each biopsy specimen and the level of visual fluorescence, and again a highly significant correlation coefficient of 0.49 was found (P<.001). When a measure of the extent of necrosis was analyzed with respect to visual fluorescence, no statistical correlation was found (correlation coefficient –0.02; P = .79).[6]

Quantitative ex vivo tissue measurements of PpIX and Ki-67 immunohistochemistry to assess tissue proliferation were the focus of another study involving 23 patients undergoing fluorescence-guided resection of either low-grade or high-grade glial tumor (**Fig. 3**). Biopsy specimens from sites showing visual fluorescence had significantly higher levels of PpIX and tissue proliferation. Quantitative PpIX concentration (C_{PpIX}) levels correlated strongly with proliferation index ($r = 0.70$, P<.0001). Increasing levels of C_{PpIX} indicated regions of increasing malignancy. Approximately 40% of biopsies that were positive for tumor histologically but nonfluorescent intraoperatively had C_{PpIX} levels greater than 0.1 µg/mL; only 2 specimens with levels greater than this threshold were negative for tumor. Showing a quantitative relationship between C_{PpIX} and increasing malignancy in both low-grade and high-grade gliomas, this study suggests an opportunity for greater use of this fluorescence technology through improved PpIX fluorescence detection.[7]

Toward this aim, a handheld fiber-optic probe for in vivo quantitative fluorescence measurement has been developed and used clinically. Connected to a spectrometer, this probe interrogates tissue with emission of a blue-violet light (405-nm wavelength)

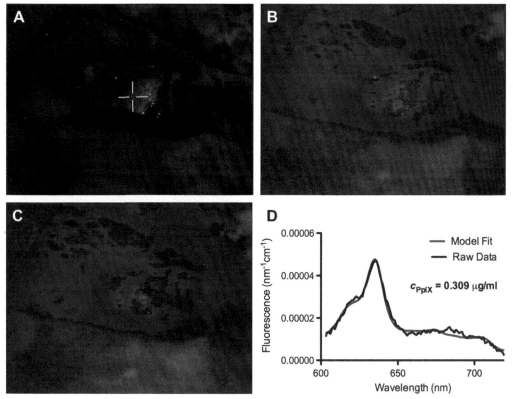

Fig. 3. (A) White-light operating microscope image at late stage of resection of a left temporal lobe GBM in a 73-year-old man. (B) Blue-violet light image corresponding to (A). (C) Handheld quantitative fluorescence probe acquiring data. (D) Raw and modeled data from probe acquisition, showing a quantitative level of the fluorophore PpIX that indicates tumor.

and with white light (450-nm to 720-nm wavelength), the latter enabling the accounting for tissue light absorption and scattering, and correction of the fluorescence spectrum. Spectral decomposition then allows determination of PpIX concentration. This device was used in a series of 14 patients harboring a variety of tumors including low-grade and high-grade gliomas as well as metastatic tumors and meningiomas, operated on using 5-ALA-induced fluorescence guidance.[8]

A statistically significant increase in C_{PpIx} ($P<.05$) was seen across all tumor types. Other spectroscopic variables (A_{615}, A_{660}, P_{635} and P_{710}) did not show similar ability to discriminate between tumor and nontumor tissue. Assessment of the diagnostic performance of this probe was then performed using a receiver operating characteristic (ROC) curve analysis and area under the curve (AUC) as a measure of performance. Comparing visual fluorescence (as used in all of the previously described clinical studies) with quantitative fluorescence by this metric, the AUC for high-grade gliomas improved from 0.78 ± 0.06 to 0.96 ± 0.03. Perhaps more important, for the implications with respect to potential application, the AUC for low-grade gliomas (which historically have not shown significant visible fluorescence) improved from 0.54 ± 0.04 to 0.75 ± 0.12, a level of performance below that of quantitative fluorescence in high-grade gliomas but comparable with that of visible fluorescence in those same high-grade tumors. For all of the tumors in this study, quantitative PpIX concentrations had a sensitivity of 84%, a specificity of 92%, a positive predictive value of 95%, and a negative predictive value of 77% (classification efficiency of 87% vs 66% for visible fluorescence). Of course, these values are dependent on the cutoff, or threshold, values chosen, which in this instance were those points on the ROC curve closest to the upper left corner; different threshold values may be chosen, should one wish to weight sensitivity and specificity differently.[8]

PROPOSED RTOG TRIAL

In an effort both to begin larger deployment of this technology in the United States as well as to acquire data required for FDA approval of 5-ALA for intracranial tumor resection, a phase III randomized, placebo-controlled, multicenter trial clinical trial using 5-ALA fluorescence guidance for resection of newly diagnosed GBM is anticipated to begin later this year. Coordinated by Emory University, this study is currently planned to determine whether fluorescence-guided resection improves extent of resection and whether improved extent of resection is associated with improved overall survival.

SUMMARY

Fluorescence guidance in resection of malignant glioma has been shown to improve extent of resection and 6-month progression-free survival in a prospective, multi-institutional clinical trial in Europe, and preliminary experience in the United States has confirmed the high correlation of this fluorescence with imaging and histologic features of malignant tumor. In this early experience, deployment of more sophisticated methods capable of increasing the diagnostic capability of this technique as well as extending the application of the technology to other tumor types have confirmed the potential of fluorescence guidance. Although the as yet unapproved FDA status of 5-ALA has slowed widespread dissemination of this technology, an increasing number of centers are using the drug under IND approvals; a large multicenter trial oriented toward providing data necessary for FDA approval is about to commence.

REFERENCES

1. Stummer W, Novotny A, Stepp H, et al. Fluorescence-guided resection of glioblastoma multiforme by using 5-aminolevulinic acid-induced porphyrins: a prospective study in 52 consecutive patients. J Neurosurg 2000;93(6):1003–13.

2. Stummer W, Pichlmeier U, Meinel T, et al. Fluorescence-guided surgery with 5-aminolevulinic acid for resection of malignant glioma: a randomised controlled multicentre phase III trial. Lancet Oncol 2006;7(5): 392–401.

3. Curran WJ Jr, Scott CB, Horton J, et al. Recursive partitioning analysis of prognostic factors in three Radiation Therapy Oncology Group malignant glioma trials. J Natl Cancer Inst 1993;85(9):704–10.

4. Pichlmeier U, Bink A, Schackert G, et al. Resection and survival in glioblastoma multiforme: an RTOG recursive partitioning analysis of ALA study patients. Neuro Oncol 2008;10(6):1025–34.

5. Stummer W, Tonn JC, Mehdorn HM, et al. Counterbalancing risks and gains from extended resections in malignant glioma surgery: a supplemental analysis from the randomized 5-aminolevulinic acid glioma resection study. J Neurosurg 2011;114(3): 613–23.

6. Roberts DW, Valdes PA, Harris BT, et al. Coregistered fluorescence-enhanced tumor resection of malignant glioma: relationships between delta-aminolevulinic acid-induced protoporphyrin IX fluorescence, magnetic resonance imaging enhancement, and neuropathological parameters. J Neurosurg 2011; 114(3):595–603.

7. Valdes PA, Kim A, Brantsch M, et al. Delta-aminolevulinic acid-induced protoporphyrin IX concentration

correlates with histopathologic markers of malignancy in human gliomas: the need for quantitative fluorescence-guided resection to identify regions of increasing malignancy. Neuro Oncol 2011;13(8):846–56.

8. Valdes PA, Leblond F, Kim A, et al. Quantitative fluorescence in intracranial tumor: implications for ALA-induced PpIX as an intraoperative biomarker. J Neurosurg 2011;115(1):11–7.

Potential Role for STAT3 Inhibitors in Glioblastoma

Christopher Jackson, BA[a,b], Jacob Ruzevick, BS[a,b], Anubhav G. Amin, BS[a,b], Michael Lim, MD[a,b,*]

KEYWORDS

- Glioblastoma multiforme • STAT3 • Signal transducers and activators of transcription • Inhibitors

KEY POINTS

- Signal transducers and activators of transcription 3 (STAT3) is a transcription factor involved in cell differentiation, proliferation, and survival.
- In a variety of tumors, including glioblastoma multiforme (GBM), constitutive activation of STAT3 has been implicated as a critical mediator of tumorigenesis and progression.
- Constitutive activation of STAT3 in the GBM microenvironment drives angiogenesis, tumor cell proliferation, invasion, and immunosuppression.
- Targeting STAT3 affords an opportunity to intervene on multiple pro-oncogenic pathways at a single molecular hub.
- Clinical implementation of STAT3 blockade in GBM awaits the identification of safe and effective strategies for inhibiting STAT3 and the development of technologies that improve delivery of these agents to the CNS.

INTRODUCTION

Signal transducers and activators of transcription (STATs) are a family of transcription factors that are activated by membrane-bound receptors and subsequently translocate to the nucleus to promote expression of a variety of genes associated with cell survival, differentiation, and proliferation.[1] The STAT family includes 7 proteins (STATs 1, 2, 3, 4, 5a, 5b, and 6) with an array of functions but a common molecular structure that reflects a highly conserved mechanism of activation and signaling.[2] Given their established role in regulating cell survival and proliferation, it is not surprising that STATs have emerged as critical mediators of oncogenesis. In particular, STAT3 has been targeted for antineoplastic therapy because of its role as molecular conversion point for several pro-oncogenic processes, including disrupted growth regulation, apoptosis, angiogenesis, invasion, and modulation of the host immune system.[3] Furthermore, STAT3 is constitutively active in a wide variety of cancers and has generally been associated with poor prognosis, although this remains controversial.[4,5] Nevertheless, the preponderance of available data support a pro-oncogenic role for STAT3 and STAT3 blockade alone is sufficient to inhibit malignant transformation in some model systems.[6,7]

Glioblastoma multiforme (GBM) is the most common and aggressive primary brain tumor. The current standard of care for GBM involves a tripartite treatment approach of cytoreductive surgery, targeted irradiation, and temozolomide.[8] Despite maximally aggressive therapy, the median survival for patients with GBM is only 14.6 months, with a 3-year survival rate of approximately 10%.[8] Hallmarks of GBM pathogenesis include the invasion of healthy brain tissue,[9] neovascularization,[10]

[a] Department of Neurosurgery, The Johns Hopkins University School of Medicine, Baltimore, MD, USA;
[b] Department of Oncology, The Johns Hopkins University School of Medicine, Baltimore, MD, USA
* Corresponding author. Department of Neurosurgery, The Johns Hopkins University School of Medicine, Phipps 123, 600 North Wolfe Street, Baltimore, MD 21287.
E-mail address: mlim3@jhmi.edu

Neurosurg Clin N Am 23 (2012) 379–389
doi:10.1016/j.nec.2012.04.002
1042-3680/12/$ – see front matter © 2012 Elsevier Inc. All rights reserved.

local hypoxia and necrosis,[11] and local and systemic immunosuppression.[12,13] Several diverse cell populations have been implicated in GBM pathogenesis. For example, cancer stem cells have been identified as a distinct cell population in GBM and are thought to be largely resistant to standard therapies.[14,15] In addition, endothelial cells of tumor-associated vasculature have been reported to harbor the same mutations as bulk tumor cells[16] and may be derived from cancer stem cells.[17,18] Coordinated interactions among these diverse cell types dictate GBM behavior and susceptibility to therapeutics. In the case of cancer stem cells, evidence suggests that GBM stem cells in culture may be susceptible to radiation[19] but acquire radioresistance within the perivascular niche.[20]

The complexity of the tumor microenvironment presents a formidable challenge to the development of effective therapies. STAT3 has emerged as an appealing target for GBM therapy because it has been implicated in several pro-oncogenic processes. In addition, constitutive activation of STAT3 has been reported in GBM and may be associated with a poor prognosis.[21] Accordingly, targeting STAT3 affords a potential therapeutic focal point, allowing a single therapy to target multiple pro-oncogenic processes. Preclinical studies suggest that STAT3 blockade has antitumor activity in vitro[22] and in vivo.[23] However, more recent evidence indicates that the role of STAT3 may be more nuanced than initially appreciated, alternately having protumor or antitumor effects depending on the genetic profile of the tumor.[5] Here the authors review the potential role of STAT3 as a therapeutic target in GBM.

STAT3 SIGNALING PATHWAY

STAT3 is a member of the STAT family of cytoplasmic transcription factors, which transmit signals from the cell surface to the nucleus in response to extracellular cytokines, growth factors, hormones, and oncoproteins.[24,25] STAT3 contains an N-terminal domain, a coiled-coil domain, a DNA-binding domain, a linker domain, an Src Homology 2 (SH2) domain, and a transactivation domain.[26] The function of each of these domains is summarized in **Table 1**.

STAT3 exists as an inactive monomer and is activated by the phosphorylation of tyrosine 705 (Y^{705}) by Janus tyrosine kinases (JAK), membrane-associated tyrosine kinases, and nonreceptor tyrosine kinases.[26–31] Another major activator of STAT3 is interleukin-6 (IL-6). When IL-6 binds to the IL-6 receptor (IL-6r), the functional subunit (gp130) facilitates the formation of a STAT3 homodimer via

Table 1
STAT3 domains

Domain	Function
N-terminal	Stabilization of STAT3 dimers and STAT3-DNA interactions
Coiled-coil	Interaction with other proteins
DNA binding	Interaction with DNA strand
SH2	Dimerization
Transactivation	Interaction with transcriptional machinery

phosphorylation of the cytoplasmic tails. The activated complex is then able to activate downstream JAK signaling proteins. The gp130 subunit of the IL6/IL6r complex also provides docking sites for STAT3 monomers using the SH2 domain.[32–34] Subsequently, STAT3 is phosphorylated by the JAK family of kinases leading to dimerization via phosphotyrosine interactions within the SH-2 domains. Following dimerization, STAT3 translocates to the nucleus where it binds to specific DNA promoters and regulates transcription.[35] STAT3 activation and signaling is reviewed in **Fig. 1**.

Increased activation of STAT3 results from the disruption of proteins that regulate STAT3 expression and activation. The critical regulators of STAT3 activity include IL-4,[36] IL-6,[37–40] epidermal growth factor receptor (EGFR),[41,42] fibroblast growth factor,[43] leptin,[44] MicroRNA-21,[45] PPARγ,[46] PIAS3,[47,48] PTPRD,[49] and SOCS3.[47] Furthermore, STAT3 activity is increased under conditions of hypoxia, infection, stress, and UV radiation.[50,51] Once bound to DNA, STAT3 influences the expression of genes involved in cell cycle regulation, apoptosis, migration, angiogenesis, and invasion via the activation of B-cell lymphoma 2 (Bcl-2), B-cell lymphoma-extra large (Bcl-xL), c-Myc, cyclin D1, Mcl-1, matrix metallopeptidase 9 (MMP9), and survivin.[52,53]

ROLE OF STAT3 IN ONCOGENESIS
Immune Evasion

GBMs have long been documented to suppress the immune system in patients, locally in the tumor microenvironment and systemically.[54] GBMs have evaded the immune system via several mechanisms. Patients with GBM have been shown to exhibit T-cell anergy, lymphopenia, impaired antibody production, impaired lymphocyte protein synthesis, and impaired lymphocyte responsiveness.[55–61] Thus, GBMs evade the immune system at the levels of antigen recognition and immune activation.

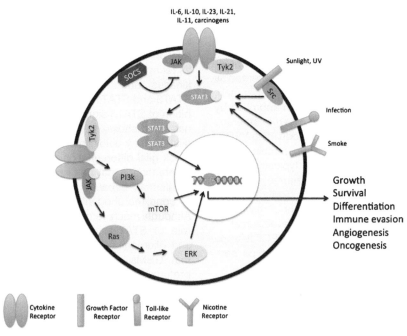

Fig. 1. Pathways involved in the activation of STAT3. STAT3 is activated when Tyrosine 705 is phosphorylated by various intracellular kinases, including JAK, Src, mTOR, and ERK. The activity of these kinases can be increased by various hormones, cytokines, and environmental factors acting at the extracellular surface.

STAT3 has been implicated as a key negative regulator of antitumor immune responses within the GBM microenvironment.[62] STAT3 activity in tumors has been shown to coordinate tumor immune evasion via multiple mechanisms. For example, STAT3 activity restricts immune surveillance by suppressing the release of proinflammatory cytokines and chemokines. Furthermore, constitutive activation of STAT3 in tumors cells has been shown to increase the secretion of soluble immunosuppressive factors,[63] such as IL-10, which negatively affects the Th1 immune response,[64] and vascular endothelial growth factor (VEGF), which feeds back to further activate STAT3 in immature dendritic cells. STAT3 expression in immature dendritic cells subsequently leads to the inhibition of dendritic maturation and activation[65] by suppressing the expression of major histocompatibility complex (MHC) class II, costimulatory molecules, and IL-12.[63] Because mature dendritic cells are the primary antigen presenting cells, STAT3-mediated inhibition of dendritic cell maturation effectively disrupts both the innate and adaptive immune responses. Conversely, inducible ablation of STAT3 in hematopoietic cells enhances dendritic cell maturation.[66]

In addition to inhibiting dendritic cell maturation, STAT3 seems to modulate multiple elements of innate and adaptive immunity. STAT3 is constitutively activated in natural killer cells, neutrophils,

and macrophages present in the tumor stroma, and STAT3 ablation results in enhanced antitumor activity in these cell types and in T lymphocytes.[66] Thus, it seems that constitutive STAT3 activation in the tumor drives a feed-forward mechanism of constitutive STAT3 activation in tumor-interacting immune cells, which drives widespread immune suppression.[67]

STAT3 expression also plays a role in the proliferation and function of regulatory T (Treg) cells,[66] a population of CD4+ T cells that accumulates inside tumors[68] and has suppressive activity toward effector T cells and other immune cell types.[69] Treg cell activation and expansion has been repeatedly shown to require direct contact with dendritic cells residing in tumors.[70–74] Subsequently, Treg cells secrete transforming growth factor β (TGFβ), leading to the suppression of CD8+ T-cell activation.[73,75]

STAT3 activity has been associated with the expansion of a lineage of T-helper cells characterized by the expression of IL-17 (Th17 cells).[76] Several studies indicate that STAT3 is critical for Th17 expansion.[77–80] Although the role of Th17 cells in immune evasion has not been clearly established, emerging evidence suggests that skewing of the T-helper cell response toward Th17 differentiation mutes the antitumor Th1 response and facilitates tumor progression.[81]

Angiogenesis

Angiogenesis has been shown to play a critical role in GBM progression.[82] The formation of new blood vessels in GBM is mediated by the elevated expression of VEGF.[83] Accordingly, VEGF has emerged as a prominent antiangiogenesis target; bevacizumab, an antibody against VEGF, has been approved by the Food and Drug Administration as monotherapy for recurrent GBM.[84,85] Factors modulating VEGF-mediated angiogenesis, however, remain poorly understood; although patients typically exhibit radiographic regression on bevacizumab, an overall survival benefit has not been clearly demonstrated.[86] Although the development of resistance plays a role in progression on bevacizumab,[87] some investigators suggest that anti-VEGF therapy induces a more invasive tumor phenotype secondary to local hypoxia.[88]

STAT3 has been implicated as a downstream effector in the VEGF angiogenesis signaling pathway. Yahata and colleagues[89] demonstrated that exposing human endothelial cells to VEGF in vitro results in nuclear translocation of phosphorylated-STAT3 (p-STAT3) and that blocking STAT3 activity leads to a reduction in endothelial cell migration and tube formation. STAT3 has also been shown to localize to glioma endothelial cells.[90] Furthermore, hypoxia induces STAT3 activation and nuclear translocation and enhances endothelial tube formation and tumor cell migration in GBM cell lines.[91] STAT3 also acts reciprocally to upregulate VEGF expression.[90] Although the connection between STAT3 and VEGF has been most extensively studied in GBM cell lines, in vivo studies in other tumors have demonstrated a correlation between STAT3 activity, VEGF expression, and tumor progression.[92] Based on these data, blocking STAT3 in GBM may have potent effects as an antiangiogenesis therapy. Additional research is needed to determine if STAT3 blockade elicits similar escape mechanisms and induces the invasive phenotype observed with VEGF inhibitors.

Differentiation

GBMs are characterized by a high degree of molecular,[93] histologic, and phenotypic diversity, suggesting that the inciting events in GBM pathogenesis likely occur early in the process of glial differentiation.[94,95] Neural stem cells give rise to all components of the nervous system. Although GBM cells share few characteristics with differentiated glia, some of the defining characteristics of neural stem cells, such as migration[96] and milieu-dependent differentiation,[97] are hallmarks of gliomagenesis.

Evidence suggests that STAT3 may play a crucial role in normal and pathologic glial differentiation through interactions with the ciliary neurotrophic factor (CNTF).[98,99] Binding of CNTF to its receptor leads to the activation of JAK tyrosine kinases and subsequent phosphorylation of STAT3 and STAT1 via their SH2 domains.[100] Inhibition of STAT3 signaling in neural precursor cells has been shown to prevent the activation of the glial fibrillary acidic protein (GFAP) promoter and block glial differentiation.[98] STAT3-mediated glial differentiation may be disrupted in at least a subset of gliomas because of the epigenetic silencing of bone morphogenic protein receptor-1B.[101,102] Although much remains to be learned about the role of STAT3 activation in glial differentiation and gliomagenesis, available evidence indicates that GBMs may be able to capitalize on the protumorigenic effects of constitutive STAT3 activation without compromising their undifferentiated phenotype. Therefore, it may be reasonable to speculate that STAT3 activation can be therapeutically blocked with relative impunity regarding glial differentiation. Conversely, some studies indicate that STAT3 blockade may induce differentiation of GBM stem cells.[103] Future studies are needed to clearly elucidate the relationship between STAT3 activation, glial differentiation, and GBM pathogenesis.

Survival and Proliferation

STAT3 plays a central role in cell survival and cell cycle progression via its interactions with the gp130 subunit of the IL-6 receptor.[104] There seems to be 2 distinct pathways for IL-6–mediated survival and proliferation. Tyrosine 759 of gp130 has been shown to be critical for facilitating the S to G2 cell cycle progression but not for preventing apoptosis. Tyrosines in the YXXQ motif, however, induce antiapoptotic signaling via Bcl-2.[105] These data indicate that STAT3 may be especially important for preventing apoptosis and involved to a lesser degree in cell cycle progression in the IL-6–dependent survival and proliferation pathways.

STAT3 is also involved in several other antiapoptotic and mitogenic pathways. The oncogene v-Src has been shown to activate STAT3, representing a critical step in v-Src's modulation of cyclin D1, cyclin D2, cyclin E, and c-Myc expression.[106,107] STAT3 has also been shown to inhibit apoptosis via upregulation of Bcl-xL,[108] Mcl-1,[109] and survivin.[110] In addition, STAT3 disrupts p53 function by binding to the p53 promoter and subsequently inducing downregulation of p53 expression.[111] In vitro studies of STAT3 inhibitors have shown that STAT3 blockade leads to cell cycle arrest and the induction of apoptosis in a dose-dependent manner.[112] Furthermore, studies of STAT3 inhibitors in GBM xenograft models have demonstrated a significant impact on tumor growth.[113,114] Taken together, these studies indicate that STAT3 inhibitors may have in vivo antitumor activity independent of an antitumor immune response.

Invasion

GBMs are highly invasive, frequently infiltrating normal brain and precluding complete surgical resection. Although several factors are involved in GBM cell migration, STAT3 has recently emerged as a potential target for inhibiting invasion because STAT3 inhibitors have been shown to decrease the migratory behavior of GBM cells in vitro.[115] This result was observed regardless of PTEN expression. Although the precise mechanism is unknown, STAT3 has been observed to induce the expression of the proinvasive factors matrix metalloproteinase-2 (MMP-2) and fascin-1.[37,38] STAT3 may also play a role in HIF- and VEGF-mediated cell migration in response to hypoxia.[88,116] Studies in other tumor types suggest that blocking STAT3 and HIF together may increase the susceptibility to antineoplastic therapies working through separate mechanisms.[117] Because local tumor hypoxia has been shown to induce a more invasive phenotype,[88] STAT3 has been suggested as a potential biomarker of VEGF activity[118] and may represent a valuable target for augmenting anti-VEGF therapy.

Antitumor Activity of STAT3

Although most studies have highlighted STAT3's role in oncogenesis, some evidence suggests that the role of STAT3 may be context dependent.[119] STAT3 has been shown to inhibit proliferation in leukemia cells,[120] prostate cells,[121] and melanoma cells.[122] Furthermore, STAT3 may actually promote differentiation in some contexts.[120,123] In GBM, an interest in STAT3's antitumor activity first emerged from evidence suggesting that STAT3 can regulate gliogenesis by promoting the differentiation of cortical precursor cells into astrocytes.[98] STAT3's antitumor properties were further explored by Iglesia and colleagues[5]; they noted that experimental ablation of STAT3 in PTEN mutations unexpectedly led to increased astrocyte proliferation, invasiveness, and tumorigenesis. This finding indicates that STAT3 may have a role in suppressing malignant transformation of astrocytes in the context of PTEN pathway disruption, and future STAT3-

targeted therapies should take into consideration the genetic background of the tumor.

APPROACHES TO STAT3 INHIBITION

STAT3 overexpression is typically driven by an impairment of inhibitory molecules. Although several drugs have been shown to be active in vitro, significant challenges in the form of administration, toxicity, cell permeability, and nonselective activity have limited the translation of STAT3 inhibitors to clinical practice.

Preventing STAT3 Activation

One approach to preventing the activation of STAT3 is disrupting upstream tyrosine kinases. These include but are not limited to JAKs, growth factor receptors, and cytokines receptors. A fundamental challenge to this strategy is the multitude of signaling pathways that converge to activate STAT3. Efforts at disrupting the activation of STAT3 have targeted several kinases, including EGFR (head and neck squamous cell carcinoma), receptor tyrosine kinases (RTK; pancreatic cancer and non–small cell lung cancer), JAK (myelofibrosis and acute lymphoblastic leukemia), and SRC (head and neck squamous cell carcinoma). A summary of therapeutics targeting upstream kinases is presented in **Table 2**.

Monoclonal antibodies against EGFR have been used to block the interaction between VEGF and its receptor (cetuximab, panitumumab). Compounds have also been developed to target the tyrosine kinase activity of the EGFR (gefitinib, erlotinib, lapatinib). Although these drugs have shown efficacy in other tumors, GBM has demonstrated resistance to EGFR therapy, thought to arise from mutations of the extracellular domain of EGFR (preventing the efficacy of monoclonal antibody therapy), increases in cytoplasmic tyrosine kinase activity, or increased activity of parallel signaling pathways.[124]

Sorafenib, a tyrosine kinase inhibitor, has been shown to decrease GBM growth both in vitro and

Table 2
Therapeutics targeting STAT3 activation

Target	Drug
EGFR	Cetuximab, panitumumab
RTK	Gefitinib, erlotinib, lapatinib, sorafenib
JAK	AG490, LS-104, ICN1824, CEP-701, JSI-124
SRC	Dasatinib, AZD0530, bosutinib

in vivo.[125] Attempts at disrupting signaling through JAK proteins have been shown to be effective in vitro, with AG490 disrupting the IL-6 activation of STAT3 in U251 cell lines.[126] JSI-124 has also been shown to arrest cells in the G2/M phase and induce apoptosis in the U251 glioma cell line.[127] Finally, Liu and colleagues[128] reported that the introduction of adenovirus-vector carrying basic fibroblast growth factor siRNA decreased the activation of extracellular signal-regulated kinases 1/2 and JAK2 and decreased IL-6 secretion, leading to reduced STAT3 phosphorylation and decreased expression of the downstream molecules cyclin D1 and Bcl-xL.

Preventing Homodimerization of STAT3

After STAT3 is phosphorylated, it forms a functional homodimer via interactions between the SH2 domains. This complex allows for translocation of the homodimer complex to the nucleus, where STAT3 modulates gene expression. Efforts aimed at preventing STAT3 dimerization have been directed against the SH2 domain.[53,129–131] Using a pY-containing peptide, the first efforts at blocking the Y^{705} residue found that this strategy was able to inhibit the binding of STAT3 to DNA in vitro.[130,131]

The SH2 domain of STAT3 also interacts with upstream signaling proteins, including EGFR and the IL-6/IL6r complex. Attempts to disrupt the interaction between EGFR and SH2 have focused on preventing the phosphorylation of 2 tyrosine residues in the EGFR (Y^{1068} and Y^{1086}), which are required for recruiting STAT3 to the activated EGF-EGFR complex.[132] A phosphodecapeptide, which was synthesized based on the amino acids surround the Y^{1068} motif, has also been shown to inhibit the binding of STAT3 to DNA. Efforts targeted at disrupting the interaction between the gp130 subunit of the IL-6/IL-6r complex and STAT3 have also shown inhibition of STAT3 binding to DNA in vitro.[32] Therapies preventing the homodimerization of STAT3 in high-grade glioma are limited to in vitro studies. Kim and colleagues[133] reported that aspirin inhibited IL-6/STAT3 signaling in A172 cells. Tocilizumab, a humanized anti–IL-6r antibody decreased proliferation in U87MG cells.[134] Furthermore, STAT3 inhibition may effectively target tumor stem cells, which are frequently resistant to standard therapies; it has been shown to be a critical regulator of growth, proliferation, and maintenance of the GBM stem cell phenotype.[135] Villalva and colleagues[136] reported a small molecule inhibitor of STAT3, Stattic, was able to both block STAT3 activity in GBM stem cell lines as well as sensitize cells to temozolomide in vitro.

Table 3
Roles of STAT3 in oncogenesis and primary downstream mediators

Oncogenic Process	Mediators
Immune evasion	↑ IL-10, VEGF ↑ Treg expansion ↑ TGFβ ↑ Th17 differentiation ↓ MHC expression ↓ Dendritic cell maturation, IL-12 ↓ Costimulatory molecules
Angiogenesis	↑ VEGF ↑ Vascular tube formation
Invasion	↑ MMP-2, MMP-9 ↑ Fascin-1
Proliferation/survival	↑ Bcl-2 ↑ Bcl-xL ↑ Mcl-1 ↑ Survivin ↑ Cyclin D1, cyclin D2, cyclin E, ↑ C-myc
Differentiation	↑ GFAP

SUMMARY

STAT3 plays multiple roles in GBM tumorigenesis and has emerged as a promising therapeutic target. The putative roles of STAT3 in oncogenesis are summarized in **Table 3**. Blocking STAT3 activity in preclinical studies has been shown to inhibit angiogenesis, promote antitumor immune responses, and inhibit the invasion of normal brain tissue. Although several approaches have been developed to block STAT3 activity in vivo, no strategy has yet emerged as a viable candidate for clinical translation. In addition, emerging evidence suggests that the role of STAT3 in tumorigenesis may be more nuanced than initially appreciated, alternately exhibiting proneoplastic or antineoplastic activity depending on the genetic background of the tumor. Future research is needed to more clearly delineate the roles of STAT3 in GBM and develop effective strategies for targeting tumor-induced STAT3 activation.

REFERENCES

1. Silva CM. Role of STATs as downstream signal transducers in Src family kinase-mediated tumorigenesis. Oncogene 2004;23:8017–23.
2. Kisseleva T, Bhattacharya S, Braunstein J, et al. Signaling through the JAK/STAT pathway, recent advances and future challenges. Gene 2002;285:1–24.

3. Johnston PA, Grandis JR. STAT3 signaling: anticancer strategies and challenges. Mol Interv 2011;11:18–26.

4. Sato T, Neilson LM, Peck AR, et al. Signal transducer and activator of transcription-3 and breast cancer prognosis. Am J Cancer Res 2011;1:347–55.

5. de la Iglesia N, Konopka G, Lim KL, et al. Identification of a PTEN-regulated STAT3 brain tumor suppressor pathway. Genes Dev 2008;22:449–62.

6. Turkson J, Bowman T, Garcia R, et al. Stat3 activation by Src induces specific gene regulation and is required for cell transformation. Mol Cell Biol 1998;18:2545–52.

7. Bromberg JF, Horvath CM, Besser D, et al. Stat3 activation is required for cellular transformation by v-src. Mol Cell Biol 1998;18:2553–8.

8. Stupp R, Mason WP, van den Bent MJ, et al. Radiotherapy plus concomitant and adjuvant temozolomide for glioblastoma. N Engl J Med 2005;352:987–96.

9. Brat DJ, Castellano-Sanchez AA, Hunter SB, et al. Pseudopalisades in glioblastoma are hypoxic, express extracellular matrix proteases, and are formed by an actively migrating cell population. Cancer Res 2004;64:920–7.

10. Kaur B, Tan C, Brat DJ, et al. Genetic and hypoxic regulation of angiogenesis in gliomas. J Neurooncol 2004;70:229–43.

11. Oliver L, Olivier C, Marhuenda FB, et al. Hypoxia and the malignant glioma microenvironment: regulation and implications for therapy. Curr Mol Pharmacol 2009;2:263–84.

12. Waziri A. Glioblastoma-derived mechanisms of systemic immunosuppression. Neurosurg Clin N Am 2010;21:31–42.

13. Bodmer S, Strommer K, Frei K, et al. Immunosuppression and transforming growth factor-beta in glioblastoma. Preferential production of transforming growth factor-beta 2. J Immunol 1989;143:3222–9.

14. Tamura K, Aoyagi M, Wakimoto H, et al. Accumulation of CD133-positive glioma cells after high-dose irradiation by Gamma Knife surgery plus external beam radiation. J Neurosurg 2010;113:310–8.

15. Mannino M, Chalmers AJ. Radioresistance of glioma stem cells: intrinsic characteristic or property of the 'microenvironment-stem cell unit'? Mol Oncol 2011;5:374–86.

16. Ricci-Vitiani L, Pallini R, Biffoni M, et al. Tumour vascularization via endothelial differentiation of glioblastoma stem-like cells. Nature 2010;468:824–8.

17. Wang R, Chadalavada K, Wilshire J, et al. Glioblastoma stem-like cells give rise to tumour endothelium. Nature 2010;468:829–33.

18. Soda Y, Marumoto T, Friedmann-Morvinski D, et al. Transdifferentiation of glioblastoma cells into vascular endothelial cells. Proc Natl Acad Sci U S A 2011;108:4274–80.

19. McCord AM, Jamal M, Williams ES, et al. CD133+ glioblastoma stem-like cells are radiosensitive with a defective DNA damage response compared with established cell lines. Clin Cancer Res 2009;15:5145–53.

20. Calabrese C, Poppleton H, Kocak M, et al. A perivascular niche for brain tumor stem cells. Cancer Cell 2007;11:69–82.

21. Birner P, Toumangelova-Uzeir K, Natchev S, et al. STAT3 tyrosine phosphorylation influences survival in glioblastoma. J Neurooncol 2010;100:339–43.

22. Ball S, Li C, Li PK, et al. The small molecule, LLL12, inhibits STAT3 phosphorylation and induces apoptosis in medulloblastoma and glioblastoma cells. PLoS One 2011;6:e18820.

23. Zhang L, Alizadeh D, Van Handel M, et al. Stat3 inhibition activates tumor macrophages and abrogates glioma growth in mice. Glia 2009;57:1458–67.

24. Levy DE, Darnell JE Jr. Stats: transcriptional control and biological impact. Nat Rev Mol Cell Biol 2002;3:651–62.

25. Battle TE, Frank DA. The role of STATs in apoptosis. Curr Mol Med 2002;2:381–92.

26. Haura EB, Turkson J, Jove R. Mechanisms of disease: insights into the emerging role of signal transducers and activators of transcription in cancer. Nat Clin Pract Oncol 2005;2:315–24.

27. Zhong Z, Wen Z, Darnell JE Jr. Stat3: a STAT family member activated by tyrosine phosphorylation in response to epidermal growth factor and interleukin-6. Science 1994;264:95–8.

28. Yu CL, Meyer DJ, Campbell GS, et al. Enhanced DNA-binding activity of a Stat3-related protein in cells transformed by the Src oncoprotein. Science 1995;269:81–3.

29. Yu H, Jove R. The STATs of cancer–new molecular targets come of age. Nat Rev Cancer 2004;4:97–105.

30. Bowman T, Garcia R, Turkson J, et al. STATs in oncogenesis. Oncogene 2000;19:2474–88.

31. Wen Z, Zhong Z, Darnell JE Jr. Maximal activation of transcription by Stat1 and Stat3 requires both tyrosine and serine phosphorylation. Cell 1995;82:241–50.

32. Heinrich PC, Behrmann I, Muller-Newen G, et al. Interleukin-6-type cytokine signaling through the gp130/Jak/STAT pathway. Biochem J 1998;334(Pt 2):297–314.

33. Hibi M, Murakami M, Saito M, et al. Molecular cloning and expression of an IL-6 signal transducer, gp130. Cell 1990;63:1149–57.

34. Murakami M, Hibi M, Nakagawa N, et al. IL-6-induced homodimerization of gp130 and associated

activation of a tyrosine kinase. Science 1993;260:1808–10.

35. Zhang X, Wrzeszczynska MH, Horvath CM, et al. Interacting regions in Stat3 and c-Jun that participate in cooperative transcriptional activation. Mol Cell Biol 1999;19:7138–46.

36. Rahaman SO, Vogelbaum MA, Haque SJ. Aberrant Stat3 signaling by interleukin-4 in malignant glioma cells: involvement of IL-13Ralpha2. Cancer Res 2005;65:2956–63.

37. Liu Q, Li G, Li R, et al. IL-6 promotion of glioblastoma cell invasion and angiogenesis in U251 and T98G cell lines. J Neurooncol 2010;100:165–76.

38. Li R, Li G, Deng L, et al. IL-6 augments the invasiveness of U87MG human glioblastoma multiforme cells via up-regulation of MMP-2 and fascin-1. Oncol Rep 2010;23:1553–9.

39. Loeffler S, Fayard B, Weis J, et al. Interleukin-6 induces transcriptional activation of vascular endothelial growth factor (VEGF) in astrocytes in vivo and regulates VEGF promoter activity in glioblastoma cells via direct interaction between STAT3 and Sp1. Int J Cancer 2005;115:202–13.

40. Weissenberger J, Loeffler S, Kappeler A, et al. IL-6 is required for glioma development in a mouse model. Oncogene 2004;23:3308–16.

41. Lo HW, Cao X, Zhu H, et al. Constitutively activated STAT3 frequently coexpresses with epidermal growth factor receptor in high-grade gliomas and targeting STAT3 sensitizes them to Iressa and alkylators. Clin Cancer Res 2008;14:6042–54.

42. Ghosh MK, Sharma P, Harbor PC, et al. PI3K-AKT pathway negatively controls EGFR-dependent DNA-binding activity of Stat3 in glioblastoma multiforme cells. Oncogene 2005;24:7290–300.

43. Cuevas P, Díaz-González D, Sánchez I, et al. Dobesilate inhibits the activation of signal transducer and activator of transcription 3, and the expression of cyclin D1 and bcl-XL in glioma cells. Neurol Res 2006;28:127–30.

44. Riolfi M, Ferla R, Del Valle L, et al. Leptin and its receptor are overexpressed in brain tumors and correlate with the degree of malignancy. Brain Pathol 2010;20:481–9.

45. Ren Y, Zhou X, Mei M, et al. MicroRNA-21 inhibitor sensitizes human glioblastoma cells U251 (PTEN-mutant) and LN229 (PTEN-wild type) to Taxol. BMC Cancer 2010;10:27.

46. Chearwae W, Bright JJ. PPARgamma agonists inhibit growth and expansion of CD133+ brain tumour stem cells. Br J Cancer 2008;99:2044–53.

47. Ehrmann J, Strakova N, Vrzalikova K, et al. Expression of STATs and their inhibitors SOCS and PIAS in brain tumors. In vitro and in vivo study. Neoplasma 2008;55:482–7.

48. Brantley EC, Nabors LB, Gillespie GY, et al. Loss of protein inhibitors of activated STAT-3 expression in glioblastoma multiforme tumors: implications for STAT-3 activation and gene expression. Clin Cancer Res 2008;14:4694–704.

49. Veeriah S, Brennan C, Meng S, et al. The tyrosine phosphatase PTPRD is a tumor suppressor that is frequently inactivated and mutated in glioblastoma and other human cancers. Proc Natl Acad Sci U S A 2009;106:9435–40.

50. Jung JE, Lee HG, Cho IH, et al. STAT3 is a potential modulator of HIF-1-mediated VEGF expression in human renal carcinoma cells. FASEB J 2005;19:1296–8.

51. Yu H, Pardoll D, Jove R. STATs in cancer inflammation and immunity: a leading role for STAT3. Nat Rev Cancer 2009;9:798–809.

52. Groner B, Lucks P, Borghouts C. The function of Stat3 in tumor cells and their microenvironment. Semin Cell Dev Biol 2008;19:341–50.

53. Germain D, Frank DA. Targeting the cytoplasmic and nuclear functions of signal transducers and activators of transcription 3 for cancer therapy. Clin Cancer Res 2007;13:5665–9.

54. Heimberger AB, Sampson JH. The PEPvIII-KLH (CDX-110) vaccine in glioblastoma multiforme patients. Expert Opin Biol Ther 2009;9:1087–98.

55. Brooks WH, Caldwell HD, Mortara RH. Immune responses in patients with gliomas. Surg Neurol 1974;2:419–23.

56. Mahaley MS Jr, Brooks WH, Roszman TL, et al. Immunobiology of primary intracranial tumors. Part 1: studies of the cellular and humoral general immune competence of brain-tumor patients. J Neurosurg 1977;46:467–76.

57. Thomas DG, Lannigan CB, Behan PO. Letter: impaired cell-mediated immunity in human brain tumours. Lancet 1975;1:1389–90.

58. Roszman TL, Brooks WH. Immunobiology of primary intracranial tumours. III. Demonstration of a qualitative lymphocyte abnormality in patients with primary brain tumours. Clin Exp Immunol 1980;39:395–402.

59. Elliott LH, Brooks WH, Roszman TL. Inability of mitogen-activated lymphocytes obtained from patients with malignant primary intracranial tumors to express high affinity interleukin 2 receptors. J Clin Invest 1990;86:80–6.

60. Menzies CB, Gunar M, Thomas DG, et al. Impaired thymus-derived lymphocyte function in patients with malignant brain tumour. Clin Neurol Neurosurg 1980;82:157–68.

61. Brooks WH, Netsky MG, Normansell DE, et al. Depressed cell-mediated immunity in patients with primary intracranial tumors. Characterization of a humoral immunosuppressive factor. J Exp Med 1972;136:1631–47.

62. Yu H, Kortylewski M, Pardoll D. Crosstalk between cancer and immune cells: role of STAT3 in the

tumour microenvironment. Nat Rev Immunol 2007; 7:41–51.

63. Wang T, Niu G, Kortylewski M, et al. Regulation of the innate and adaptive immune responses by Stat-3 signaling in tumor cells. Nat Med 2004;10: 48–54.

64. Williams L, Bradley L, Smith A, et al. Signal transducer and activator of transcription 3 is the dominant mediator of the anti-inflammatory effects of IL-10 in human macrophages. J Immunol 2004; 172:567–76.

65. Gabrilovich DI, Chen HL, Girgis KR, et al. Production of vascular endothelial growth factor by human tumors inhibits the functional maturation of dendritic cells. Nat Med 1996;2:1096–103.

66. Kortylewski M, Kujawski M, Wang T, et al. Inhibiting Stat3 signaling in the hematopoietic system elicits multicomponent antitumor immunity. Nat Med 2005;11:1314–21.

67. Kortylewski M, Yu H. Role of Stat3 in suppressing anti-tumor immunity. Curr Opin Immunol 2008;20: 228–33.

68. Zou W. Immunosuppressive networks in the tumour environment and their therapeutic relevance. Nat Rev Cancer 2005;5:263–74.

69. Nishikawa H, Kato T, Tawara I, et al. IFN-gamma controls the generation/activation of CD4+ CD25+ regulatory T cells in antitumor immune response. J Immunol 2005;175:4433–40.

70. Yamazaki S, Bonito AJ, Spisek R, et al. Dendritic cells are specialized accessory cells along with TGF- for the differentiation of Foxp3+ CD4+ regulatory T cells from peripheral Foxp3 precursors. Blood 2007;110:4293–302.

71. Luo X, Tarbell KV, Yang H, et al. Dendritic cells with TGF-beta1 differentiate naive CD4+CD25- T cells into islet-protective Foxp3+ regulatory T cells. Proc Natl Acad Sci U S A 2007;104:2821–6.

72. Liu VC, Wong LY, Jang T, et al. Tumor evasion of the immune system by converting CD4+CD25- T cells into CD4+CD25+ T regulatory cells: role of tumor-derived TGF-beta. J Immunol 2007;178:2883–92.

73. Chen W, Jin W, Hardegen N, et al. Conversion of peripheral CD4+CD25- naive T cells to CD4+ CD25+ regulatory T cells by TGF-beta induction of transcription factor Foxp3. J Exp Med 2003;198: 1875–86.

74. Yamazaki S, Iyoda T, Tarbell K, et al. Direct expansion of functional CD25+ CD4+ regulatory T cells by antigen-processing dendritic cells. J Exp Med 2003;198:235–47.

75. Zou W. Regulatory T cells, tumour immunity and immunotherapy. Nat Rev Immunol 2006;6:295–307.

76. Kryczek I, Wei S, Zou L, et al. Cutting edge: Th17 and regulatory T cell dynamics and the regulation by IL-2 in the tumor microenvironment. J Immunol 2007;178:6730–3.

77. Harris TJ, Grosso JF, Yen HR, et al. Cutting edge: an in vivo requirement for STAT3 signaling in TH17 development and TH17-dependent autoimmunity. J Immunol 2007;179:4313–7.

78. Chen Z, Laurence A, Kanno Y, et al. Selective regulatory function of Socs3 in the formation of IL-17-secreting T cells. Proc Natl Acad Sci U S A 2006; 103:8137–42.

79. Cho ML, Kang JW, Moon YM, et al. STAT3 and NF-kappaB signal pathway is required for IL-23-mediated IL-17 production in spontaneous arthritis animal model IL-1 receptor antagonist-deficient mice. J Immunol 2006;176:5652–61.

80. Mathur AN, Chang HC, Zisoulis DG, et al. Stat3 and Stat4 direct development of IL-17-secreting Th cells. J Immunol 2007;178:4901–7.

81. Wang L, Yi T, Kortylewski M, et al. IL-17 can promote tumor growth through an IL-6-Stat3 signaling pathway. J Exp Med 2009;206:1457–64.

82. Fischer I, Gagner JP, Law M, et al. Angiogenesis in gliomas: biology and molecular pathophysiology. Brain Pathol 2005;15:297–310.

83. Plate KH, Breier G, Weich HA, et al. Vascular endothelial growth factor is a potential tumour angiogenesis factor in human gliomas in vivo. Nature 1992; 359:845–8.

84. Raizer JJ, Grimm S, Chamberlain MC, et al. A phase 2 trial of single-agent bevacizumab given in an every-3-week schedule for patients with recurrent high-grade gliomas. Cancer 2010;116: 5297–305.

85. Vredenburgh JJ, Desjardins A, Herndon JE 2nd, et al. Phase II trial of bevacizumab and irinotecan in recurrent malignant glioma. Clin Cancer Res 2007;13:1253–9.

86. Friedman HS, Prados MD, Wen PY, et al. Bevacizumab alone and in combination with irinotecan in recurrent glioblastoma. J Clin Oncol 2009;27:4733–40.

87. Lucio-Eterovic AK, Piao Y, de Groot JF. Mediators of glioblastoma resistance and invasion during antivascular endothelial growth factor therapy. Clin Cancer Res 2009;15:4589–99.

88. Keunen O, Johansson M, Oudin A, et al. Anti-VEGF treatment reduces blood supply and increases tumor cell invasion in glioblastoma. Proc Natl Acad Sci U S A 2011;108:3749–54.

89. Yahata Y, Shirakata Y, Tokumaru S, et al. Nuclear translocation of phosphorylated STAT3 is essential for vascular endothelial growth factor-induced human dermal microvascular endothelial cell migration and tube formation. J Biol Chem 2003; 278:40026–31.

90. Schaefer LK, Ren Z, Fuller GN, et al. Constitutive activation of Stat3alpha in brain tumors: localization to tumor endothelial cells and activation by the endothelial tyrosine kinase receptor (VEGFR-2). Oncogene 2002;21:2058–65.

91. Kang SH, Yu MO, Park KJ, et al. Activated STAT3 regulates hypoxia-induced angiogenesis and cell migration in human glioblastoma. Neurosurgery 2010;67:1386–95 [discussion: 1395].

92. Wei D, Le X, Zheng L, et al. Stat3 activation regulates the expression of vascular endothelial growth factor and human pancreatic cancer angiogenesis and metastasis. Oncogene 2003;22:319–29.

93. Goodwin CR, Laterra J. Neuro-oncology: unmasking the multiforme in glioblastoma. Nat Rev Neurol 2010;6:304–5.

94. Uhrbom L, Dai C, Celestino JC, et al. Ink4a-Arf loss cooperates with KRas activation in astrocytes and neural progenitors to generate glioblastomas of various morphologies depending on activated Akt. Cancer Res 2002;62:5551–8.

95. Kwon CH, Zhao D, Chen J, et al. Pten haploinsufficiency accelerates formation of high-grade astrocytomas. Cancer Res 2008;68:3286–94.

96. Cayre M, Canoll P, Goldman JE. Cell migration·in the normal and pathological postnatal mammalian brain. Prog Neurobiol 2009;88:41–63.

97. Gilbertson RJ, Gutmann DH. Tumorigenesis in the brain: location, location, location. Cancer Res 2007;67:5579–82.

98. Bonni A, Sun Y, Nadal-Vicens M, et al. Regulation of gliogenesis in the central nervous system by the JAK-STAT signaling pathway. Science 1997; 278:477–83.

99. Lee HS, Han J, Lee SH, et al. Meteorin promotes the formation of GFAP-positive glia via activation of the Jak-STAT3 pathway. J Cell Sci 2010;123: 1959–68.

100. Lutticken C, Wegenka UM, Yuan J, et al. Association of transcription factor APRF and protein kinase Jak1 with the interleukin-6 signal transducer gp130. Science 1994;263:89–92.

101. Lee J, Son MJ, Woolard K, et al. Epigenetic-mediated dysfunction of the bone morphogenetic protein pathway inhibits differentiation of glioblastoma-initiating cells. Cancer Cell 2008;13: 69–80.

102. Fukuda S, Abematsu M, Mori H, et al. Potentiation of astrogliogenesis by STAT3-mediated activation of bone morphogenetic protein-Smad signaling in neural stem cells. Mol Cell Biol 2007;27:4931–7.

103. Yang YP, Chang YL, Huang PI, et al. Resveratrol suppresses tumorigenicity and enhances radiosensitivity in primary glioblastoma tumor initiating cells by inhibiting the STAT3 axis. J Cell Physiol 2012;227(3):976–93.

104. Hirano T, Ishihara K, Hibi M. Roles of STAT3 in mediating the cell growth, differentiation and survival signals relayed through the IL-6 family of cytokine receptors. Oncogene 2000;19:2548–56.

105. Fukada T, Hibi M, Yamanaka Y, et al. Two signals are necessary for cell proliferation induced by a cytokine receptor gp130: involvement of STAT3 in anti-apoptosis. Immunity 1996;5:449–60.

106. Odajima J, Matsumura I, Sonoyama J, et al. Full oncogenic activities of v-Src are mediated by multiple signaling pathways. Ras as an essential mediator for cell survival. J Biol Chem 2000;275: 24096–105.

107. Sinibaldi D, Wharton W, Turkson J, et al. Induction of p21WAF1/CIP1 and cyclin D1 expression by the Src oncoprotein in mouse fibroblasts: role of activated STAT3 signaling. Oncogene 2000;19: 5419–27.

108. Thiel JH, Treurniet N. Panel on "the implications of recent advances in the knowledge of child development for the treatment of adults". Int J Psychoanal 1976;57:429–39.

109. Epling-Burnette PK, Liu JH, Catlett-Falcone R, et al. Inhibition of STAT3 signaling leads to apoptosis of leukemic large granular lymphocytes and decreased Mcl-1 expression. J Clin Invest 2001;107: 351–62.

110. Aoki Y, Feldman GM, Tosato G. Inhibition of STAT3 signaling induces apoptosis and decreases survivin expression in primary effusion lymphoma. Blood 2003;101:1535–42.

111. Niu G, Wright KL, Ma Y, et al. Role of Stat3 in regulating p53 expression and function. Mol Cell Biol 2005;25:7432–40.

112. Yang F, Brown C, Buettner R, et al. Sorafenib induces growth arrest and apoptosis of human glioblastoma cells through the dephosphorylation of signal transducers and activators of transcription 3. Mol Cancer Ther 2010;9:953–62.

113. Lin L, Hutzen B, Li PK, et al. A novel small molecule, LLL12, inhibits STAT3 phosphorylation and activities and exhibits potent growth-suppressive activity in human cancer cells. Neoplasia 2010; 12:39–50.

114. Fuh B, Sobo M, Cen L, et al. LLL-3 inhibits STAT3 activity, suppresses glioblastoma cell growth and prolongs survival in a mouse glioblastoma model. Br J Cancer 2009;100:106–12.

115. Senft C, Priester M, Polacin M, et al. Inhibition of the JAK-2/STAT3 signaling pathway impedes the migratory and invasive potential of human glioblastoma cells. J Neurooncol 2011;101:393–403.

116. Wei J, Wu A, Kong LY, et al. Hypoxia potentiates glioma-mediated immunosuppression. PLoS One 2011;6:e16195.

117. Reddy KR, Guan Y, Qin G, et al. Combined treatment targeting HIF-1alpha and Stat3 is a potent strategy for prostate cancer therapy. Prostate 2011;71:1796–809.

118. Tran PT, Felsher DW. The current STATe of biomarkers to predict the response to anti-angiogenic therapies. Cancer Biol Ther 2008;7: 2004–6.

119. de la Iglesia N, Puram SV, Bonni A. STAT3 regulation of glioblastoma pathogenesis. Curr Mol Med 2009;9:580–90.

120. Nakajima K, Yamanaka Y, Nakae K, et al. A central role for Stat3 in IL-6-induced regulation of growth and differentiation in M1 leukemia cells. EMBO J 1996;15:3651–8.

121. Spiotto MT, Chung TD. STAT3 mediates IL-6-induced growth inhibition in the human prostate cancer cell line LNCaP. Prostate 2000;42:88–98.

122. Kortylewski M, Heinrich PC, Mackiewicz A, et al. Interleukin-6 and oncostatin M-induced growth inhibition of human A375 melanoma cells is STAT-dependent and involves upregulation of the cyclin-dependent kinase inhibitor p27/Kip1. Oncogene 1999;18:3742–53.

123. Spiotto MT, Chung TD. STAT3 mediates IL-6-induced neuroendocrine differentiation in prostate cancer cells. Prostate 2000;42:186–95.

124. Chen LF, Cohen EE, Grandis JR. New strategies in head and neck cancer: understanding resistance to epidermal growth factor receptor inhibitors. Clin Cancer Res 2010;16:2489–95.

125. Siegelin MD, Raskett CM, Gilbert CA, et al. Sorafenib exerts anti-glioma activity in vitro and in vivo. Neurosci Lett 2010;478:165–70.

126. Rahaman SO, Harbor PC, Chernova O, et al. Inhibition of constitutively active Stat3 suppresses proliferation and induces apoptosis in glioblastoma multiforme cells. Oncogene 2002;21:8404–13.

127. Su Y, Li G, Zhang X, et al. JSI-124 inhibits glioblastoma multiforme cell proliferation through G(2)/M cell cycle arrest and apoptosis augment. Cancer Biol Ther 2008;7:1243–9.

128. Liu J, Xu X, Feng X, et al. Adenovirus-mediated delivery of bFGF small interfering RNA reduces STAT3 phosphorylation and induces the depolarization of mitochondria and apoptosis in glioma cells U251. J Exp Clin Cancer Res 2011;30:80.

129. Leeman RJ, Lui VW, Grandis JR. STAT3 as a therapeutic target in head and neck cancer. Expert Opin Biol Ther 2006;6:231–41.

130. Jing N, Tweardy DJ. Targeting Stat3 in cancer therapy. Anticancer Drugs 2005;16:601–7.

131. Fletcher S, Drewry JA, Shahani VM, et al. Molecular disruption of oncogenic signal transducer and activator of transcription 3 (STAT3) protein. Biochem Cell Biol 2009;87:825–33.

132. Shao H, Cheng HY, Cook RG, et al. Identification and characterization of signal transducer and activator of transcription 3 recruitment sites within the epidermal growth factor receptor. Cancer Res 2003;63:3923–30.

133. Kim SR, Bae MK, Kim JY, et al. Aspirin induces apoptosis through the blockade of IL-6-STAT3 signaling pathway in human glioblastoma A172 cells. Biochem Biophys Res Commun 2009;387: 342–7.

134. Kudo M, Jono H, Shinkriki S, et al. Antitumor effect of humanized anti-interleukin-6 receptor antibody (tocilizumab) on glioma cell proliferation. Laboratory investigation. J Neurosurg 2009; 111:219–25.

135. Sherry MM, Reeves A, Wu JK, et al. STAT3 is required for proliferation and maintenance of multipotency in glioblastoma stem cells. Stem Cells 2009;27:2383–92.

136. Villalva C, Martin-Lanneree S, Cortes U, et al. STAT3 is essential for the maintenance of neurosphere-initiating tumor cells in patients with glioblastomas: a potential for targeted therapy? Int J Cancer 2011;128:826–38.

CD133 as a Marker for Regulation and Potential for Targeted Therapies in Glioblastoma Multiforme

Winward Choy, BA[a], Daniel T. Nagasawa, MD[a],
Andy Trang, BS[a], Kimberly Thill, BS[a], Marko Spasic, BA[a],
Isaac Yang, MD[a,b,*]

KEYWORDS

- Cancer stem cell • CD133 • Glioblastoma • Glioma

KEY POINTS

- CD133 is a reliable and widely studied tumor marker for glioblastoma multiforme (GBM) cells with cancer stem cell (CSC)-associated phenotypes.
- Tumorigenic capacity is not limited in the CD133[+] subpopulation, and several models bridging the relationship between CD133[+] and CD133[−] tumorigenic cells in GBMS have been proposed.
- Many of the studies examining CD133[+] GBM cells as putative CSCs are complicated by the complex regulation of CD133, lack of a uniform protocol, and ability of in vivo and in vitro studies to replicate the true physiologic role of CD133 in patients.
- Associations between the presence of CD133[+] cells within resected tumors and clinical outcomes, including poorer prognosis and resistance to adjuvant therapies, have been demonstrated, and CD133[+] cells remain a promising target for future GBM therapies.

INTRODUCTION

Glioblastoma multiforme (GBM) is the most common primary malignant brain tumor found in adults. Despite standard treatment comprising surgical resection followed by concomitant radiotherapy and adjuvant temozolomide chemotherapy, the prognosis for GBM is poor, with a median survival of 14.6 months.[1] The major challenge for current treatment paradigms stems from the characteristically diffuse patterns of tumor infiltration throughout healthy brain parenchyma.[2] Most therapeutic efforts and glioma research to date have focused on the tumor in its entirety; however, recent findings have highlighted the incredible heterogeneity of GBM cells, denoted by the term *multiforme*, in terms of not only their immunogenic, histologic, and genetic profile but also their proliferative and tumorigenic potential. Thus, the characterization and identification of the different GBM cell types, particularly

Disclosure of interests: Marko Spasic was partially supported by an American Association of Neurological Surgeons Fellowship grant. Isaac Yang (senior author) was partially supported by a Visionary Fund Grant, an Eli and Edythe Broad Center of Regenerative Medicine and Stem Cell Research UCLA Scholars in Translational Medicine Program Award, the Stein Oppenheimer Endowment Award, and the STOP CANCER Jason Dessel Memorial Seed Grant.
[a] Department of Neurosurgery, David Geffen School of Medicine, University of California–Los Angeles, Los Angeles, CA, USA; [b] Jonsson Comprehensive Cancer Center, University of California–Los Angeles, Los Angeles, CA, USA
* Corresponding author. UCLA Department of Neurosurgery, UCLA Jonsson Comprehensive Cancer Center, University of California, Los Angeles, David Geffen School of Medicine at UCLA, 695 Charles East Young Drive South, UCLA Gonda 3357, Los Angeles, CA 90095-1761.
E-mail address: iyang@mednet.ucla.edu

Neurosurg Clin N Am 23 (2012) 391–405
doi:10.1016/j.nec.2012.04.011
1042-3680/12/$ – see front matter © 2012 Elsevier Inc. All rights reserved.

those involved with driving tumor growth, are critical not only in the understanding of GBM formation and pathogenesis but also in the advancement of more effective cancer therapies.

Cancer Stem Cells

The cancer stem cell (CSC) model has provided a new paradigm in understanding what predominant cellular mechanisms drive tumor growth. Similar to the organization of growth processes within normal tissue such as bone marrow or intestinal epithelium, the CSC concept postulates the presence of a functional and cellular hierarchy within the heterogeneous tumor body.[3] Within this hierarchical model, the vast majority of the tumor bulk comprises rapidly dividing, partially or terminally differentiated cells with limited replicative potential, while neoplastic growth is driven by a small population of cancer cells with stemlike properties.[3] Similar to the properties of normal stem cells, CSCs represent a population of neoplastic cells that have the capacity to initiate and maintain tumors and are characterized by self-renewal, resistance to chemical insults and radiation, and ability to produce new tumors even after periods of dormancy.[3]

To be defined as CSCs, the cells must have the following characteristics: (1) self-renewal and proliferation, (2) multilineage differentiation into mature fates resembling tissue of origin, and (3) capacity to form new tumors resembling the original tumor. To date, studies have used similar procedures to identify and characterize the stemness of putative CSCs. A differentially expressed marker or set of markers is used to isolate a small subset of tumor cells within the tumor bulk.[3] The capacity to form nonadherent tumorspheres by limiting dilution in culture conditions permissive for stem cell proliferation is assessed to demonstrate properties of clonal expansion and self-renewal and is used to identify and expand potential CSCs. In vivo demonstration of CSC behavior is confirmed by the ability of putative CSCs transplanted into immunodeficient mice to form tumors resembling the original tumor.[4]

DISCOVERY OF CD133

CD133 was first identified by Yin and colleagues[5] in 1997 through generating a monoclonal antibody–recognizing AC133, a glycosylated CD133 epitope. AC133 expression was restricted to the CD34[+] subset of hematopoietic stem cells derived from human fetal liver, adult blood, and bone marrow, suggesting that AC133 is a novel marker for human hematopoietic stem cells and progenitor cells. Unlike CD34, the AC133 antigen is not found in other blood cells, endothelial cells (ECs), or fibroblasts and may be an important marker of more primitive progenitor cells.[5,6] In xenograft models, AC133[+] cells obtained from primary fetal sheep recipients demonstrated sustained proliferative and self-renewal potential when transplanted into secondary recipients.[5] Of note, a second glycosylated CD133 epitope, AC141, distinct from AC133, has also been characterized, and both AC141 and AC133 are commonly used to identify and purify CD133[+] cells.[7,8]

The gene for human CD133, located on chromosome 4p15.33, encodes a 120-kD protein with 865 amino acids and shares 60% homology with mouse prominin, which is localized to neuroepithelial stem cells.[9,10] Structurally, CD133 comprises 5 transmembrane domains, an extracellular N-terminus, a cytoplasmic C-terminus, 2 large extracellular loops containing 8 putative N-glycosylation sites, and 2 smaller cytoplasmic loops.[10] Although the precise function of CD133 is unclear, the localization of AC133 antigen expression on epithelial microvilli suggests a possible role in the organization of plasma membrane topography and the maintenance of apical-basal cell polarity.[6,11] Associations between CD133 and plasma membrane cholesterol have alluded to a role in the regulation of lipid composition within the cell membrane.[6,7] Loss of CD133 has been associated with degeneration of photoreceptors associated with improper retinal disk formation, suggesting a possible role in the regulation of phototransduction and neural retinal development.[12,13] In addition, CD133[+] progenitor cells obtained from human fetal aorta have also been shown to stimulate Wnt pathway–dependent angiogenesis during wound healing of ischemic diabetic ulcers.[14,15]

CD133 AS A STEM CELL MARKER

Following the initial characterization in CD34[+] hematopoietic stem cells, CD133 has been used to purify several progenitor and stemlike cell populations within both healthy and neoplastic tissues. CD133[+] neural progenitor cells have been identified in human fetal and postmortem brain tissue.[16–19] Neural stemlike cells have been isolated from human fetal brain tissue through flow cytometry. These CD133[+], CD34[−], CD45[−] cells demonstrated characteristic stem cell activity, including clonal expansion, serial neurosphere culture initiation, and differentiation.[17,18] On intracranial transplantation into neonatal nonobese diabetic, severe combined immunodeficient (NOD-SCID) mice, the sorted cells successfully engrafted, migrated, proliferated, and differentiated along neuronal and glial fates.[8,17]

Human epithelial-derived CD133[20] cells and fetal liver-derived CD133+, CD34+, CD3− hematopoietic cells[21] have been shown to differentiate into neurons and astrocytes on transplantation into intracranial mouse and in culture with differentiation-promoting media. Vascular endothelial growth factor receptor 2–positive circulating human endothelial progenitor cells coexpress CD133, and plating of these nonadherent cells in vascular endothelial growth factor (VEGF) and fibroblast growth factor 2 led to rapid differentiation, loss of CD133 expression, and formation of adherent colonies.[22] Similar downregulation of CD133 on differentiation was observed in the colon carcinoma–derived epithelial cell line Caco-2.[23]

Some studies have demonstrated the ability of these progenitor cells to reconstitute the original tissue.[16,24,25] CD133+ human prostate basal cells showed increased proliferation in vitro and, on transplantation, formed fully differentiated prostate epithelium–expressing prostatic secretions.[24] CD133 expression either independently or in conjunction with other stem and progenitor cell markers has also been used to identify CSC subpopulations within a wide range of human cancers, including osteosarcomas,[26,27] laryngeal carcinomas,[26,28] melanomas,[26,29–32] breast cancers,[26,33] hepatocellular carcinomas,[26,34] prostate tumors,[26,35,36] retinoblastomas,[10] leukemias,[37–39] and non–small cell lung cancer.[40] In addition, CD133 expression has been used to purify CSC populations in a number of brain tumors, including medulloblastomas[5,26] and ependymomas.[26,41]

Gliomas

Initial evidence suggesting the presence of brain tumor cells with stemlike potential came from the isolation of a clonogenic subpopulation of cells from resected gliomas through neurosphere assays.[42,43] These neurospheres possessed the capacity for self-renewal and demonstrated intraclonal neuronal and glial cell lineage heterogeneity. Among the several markers associated with CSCs, CD133 is one of the most widely studied in brain tumors.[15] Singh and colleagues[44] first identified a subpopulation of brain tumor cells within medulloblastomas and gliomas coexpressing CD133 and nestin, a marker for undifferentiated neural stem cells. Unlike the CD133− population, CD133+ cells, representing 0.3% to 25.1% of the tumor bulk, were capable of neurosphere formation in serum-free media following addition of the stem cell growth factors bFGF and EGF. These tumorspheres had greater proliferative capacity relative to neural stem cell controls and formed secondary tumorspheres with immunoreactivity for nestin and CD133. Tumorspheres resembled a more primitive state and were devoid of glial fibrillary acidic protein (GFAP) and β-tubulin III, markers of differentiated neural cells and glial cells, respectively. However, CD133+ cells were capable of multilineage differentiation into oligodendrocytes, astrocytes, and neurons and expressed differentiated markers mirroring that of the parent tumor.[6] Although many xenograft assays require up to 10^6 tumor cells for successful engraftment,[45–47] as few as 100 purified CD133+ tumor cells have been reported to be sufficient for intracranial tumor formation when transplanted into NOD-SCID mice. In contrast, injection of 10^5 CD133− cells failed to form tumors.[45] Engrafted CD133+ GBM cells produced tumors with classic GBM features that were phenotypically identical to the patient's original tumor and could be serially transplanted.[45] In addition, engrafted tumors were widely infiltrating and comprised differential expression of CD133 and GFAP, suggesting that CD133+ cells were capable of self-renewal and differentiation in vivo.[45]

Subsequently, 2 groups identified tumorsphere-forming subpopulations within tumor specimens obtained from patients with primary and secondary GBMs.[48,49] Spheres arising from less than 1% of all GBM cells coexpressed nestin and CD133. Unlike the progeny of normal neural stem cell (NSC)-derived neurospheres, differentiation of GBM tumorspheres led to progeny that closely mirrored the parental tumor phenotype, comprising 80% β-tubulin III+ cells and 25% oligodendrocytes. In addition, tumorspheres demonstrated greater proliferative potential and the ability to retain stemlike features following differentiation, suggesting a role in the maintenance of the stem cell pool and production of differentiated cells within the tumor bulk.[49] Unlike the non–sphere-forming population, the sphere-forming GBM cells were able to form tumors following transplantation in nude mice, and the new tumors expressed both neural and glial markers.[49] Expression of CD133 is restricted to a subpopulation of tumor cells positive for the neural stem and progenitor cell marker nestin, which suggests that this subpopulation may represent a less-differentiated subset of tumor cells.[50] Consistent with CSC model, which proposes that CSCs represent a rare fraction of tumor cells, the extent of CD133 expression within gliomas is typically low or barely detectable, as demonstrated by quantitative analysis using flow cytometry.[7,45,51–54] However, some immunohistochemical reports have suggested that the CD133+ glioma fraction comprises up to 25% of the tumor bulk.[50]

Recently, transcriptome profiling of purified CD133$^+$ and CD133$^-$ GBM cells identified a CD133 gene expression profile comprising 214 differentially expressed genes.[55] Computational comparison with established stem cell and cancer cell profiles demonstrated a close association of the CD133 gene expression signature with that of human embryonic stem cells. The CD133 gene signature distinctly differentiated between NSC-like GBM cells cultured in stem cell medium and GBM cells cultured in serum. Enrichment of the CD133 gene signature was closely associated with increasing glioma grade, with greatest resemblance in grade IV GBMs. The CD133 gene signature was associated with a more aggressive GBM subtype and significantly shorter median patient survival. In addition, the GBMs enriched for the CD133 gene signature were associated with a greatly increased number of genetic mutations. Overall, the CD133 gene signature, obtained from sorted CD133$^+$ populations, is characteristic of a stemlike cell population of tumor cells as well as more clinically aggressive and hypermutated subtypes of GBM cells.[55]

There exists a functional hierarchy within the heterogeneous GBM cell population consisting of a small CD133$^+$ fraction of GBM cells that formed tumorspheres in stem cell media, generated serial tumorspheres on dissociation, was enriched for several stem cell markers (nestin, Musashi 1, and SOX2), and gave rise to progeny-expressing neuronal, oligodendrocytic, and astrocytic markers on culturing under prodifferentiation conditions.[56] Consistent with in vitro features of stem cells, CD133$^+$ GBM cells demonstrated a heightened capacity for proliferation, self-renewal, and multilineage differentiation.[56] Transplantation led to the formation of highly invasive and angiogenic tumors that histologically and morphologically resembled the original patient GBM.[4,45] Altogether, these findings suggest that the CD133$^+$ GBM subpopulation contains putative stemlike cells that can initiate and maintain tumors that phenotypically resemble the original GBM and are capable of driving tumor growth even when challenged with serial transplantations.[56]

CD133$^-$ CELLS IN GLIOMAS

Although there has been mounting evidence for a selected population of cells with stemlike properties, the role of CD133 as a definitive marker for tumor-initiating cells is contentious. Studies have demonstrated that CD133$^+$ cells are absent from select GBM specimens and glioma cell lines that are capable of tumor formation in vivo.[7,52,57,58] Following initial studies characterizing

the stemness of CD133$^+$ glioma cells and the lack of tumorigenicity in CD133$^-$ cells, several investigators demonstrated that CD133$^-$ glioma cells were also capable of in vivo tumor initiation and maintenance.[54,57] Beier and colleagues[57] demonstrated that both CD133$^+$ and CD133$^-$ populations obtained from primary GBM cell cultures formed tumorspheres in stem cell–permissive media. Although the CD133$^-$ sphere-forming population represented a smaller fraction than the CD133$^+$ sphere-forming cells, both subpopulations demonstrated stemlike features in vitro, including sustained proliferative ability and formation of tumorspheres containing cells expressing differentiated markers from all 3 neural lineages.[57] Transplantation of both CD133$^+$ and CD133$^-$ GBM cells formed GBM-resembling tumors within mice. Transplantation of CD133$^-$ cells derived from CD133$^+$ cell lines failed to produce tumors,[57] suggesting a functional heterogeneity between tumorigenic CD133$^-$ cells and CD133$^+$-derived CD133$^-$ cells.

Studies using marker-independent sorting methods have further demonstrated the presence of putative CD133$^-$ GBM CSCs. Using fluorescence-activated cell sorting (FACS) based on specific tumor cell autofluorescence, Clément and colleagues[51] isolated a subpopulation of glioma cells (FL1$^+$) with high nuclear:cytoplasmic ratios capable of multipassage tumorsphere formation. FL1$^+$ cells demonstrated marked capacity for self-renewal, differentiation associated with a loss of FL1 properties, and tumorigenicity when as few as 10^3 FL1$^+$ cells were transplanted into mice. FL1$^+$ cells displayed a heightened expression of several stemness-related genes, including POU5F1/OCT4, SOX2, NOTCH1, and NANOG. However, CD133 expression was not correlated with tumorigenicity, and differences in CD133 expression between FL1$^+$ cells and the remaining tumor block were not statistically significant. The side population (SP), sorted based on the ability to extrude Hoechst 33342 dye, represented a rare stemlike fraction of highly tumorigenic glioma cells that, unlike non-SP cells, can give rise to both SP and non-SP cells.[16,59] While studies examining the SP and CD133 expression have been scarce, a single murine glioma cell line (GL261) study found that sphere-forming and highly tumorigenic CD133$^+$ glioma cells demonstrating stemlike features did not reside within the SP.[16,60] Although this may suggest the presence of a tumorigenic CD133$^-$ SP cells, recent data from Broadley and colleagues[61] demonstrated that cells within the GBM SP could not self-renew and form tumors.

Son and colleagues[58] used stage-specific embryonic antigen 1 (SSEA-1), a marker for embryonic stem cells, to purify a subpopulation of patient-derived GBMs with high tumorigenic potential. Although CD133 expression was present in only half of the 24 GBM samples, SSEA-1 immunoreactivity was present in all but one. Relative to the SSEA-1⁻ population, SSEA-1⁺ cells expressed higher levels of established stem cell makers, including SOX2, Bmi2, L1CAM, Olig2, and Ezh2. Independent of CD133 expression, SSEA-1 allowed enrichment of a tumorsphere-forming population with increased clonogenic potential and the ability to differentiate down neuronal lineages. In addition, SSEA-1⁺ cells could generate both SSEA-1⁻ and SSEA-1⁺ cells, suggesting a hierarchal organization underlying a heterogeneous population.[58] Unlike SSEA-1⁻ cells, transplantation of as few as 10^4 SSEA-1⁺ cells successfully formed tumors in mice that retained their tumorigenic capacity following serial transplantations.[58] Similarly, other investigators have successfully identified putative GBM CSCs expressing alternative markers, including integrin $\alpha6$[62] and A2B5,[63] that displayed heightened tumorigenicity and distinct stemlike phenotypes that either lacked or were independent of CD133 immunoreactivity.[16,64] In addition, alternative methods and parameters have been used to identify putative CSCs within gliomas.[48,59,64–66]

Limitations

The variable protocols used in the purification of CD133⁺ cells and the assessment of stemness make comparing study results difficult.[67] Tumor samples have been obtained from a variety of sources (eg, fresh resections from patients,[50] glioma cell lines[60]) and cultured in variable conditions, including serum-free media[16,44] and in the presence of fetal calf serum.[16,68] Because serum has been shown to induce differentiation, culture media should be taken into account when assessing results from studies examining CD133 expression.[16,67,69]

Furthermore, many of the CD133 studies use AC133 monoclonal antibodies, which recognize glycosylated CD133 epitopes. Accurate detection of CD133 may be limited because of the unknown specificity of AC133 binding to differential glycosylation patterns of the 8 potential glycosylation sites on CD133.[5,16] Furthermore, studies have characterized several different tissue-dependent isoform tissue produced by alternative splicing of the CD133 transcript within human[37] and murine models.[8,70] It is possible that AC133 monoclonal antibodies, unable to uniformly recognize different

isoforms, would provide an underestimate of true CD133 protein expression levels within gliomas.[8,71] Recently, Osmond and colleagues[71] reported that GBM cells found to be AC133⁻ contained a truncated and possibly functional CD133 variant that was localized within the cytoplasm. It is unclear whether the isoform type, the extent of protein expression, or the specific glycosylation status is the more biologically relevant marker of CD133 expression.[8] Tissue distribution of CD133 messenger RNA is much more prevalent than expression of AC133,[10] as the downregulation of the AC133 epitope is independent of intracellular levels of CD133 messenger RNA.[8,23,72] Thus, the presence of AC133 epitopes is not necessarily equivalent to CD133 expression.

Although transplantation of sorted cells into immunodeficient mice remains the gold standard of assessing tumorigenicity, it has several limitations. The process of sorting and transplanting tumor cells into mice subjects the cells to several procedural insults and places them in a foreign environment vastly different from the original tumor niche.[3] Inherent differences between the patient and mice microenvironment due to various species barriers (eg, differences in cytokines and growth factors important in tumor growth) may drastically alter proliferation potential.[3] In addition, the xenographic immune response in mice receiving transplants is significantly more robust than the native immune response within the patient.[73] Fundamentally, the issue is the applicability of tumor xenograft assays in immunocompromised mice in studying the clinical behavior of human cancers.

LINKING CD133⁻ AND CD133⁺ SUBPOPULATIONS

Despite the limitations, there is still strong support for the role of both CD133⁺ and CD133⁻ cells in driving GBM tumorigenesis and maintenance. Progress in understanding the multifaceted mechanisms regulating CD133⁺ expression has led to several models proposed to bridge the functional relationship between these 2 cell types.

The Multiple CSC Model

Recent data have suggested that CD133⁺ and CD133⁻ tumorigenic glioma cells may represent distinct CSC populations associated with different GBM subtypes.[65,74] Following the initial characterization of CD133⁻ glioma cells with stemlike properties,[57] Lottaz and colleagues[74] compared gene expression profiles in various GBM CSC lines and identified a 24-gene signature that faithfully distinguished 2 distinct subgroups of GBM CSC cells. Compared with a previously established gene signature differentiating different GBM subtypes,[74,75] type I CSCs showed a proneural transcriptional profile, whereas type II CSCs displayed a mesenchymal profile. Type I CSCs resembled fetal NSCs and were strongly CD133 positive, whereas type II CSC lines resembled adult NSCs and were mainly CD133 negative. In accord with previous studies reporting different growth capacities and extent of stemlike phenotypes between the 2 CSC types,[57,65] CD133+ type I CSCs formed tumorspheres in culture, whereas type II cells displayed semiadherent growth. Key molecular differences among the 2 types included differences in TGF-β/BMP pathway activation and expression of extracellular matrix and adhesion molecules.[65,74] Compared with their presumed cells of origin, both CSC types demonstrated heightened metabolic and proliferative activity as well as greatly impaired differentiation capacity. As suggested in previous studies of genetically engineered medulloblastoma and glioma models,[76–81] tumorigenic CSCs are derived through distinct mechanisms from cells that have either preserved or gained (eg, trough dedifferentiation) features reminiscent of fetal NSCs and adult NSCs.[16,74] The findings, corroborated by an earlier array-based classification system by Gunther and colleagues,[65] suggest that CD133+ and CD133− CSCs represents at least 2 different GBM subtypes with distinct molecular and phenotypic characteristics.

The Hierarchical Model

Other studies have demonstrated the ability of CD133− glioma cells to give rise to both CD133+ and CD133− progeny. Intracranial transplanted glioma spheroids obtained from human GBM biopsies in nude rats gave rise to invasive CD133-negative tumors with minor signs of angiogenesis.[54,82] Successive serial transplantation of these initial tumors gave rise to tumors with increasing CD133 immunoreactivity, which was closely correlated with an increased angiogenic phenotype and decreased survival in the host rats. Transplantation of CD133− cells, purified via FACS of the serially transplanted tumors, into nude rat brains gave rise to tumors with both CD133+ and CD133− cells. Tumors derived from CD133− GBM cells contained up to 5% CD133+ cells, suggesting that a subset of CD133− cells can not only initiate and support tumor growth but also recapitulate the initial tumor heterogeneity.[54]

Similarly, Chen and colleagues[76] demonstrated that both CD133+ and CD133− GBM cell fractions are capable of neurosphere formation and also demonstrate varying degrees of tumorigenicity in vivo. Accounting for all clonogenic GBM cells within neurosphere cultures, the investigators proposed 3 categories of GBM CSCs organized within a lineage hierarchy representing different stages of differentiation. CD133− type I cells give rise to a mixture of CD133+ and CD133− cells, CD133+ type II cells also give rise to a mixture of CD133+ and CD133− cells, but CD133− type III cells only give rise to a population of self-renewing CD133− cells. All 3 cell types expressed the NSC marker nestin, were capable of multilineage differentiation, and formed tumors following serial transplantation in mice. Much of the histologic and molecular differences between the 3 types place types I and III at 2 extremes, whereas type II cells possessed intermediate features. Although CD133− type III cells were restricted to only producing CD133− tumors, type I cells could produce type I, II, and III cells. Tumors derived from type III cells grew the slowest and gave rise to well-circumscribed tumors, whereas type I cells were more elongated and generated more aggressive and invasive tumors with diffuse borders. Consistent with the observed histologic characteristics, type I and II clones expressed significantly higher levels of the radial glial marker, FABP7, among several other NSC markers in comparison with type III clones. FABP expression has been established as a GBM marker for increased invasion and shorter survival[76,83,84] and is associated with maintaining the stem cell features during neural development.[76,85] In contrast, type III grafts displayed higher levels of intermediate progenitor markers such as TBR2, DLX1, DLX2, and CUTL2.[76] Within this model, type I and III CD133− cells represent the most primitive and differentiated states along a spectrum. Taken together, CD133− progenitor cells are capable of forming both CD133+ and CD133− cells, supporting the presence of a lineal hierarchy of self-renewing cells that support GBM growth.

Enrichment of neurosphere-forming GBM cells have identified 2 lineally related but distinct populations of CD133− cells (type I and III) with unique gene signatures and in vivo phenotypes representing differing stages of differentiation. These differences within the CD133− population, comprising both type I and type III CD133− cells, may account for the discordant results of previous studies examining the ability of CD133− cells to demonstrate in vitro or in vivo stem cell properties.[76]

The Dynamic Model

In addition, the cancer stem–like phenotype associated with CD133 expression may actually represent a dynamic and plastic trait that responds to the changing signals and stresses. Oxygen has been the well-characterized signaling molecule involved with mediating various signaling pathways and regulating gene expression,[86,87] and availability of oxygen within the tumor microenvironment has been thought to influence the proliferative phase underlying neoplastic growth.[88] Although oxygen tensions within the normal brain range from 5% to 10% and likely lower within the tumor bulk, in vitro studies typically culture glioma cells under normoxic conditions of 20% O_2.[86,89,90] Platet and colleagues[91] demonstrated that culturing of GBM resection specimens at 3% O_2, representing a more physiologically relevant concentration, was associated with a significant increase in CD133 expression in comparison with GBM cells cultured at atmospheric concentrations of 20% O_2. McCord and colleagues[86] demonstrated similar results with more mild reductions of oxygen concentration and that disaggregated GBM spheres derived from surgical resection samples had a 2-fold increase in percentage of CD133+ cells when recultured and allowed to form neurospheres in 7% O_2 compared with normoxic 20% O_2 conditions. CD133+ cells cultured in 7% O_2 had a higher frequency of colony formation, shorter doubling time, and enhanced ability to differentiate along glial and neuronal lines, suggesting that hypoxic conditions not only increase the CD133+ cell composition but also modify and enhance the associated tumorigenic and stemlike phenotype. CD133+ neurospheres cultured in hypoxic conditions demonstrated increased expression of other stem cell markers, including nestin, Oct4, and SOX2. Levels of HIF-2α were increased in CD133+ cells cultured in 7% O_2, and consequent small interfering RNA silencing of HIF-2α led to decreased Oct4 and SOX2.[86] Consistent with the induction of the stemlike phenotype, growth in 7% O_2 induced alterations in global gene expression patterns with the upregulation of critical stem cell–associated genes including those involved with the notch and frizzled-2 signaling pathway, angiogenesis, and transforming growth factor β.[86] When CD133+ cells were moved from 7% to 20% O_2, rates of colony formation and expression of HIF-2α and stem cell markers reversed to levels originally observed in normoxic conditions. Oxygen-induced stemlike features, partially mediated by HIF-2α, are reversible and mediated by epigenetic changes and are not the result of the hypoxic selection of a CD133+ subpopulation of tumorigenic cells.[86]

In their studies with the established human glioma cell line U251MG, Griguer and colleagues[92] further proposed that mechanisms underlying hypoxia-induced CD133 upregulation and functional changes partly involved loss of mitochondrial function. In accord with previous studies, U251MG glioma cells, containing undetectable levels of CD133 above background in 21% O_2 culture conditions, became strongly CD133 positive when changed to 1% O_2. Following exposure, 20% of U251MG cells were CD133+ within 24 hours and up to 60% were CD133+ within 72 hours. On return to 21% O_2, levels of CD133 expression decreased to original normoxic levels. In addition, treatment of U251MG glioma cells with rotenone, an electron transport chain blocker, resulted in a significant and dose-dependent increase in CD133+ expression, reminiscent of exposure to hypoxic conditions. Depletion of mitochondrial DNA similarly led to constitutive and substantial increases in CD133 expression that persisted through multiple cell passages. Relative to controls, mitochondrial DNA–depleted glioma cells demonstrated a more aggressive phenotype of increased anchorage-independent growth and invasiveness. These cells readily initiated and expanded as tumorspheres in serum-free media that expressed the stem cell markers nestin and CD133 and had multilineage differentiation potential. In addition, rescue of mitochondrial function by transfer of parental mitochondrial DNA reversed the elevated CD133 expression levels. In their proposed model of glioma progression, Griguer and colleagues[92] suggest that tumor growth is driven by a dynamic and adaptive biological response to oxygen and metabolic demands in reaction to a changing tumor microenvironment. Stringent nutrient and oxygen barriers selectively signal a switch within glioma cells in hypoxic regions to gain phenotypic changes associated with increased survival and migration.

Overall, the data support a critical role of reduced oxygen tension and disruption of mitochondrial function in mediating an in vitro response within glioma cells characterized by upregulated CD133 expression.[16,86,91–95] These hypoxia-induced changes are associated with global alterations in the expression of stem cell–associated genes and promote CSC phenotypes, including increased clonogenicity, proliferation, invasiveness, capacity for multilineage differentiation, and tumorigenicity in xenograft models. While it is unclear if the extent of fluidity is present in vivo, the sensitivity of glioma cells toward changes in oxygen levels and the reversibility of hypoxia-induced characteristics suggest a dynamic regulatory component of CD133 expression and stemlike features. In addition, the low frequency of CD133+ glioma cells reported in literature may be linked to normoxic culture oxygen concentrations that do not reflect physiologic levels.

Recent studies have begun to provide further insight into the complex mechanisms regulating the expression of CD133 and its associated phenotype in gliomas. Differential methylation patterns have been identified as transcriptional regulators of CD133 in several cancers.[96,97] CD133 promoter methylation, not present within normal brain tissue, represents an abnormal epigenetic regulator of differential CD133 expression in glioma cells.[97] Yi and colleagues[97] reported a high frequency of CD133 promoter hypermethylation in both GBM and colon cancer cells lines and primary tumor samples; however, such methylation patterns were absent in CD133+ cells. Upregulation of CD133 expression was strongly associated with genetic and drug-induced inhibition of DNA methyltransferase activity. This mode of regulation is unique to CD133, as hypermethylation profiles of other genes do not vary between CD133+ and CD133- populations.[97] In addition, Jaksch and colleagues[98] demonstrated that the extent of AC133 immunoreactivity is cycle dependent in embryonic stem cells, colon cancer, and melanomas. Specifically, AC133 immunoreactivity was highest in the actively dividing cell subpopulation with 4N DNA content and lowest in cells in the G_0 and G_1 phases with 2N DNA content. MELK protein expression, which has been demonstrated to be cell cycle dependent,[98,99] mirrored AC133 immunoreactivity with respect to cell cycle status. Prolonged culturing of purified CD133- and purified CD133+ cells produced similarly heterogeneous cell populations comprising both CD133+ and CD133- cells. The ability of cells at either extremes of CD133 immunoreactivity to produce CD133-heterogeneous populations suggests that CD133 immunoreactivity may not be unique to a discrete and stable population.[98] Overall, although it does appear that CD133 expression may be used to enrich a glioma population with increased tumorigenicity, it is possible that CD133 expression and the associated phenotype are fluid traits responding to dynamic extracellular and intracellular processes.

CONTRIBUTION TO ANGIOGENESIS

The extensive tumor vascularity, high endothelial proliferation rates, and elevated VEGF production within GBMs have provided promise for antiangiogenic therapies.[100] Indeed, in clinical trials using the anti-VEGF antibody, Avastin, roughly half of the patients responded to treatment.[101,102] However, the effect was transient, and antiangiogenic resistance developed in most patients.[102,103]

Bao and colleagues[56] reported the formation of highly vascular and hemorrhagic tumors following mice xenograft of purified CD133+ GBM cells relative to CD133- cells. CD133+ cells demonstrated a marked elevation of VEGF expression in comparison with CD133- cells in both normoxic and hypoxic conditions. CD133+ promoted EC migration and formation of vasculature in vitro, and these proangiogenic effects were blocked by treatment with anti-VEGF antibodies (bevacizumab). In addition, bevacizumab reduced the growth and vascularity of tumors derived from mice transplantation.

Recently, CD133+ GBM cells have demonstrated to contribute to tumor neoangiogenesis through direct transdifferentiation down endothelial lineages to give rise to tumor-derived ECs (TDECs).[104–106] Wang and colleagues[105] identified a subpopulation within the CD133+ fraction of GBM cells that coexpressed vascular endothelial cadherin (CD144) that were capable of giving rise to ECs. These TDECs harbored the same mutations found within the parent tumor, namely, gains in chromosome 7 and epidermal growth factor receptor.[105] He and colleagues[104] further demonstrated that CD133+ GBM CSCs are capable of forming TDECs and were localized within niches that were in close proximity to blood vessels. Blood vessels surrounding CD133+ tumor cell niches expressed tumor-specific markers, further suggesting that these ECs are of neoplastic origin and arise from the differentiation of GBM stem cells.[104]

These TDEC comprised up to 90% of ECs in the tumors and appeared to contribute to glioma angiogenesis.[105,106] Although CD133+/CD144- cells were capable of sphere formation and differentiation along neuronal lineages, cocultures of tumor cells and purified CD133+/CD144- cells generate ECs through intermediate CD133+/CD144+ progenitor cells. When cultured in EC media, CD133+/CD144+ cells lose CD144 expression and display features associated with an epithelial phenotype (eg, CD105 and CD31 expression, and DiI-AcLDL uptake). Endothelium derived from CD133+/CD144+ GBM cells formed vessels with glomeruloid features morphologically reminiscent of abnormal tumor vasculature. Unlike CD133-/CD144+ cells, transplantation of CD133+/CD144+ and CD133+/CD144- populations gave rise to highly invasive and aggressive tumors, with CD133+/CD144+-derived tumors displaying significantly increased levels of angiogenesis. In addition, CD133+/CD144- fractions were capable of maintaining its multilineage potential following serial transplantations. Elevated levels of HIF-1α in tumors exposed to hypoxic conditions lead to increased angiogenesis through VEGF production.[103,107,108] Similarly, hypoxia seems to induce the transdifferentiation of select glioma cells into ECs through elevation of HIF-1α levels in vitro.[103] However, unlike normal ECs, most TDECs lacked VEGF-R1, VEGF-R2, and VEGF-R3 expression.[103] Accordingly, treatment with anti-VEGF did not inhibit in vivo TDEC tube formation and did not produce improved survival in murine GBM models.[103] TDEC transdifferentiation is VEGF independent and may explain GBM resistance to anti-VEGF therapies.[103] Furthermore, selective targeting of TDEC in mouse xenografts led to marked tumor regression, indicating that TDECs play a critical role in maintaining tumor viability.[106]

Although tumor angiogenesis is typically thought to be driven by bone marrow–derived circulating endothelial precursors,[103,109] tumor cells appear to be closely involved with tumor angiogenesis and TDECs have been identified in other cancers, including myeloma, lymphoma, and chronic myelocytic leukemia.[103,110–112] Taken together, the data suggest that CD133+ GBM cells not only are capable of giving rise to the tumor bulk but also can contribute to tumor angiogenesis partly through transdifferentiation through a CD133+/CD144+ intermediate to generate ECs of neoplastic origin that can form functional vessels.

The Stem Cell Niche

Normal stem cells have been demonstrated to exist within a stem cell niche comprising differentiated cell types that help regulate and maintain the stem cell trait.[113–116] Coculture studies have demonstrated a role of ECs within the stem cell niche in modulating and maintaining NSCs.[117] ECs secrete pigment epithelium–derived factor, which modulates capacity for self-renewal in adult neural stem cells within the subventricular zone.[118] Similarly, other diffusible factors released by ECs within the stem cell niche, including brain-derived neurotrophic factor and leukemia inhibitory factor, have been characterized to regulate NSC proliferation and differentiation.[119,120] In addition, recent studies have suggested that a parallel interaction exists between glioma stem cells and tumor ECs within the vascular niches critical in maintaining CSCs.[113]

CD133+ brain tumor cells demonstrated a high affinity for ECs and formed close interactions along vascular tubes formed by primary human ECs (PHECs) in culture. When CD133+ tumorspheres were cocultured with PHECs, the tumorspheres demonstrated heightened capacity for proliferation and self-renewal.[113] ECs similarly enhanced the CSC phenotype in vivo, as transplantation of

tumor cells into mice in the presence of PHECs was associated with increased expansion of CD133+ cells and quicker tumor initiation and growth. Increased number of blood vessels in tumor xenografts, and consequently an increase in the release of endothelial derived factors, led to a significant expansion of self-renewing tumorigenic cells while treatment with antiangiogenic drugs blocked tumor growth and depleted the self-renewing CD133+/nestin+ tumor population.[113] A recent study of 87 resected grade II–IV glioma samples identified CSC niches characterized by CD133+ blood vessels surrounding and infiltrating CD133+ glioma cell clusters.[121] Prevalence of CD133+ niches, ranging from 11.57% to 24.81%, was correlated with increasing tumor grade and extent of CD133+ blood vessels. In accordance with previous reports of glioma CSC–derived EC cells, CD133+ cells were localized around CD31+ blood vessels that contained cells that coexpressed CD31 and CD133. In contrast to NSC maintained in predominantly quiescent states by NSC niches, a fraction of CD133+ cells within the neoplastic perivascular niche were proliferating cell nuclear antigen positive and actively proliferating.[121] Thus, ECs and the vascular niche are critical for not only nutrient supply but also providing a tumor microenvironment that supports and promotes the proliferation of CSCs.[113]

Recently endothelium-derived nitric oxide (NO) was demonstrated to regulate stemlike features of glioma cells within the perivascular niche in platelet-derived growth factor–induced mouse glioma models.[122] Charles and Holland[122] demonstrated a close correlation between endothelial NO synthase (eNOS) expression, which was limited to ECs, and Notch1 expression in adjacent nestin+ glioma stem cells within the perivascular niche. NO activation of the Notch signaling pathway heightened the stemlike features of glioma cells in vitro and enhanced tumorigenicity and tumor growth in tumor xenografts. In addition, mice lacking eNOS exhibited impaired notch pathway activation and tumor growth and improved survival. These results complement the established role of NO in mediating glioma angiogenesis and highlight the critical importance of the tumor perivascular niche in maintaining and supporting resident tumor stem cells.[122] Thus, the capacity for CD133+ CSCs to transdifferentiate and directly contribute to tumor vasculature, to modulate regulated angiogenesis, and to respond to endothelium-derived signals, among other mechanisms, represents an intricate and bidirectional cross talk between glioma CSCs and their microenvironment niche.

THERAPEUTIC POTENTIAL

The glycosylated CD133 epitope has been identified as a reliable tumor marker for the purification of a subpopulation of GBM cells demonstrating CSC phenotypes. Isolated tumorsphere-forming CD133[+] GBM cells demonstrated heightened in vitro proliferation, self-renewal, and invasive capacity. When cultured in prodifferentiation conditions, CD133[+] GBM cells were capable of differentiating along neuronal, oligodendrocytic, and astrocytic lineages. Orthotopic transplantation of CD133[+] cells led to the formation of heterogeneous tumors that were phenocopies of the original patient tumor. Thus, CD133[+] cells are highly tumorigenic and demonstrate extensive capacity for self-renewal even when challenged with serial transplantation. Given these characteristic stemlike properties of the CD133[+] population, the CSC model has been extended to GBMs. The application of the CSC model may account for the highly heterogeneous, invasive, and therapy-resistant nature of GBMs[67] and has directed investigators to identify specific cellular elements for targeted therapies.

Later CSC studies using CD133-independent means to isolate putative CSCs in GBMs have demonstrated that these in vitro and in vivo CSC features are not present in all CD133[+] GBM cells nor are they unique to the CD133[+] subpopulation. The identification and characterization of tumorigenic CD133[−] cells has led to not only a greater appreciation of the multifaceted regulation of CD133 in GBMs but also a more comprehensive understanding of the role of CD133 in GBM tumorigenesis. These findings have suggested several models that are not necessarily mutually exclusive: (1) CD133[+] and CD133[−] GBM cells comprise unique and separate CSC populations responsible for driving the growth of different GBM subtypes, (2) CD133[−] GBM cells are functionally heterogeneous and may comprise more primitive cells capable of giving rise to tumorigenic CD133[+] cells, and (3) the CD133[+] stemlike phenotype is transient and fluid, and CD133expression depends on temporally and spatially dynamic intracellular and extracellular cues.

Most of the studies analyzing CD133 expression are faced with technical challenges from accounting for the complex genetic and epigenetic regulation of CD133 to the ability of the in vitro and in vivo assays to reflect the true physiologic role of CD133 in patients' tumors. However, a growing number of studies have linked clinical outcomes with the presence of CD133[+] cells within resected tumors.[50,55,123,124] Analysis of 95 resected gliomas found that increased CD133 expression and presence of CD133[+] clusters were significant prognostic predictors of worse overall survival and progression-free survival independent of glioma grade, patient age, or extent of resection.[50] In addition, greater extent of CD133 expression is correlated with increasing glioma grade and is typically found in advanced-stage gliomas.[125] The greater reliability of CD133 expression relative to histologic analysis in predicting patient outcomes has suggested that the gain of CD133 expression may be a key step in the progression to secondary GBM.[124] Furthermore, CD133[+] cells have been found to play a critical role in mediating GBM resistance to radiation and chemotherapy. Standard cancer treatments, which mainly target rapidly dividing cells of the tumor bulk, are not effective in eradicating CSCs, which are slowly dividing and often quiescent cells. GBM CSCs preferentially activate DNA checkpoint proteins to ensure proper repair of DNA damage resulting from treatment.[126] CD133[+] glioma cells persist in greater fractions after treatment with ionizing radiation through preferentially activating Chk1 and Chk2 checkpoint kinases, and this radioresistance is lost following Chk1 and Chk2 inhibition.[126] Chemoresistance of CD133[+] glioma cells is mediated through several mechanisms, including the upregulation of adenosine triphosphate–binding cassette transporters to facilitate drug efflux,[127] elevated expression of multidrug-resistant associated proteins 1 and 3,[128] and the enrichment of the "side population" that is resistant to cytotoxic drugs.[60] In addition, CD133[+] glioma cells upregulate the DNA repair protein, O-methylguanine-DNA methyltransferase, as well as other antiapoptotic genes, including Bcl-2, Bcl-X, and FLIP.[129] Adjacent ECs within the perivascular niche, along with the activation of a number of developmental pathways, have been suggested to contribute to CD133[+] GBM resistance to radiotherapy and chemotherapy.[26,130]

While CD133's status as a stable, obvious CSC is still not established and its biological functions are unclear, CD133 remains a promising marker for targeted and personalized therapeutic intervention. Although several putative models exist, CD133 consistently identifies cells with not only stemlike properties intimately involved with tumor growth and angiogenesis but also profound clinical consequences in dictating patient outcomes and resistance to chemotherapy and radiotherapy. Thus, targeting the CD133[+] subpopulation represents a promising adjuvant in conjunction with standard therapies. Several exciting and novel approaches have been proposed, including treatment with prodifferentiation agents, drugs that target aberrant CSC signaling pathways, disruption of the perivascular niche, and the use of

CSC-targeted immunotherapies. Research into therapies targeting CSCs is still in nascent stages and must consider several challenges: (1) several different and heterogeneous glioma CSCs may exist, (2) the CSC phenotype is regulated by several complex extracellular and intracellular mechanisms, and (3) treatment of glioma CSCs may also affect healthy neural stem cells that share similar markers and phenotypes.[26] Indeed, the optimal treatment strategies likely include a combinatorial approach and rely on continued exploration of the complex regulation of GBM CSCs and their underlying biology.

ACKNOWLEDGMENTS

Marko Spasic was partially supported by an American Association of Neurological Surgeons Fellowship. Daniel Nagasawa was supported by an American Brain Tumor Association Medical Student Summer Fellowship in Honor of Connie Finc. Isaac Yang (senior author) was partially supported by a Visionary Fund Grant, an Eli and Edythe Broad Center of Regenerative Medicine and Stem Cell Research UCLA Scholars in Translational Medicine Program Award, and the STOP CANCER Jason Dessel Memorial Seed Grant.

REFERENCES

1. Stupp R, Mason WP, van den Bent MJ, et al. Radiotherapy plus concomitant and adjuvant temozolomide for glioblastoma. N Engl J Med 2005;352: 987–96.

2. Holland EC. Glioblastoma multiforme: the terminator. Proc Natl Acad Sci U S A 2000;97:6242–4.

3. Clevers H. The cancer stem cell: premises, promises and challenges. Nat Med 2011;17:313–9.

4. Dirks PB. Brain tumour stem cells: the undercurrents of human brain cancer and their relationship to neural stem cells. Philos Trans R Soc Lond B Biol Sci 2008;363:139–52.

5. Yin AH, Miraglia S, Zanjani ED, et al. AC133, a novel marker for human hematopoietic stem and progenitor cells. Blood 1997;90:5002–12.

6. Mizrak D, Brittan M, Alison MR. CD133: molecule of the moment. J Pathol 2008;214:3–9.

7. Wan F, Zhang S, Xie R, et al. The utility and limitations of neurosphere assay, CD133 immunophenotyping and side population assay in glioma stem cell research. Brain Pathol 2010;20:877–89.

8. Bidlingmaier S, Zhu X, Liu B. The utility and limitations of glycosylated human CD133 epitopes in defining cancer stem cells. J Mol Med (Berl) 2008;86:1025–32.

9. Shmelkov SV, St Clair R, Lyden D, et al. AC133/CD133/Prominin-1. Int J Biochem Cell Biol 2005; 37:715–9.

10. Miraglia S, Godfrey W, Yin AH, et al. A novel five-transmembrane hematopoietic stem cell antigen: isolation, characterization, and molecular cloning. Blood 1997;90:5013–21.

11. Corbeil D, Roper K, Fargeas CA, et al. Prominin: a story of cholesterol, plasma membrane protrusions and human pathology. Traffic 2001;2:82–91.

12. Maw MA, Corbeil D, Koch J, et al. A frameshift mutation in prominin (mouse)-like 1 causes human retinal degeneration. Hum Mol Genet 2000;9:27–34.

13. Zacchigna S, Oh H, Wilsch-Brauninger M, et al. Loss of the cholesterol-binding protein prominin-1/CD133 causes disk dysmorphogenesis and photoreceptor degeneration. J Neurosci 2009;29: 2297–308.

14. Barcelos LS, Duplaa C, Krankel N, et al. Human CD133+ progenitor cells promote the healing of diabetic ischemic ulcers by paracrine stimulation of angiogenesis and activation of Wnt signaling. Circ Res 2009;104:1095–102.

15. Ji J, Black KL, Yu JS. Glioma stem cell research for the development of immunotherapy. Neurosurg Clin N Am 2010;21:159–66.

16. Campos B, Herold-Mende CC. Insight into the complex regulation of CD133 in glioma. Int J Cancer 2011;128:501–10.

17. Uchida N, Buck DW, He D, et al. Direct isolation of human central nervous system stem cells. Proc Natl Acad Sci U S A 2000;97:14720–5.

18. Tamaki S, Eckert K, He D, et al. Engraftment of sorted/expanded human central nervous system stem cells from fetal brain. J Neurosci Res 2002; 69:976–86.

19. Schwartz PH, Bryant PJ, Fuja TJ, et al. Isolation and characterization of neural progenitor cells from post-mortem human cortex. J Neurosci Res 2003;74:838–51.

20. Belicchi M, Pisati F, Lopa R, et al. Human skin-derived stem cells migrate throughout forebrain and differentiate into astrocytes after injection into adult mouse brain. J Neurosci Res 2004;77:475–86.

21. Hao HN, Zhao J, Thomas RL, et al. Fetal human hematopoietic stem cells can differentiate sequentially into neural stem cells and then astrocytes in vitro. J Hematother Stem Cell Res 2003;12:23–32.

22. Peichev M, Naiyer AJ, Pereira D, et al. Expression of VEGFR-2 and AC133 by circulating human CD34(+) cells identifies a population of functional endothelial precursors. Blood 2000;95:952–8.

23. Corbeil D, Roper K, Hellwig A, et al. The human AC133 hematopoietic stem cell antigen is also expressed in epithelial cells and targeted to plasma membrane protrusions. J Biol Chem 2000;275: 5512–20.

24. Richardson GD, Robson CN, Lang SH, et al. CD133, a novel marker for human prostatic epithelial stem cells. J Cell Sci 2004;117:3539–45.

25. Leong KG, Wang BE, Johnson L, et al. Generation of a prostate from a single adult stem cell. Nature 2008;456:804–8.

26. Cheng JX, Liu BL, Zhang X. How powerful is CD133 as a cancer stem cell marker in brain tumors? Cancer Treat Rev 2009;35:403–8.

27. Tirino V, Desiderio V, d'Aquino R, et al. Detection and characterization of CD133+ cancer stem cells in human solid tumours. PLoS One 2008;3: e3469.

28. Zhou L, Wei X, Cheng L, et al. CD133, one of the markers of cancer stem cells in Hep-2 cell line. Laryngoscope 2007;117:455–60.

29. Frank NY, Margaryan A, Huang Y, et al. ABCB5-mediated doxorubicin transport and chemoresistance in human malignant melanoma. Cancer Res 2005;65:4320–33.

30. Frank NY, Pendse SS, Lapchak PH, et al. Regulation of progenitor cell fusion by ABCB5 P-glycoprotein, a novel human ATP-binding cassette transporter. J Biol Chem 2003;278:47156–65.

31. Klein WM, Wu BP, Zhao S, et al. Increased expression of stem cell markers in malignant melanoma. Mod Pathol 2007;20:102–7.

32. Monzani E, Facchetti F, Galmozzi E, et al. Melanoma contains CD133 and ABCG2 positive cells with enhanced tumourigenic potential. Eur J Cancer 2007;43:935–46.

33. Wright MH, Calcagno AM, Salcido CD, et al. Brca1 breast tumors contain distinct CD44+/CD24- and CD133+ cells with cancer stem cell characteristics. Breast Cancer Res 2008;10:R10.

34. Suetsugu A, Nagaki M, Aoki H, et al. Characterization of CD133+ hepatocellular carcinoma cells as cancer stem/progenitor cells. Biochem Biophys Res Commun 2006;351:820–4.

35. Collins AT, Berry PA, Hyde C, et al. Prospective identification of tumorigenic prostate cancer stem cells. Cancer Res 2005;65:10946–51.

36. Miki J, Furusato B, Li H, et al. Identification of putative stem cell markers, CD133 and CXCR4, in hTERT-immortalized primary nonmalignant and malignant tumor-derived human prostate epithelial cell lines and in prostate cancer specimens. Cancer Res 2007;67:3153–61.

37. Shmelkov SV, Jun L, St Clair R, et al. Alternative promoters regulate transcription of the gene that encodes stem cell surface protein AC133. Blood 2004;103:2055–61.

38. Kratz-Albers K, Zuhlsdorp M, Leo R, et al. Expression of a AC133, a novel stem cell marker, on human leukemic blasts lacking CD34-antigen and on a human CD34+ leukemic line:MUTZ-2. Blood 1998;92:4485–7.

39. Buhring HJ, Seiffert M, Marxer A, et al. AC133 antigen expression is not restricted to acute myeloid leukemia blasts but is also found on acute lymphoid leukemia blasts and on a subset of CD34 + B-cell precursors. Blood 1999;94:832–3.

40. Tirino V, Camerlingo R, Franco R, et al. The role of CD133 in the identification and characterisation of tumour-initiating cells in non-small-cell lung cancer. Eur J Cardiothorac Surg 2009;36:446–53.

41. Taylor MD, Poppleton H, Fuller C, et al. Radial glia cells are candidate stem cells of ependymoma. Cancer Cell 2005;8:323–35.

42. Vescovi AL, Galli R, Reynolds BA. Brain tumour stem cells. Nat Rev Cancer 2006;6:425–36.

43. Ignatova TN, Kukekov VG, Laywell ED, et al. Human cortical glial tumors contain neural stem-like cells expressing astroglial and neuronal markers in vitro. Glia 2002;39:193–206.

44. Singh SK, Clarke ID, Terasaki M, et al. Identification of a cancer stem cell in human brain tumors. Cancer Res 2003;63:5821–8.

45. Singh SK, Hawkins C, Clarke ID, et al. Identification of human brain tumour initiating cells. Nature 2004; 432:396–401.

46. Houchens DP, Ovejera AA, Riblet SM, et al. Human brain tumor xenografts in nude mice as a chemotherapy model. Eur J Cancer Clin Oncol 1983;19: 799–805.

47. Hu B, Guo P, Fang Q, et al. Angiopoietin-2 induces human glioma invasion through the activation of matrix metalloprotease-2. Proc Natl Acad Sci U S A 2003;100:8904–9.

48. Galli R, Binda E, Orfanelli U, et al. Isolation and characterization of tumorigenic, stem-like neural precursors from human glioblastoma. Cancer Res 2004;64:7011–21.

49. Yuan X, Curtin J, Xiong Y, et al. Isolation of cancer stem cells from adult glioblastoma multiforme. Oncogene 2004;23:9392–400.

50. Zeppernick F, Ahmadi R, Campos B, et al. Stem cell marker CD133 affects clinical outcome in glioma patients. Clin Cancer Res 2008;14:123–9.

51. Clément V, Dutoit V, Marino D, et al. Limits of CD133 as a marker of glioma self-renewing cells. Int J Cancer 2009;125:244–8.

52. Joo KM, Kim SY, Jin X, et al. Clinical and biological implications of CD133-positive and CD133-negative cells in glioblastomas. Lab Invest 2008; 88:808–15.

53. Shu Q, Wong KK, Su JM, et al. Direct orthotopic transplantation of fresh surgical specimen preserves CD133+ tumor cells in clinically relevant mouse models of medulloblastoma and glioma. Stem Cells 2008;26:1414–24.

54. Wang J, Sakariassen PO, Tsinkalovsky O, et al. CD133 negative glioma cells form tumors in nude rats and give rise to CD133 positive cells. Int J Cancer 2008;122:761–8.

55. Yan X, Ma L, Yi D, et al. A CD133-related gene expression signature identifies an aggressive

glioblastoma subtype with excessive mutations. Proc Natl Acad Sci U S A 2011;108:1591–6.

56. Bao S, Wu Q, Sathornsumetee S, et al. Stem cell-like glioma cells promote tumor angiogenesis through vascular endothelial growth factor. Cancer Res 2006;66:7843–8.

57. Beier D, Hau P, Proescholdt M, et al. CD133(+) and CD133(-) glioblastoma-derived cancer stem cells show differential growth characteristics and molecular profiles. Cancer Res 2007;67:4010–5.

58. Son MJ, Woolard K, Nam DH, et al. SSEA-1 is an enrichment marker for tumor-initiating cells in human glioblastoma. Cell Stem Cell 2009;4: 440–52.

59. Kondo T, Setoguchi T, Taga T. Persistence of a small subpopulation of cancer stem-like cells in the C6 glioma cell line. Proc Natl Acad Sci U S A 2004; 101:781–6.

60. Wu A, Oh S, Wiesner SM, et al. Persistence of CD133+ cells in human and mouse glioma cell lines: detailed characterization of GL261 glioma cells with cancer stem cell-like properties. Stem Cells Dev 2008;17:173–84.

61. Broadley KW, Hunn MK, Farrand KJ, et al. Side population is not necessary or sufficient for a cancer stem cell phenotype in glioblastoma multiforme. Stem Cells 2011;29:452–61.

62. Lathia JD, Gallagher J, Heddleston JM, et al. Integrin alpha 6 regulates glioblastoma stem cells. Cell Stem Cell 2010;6:421–32.

63. Ogden AT, Waziri AE, Lochhead RA, et al. Identification of A2B5+CD133- tumor-initiating cells in adult human gliomas. Neurosurgery 2008;62: 505–14 [discussion: 514–5].

64. Tabatabai G, Weller M. Glioblastoma stem cells. Cell Tissue Res 2011;343:459–65.

65. Gunther HS, Schmidt NO, Phillips HS, et al. Glioblastoma-derived stem cell-enriched cultures form distinct subgroups according to molecular and phenotypic criteria. Oncogene 2008;27:2897–909.

66. Rasper M, Schafer A, Piontek G, et al. Aldehyde dehydrogenase 1 positive glioblastoma cells show brain tumor stem cell capacity. Neuro Oncol 2010;12:1024–33.

67. Fatoo A, Nanaszko MJ, Allen BB, et al. Understanding the role of tumor stem cells in glioblastoma multiforme: a review article. J Neurooncol 2011;103:397–408.

68. Zheng X, Shen G, Yang X, et al. Most C6 cells are cancer stem cells: evidence from clonal and population analyses. Cancer Res 2007;67:3691–7.

69. Lee J, Kotliarova S, Kotliarov Y, et al. Tumor stem cells derived from glioblastomas cultured in bFGF and EGF more closely mirror the phenotype and genotype of primary tumors than do serum-cultured cell lines. Cancer Cell 2006;9: 391–403.

70. Fargeas CA, Joester A, Missol-Kolka E, et al. Identification of novel Prominin-1/CD133 splice variants with alternative C-termini and their expression in epididymis and testis. J Cell Sci 2004;117: 4301–11.

71. Osmond TL, Broadley KW, McConnell MJ. Glioblastoma cells negative for the anti-CD133 antibody AC133 express a truncated variant of the CD133 protein. Int J Mol Med 2010;25:883–8.

72. Florek M, Haase M, Marzesco AM, et al. Prominin-1/CD133, a neural and hematopoietic stem cell marker, is expressed in adult human differentiated cells and certain types of kidney cancer. Cell Tissue Res 2005;319:15–26.

73. Shackleton M, Quintana E, Fearon ER, et al. Heterogeneity in cancer: cancer stem cells versus clonal evolution. Cell 2009;138:822–9.

74. Lottaz C, Beier D, Meyer K, et al. Transcriptional profiles of CD133+ and CD133- glioblastoma-derived cancer stem cell lines suggest different cells of origin. Cancer Res 2010;70:2030–40.

75. Phillips HS, Kharbanda S, Chen R, et al. Molecular subclasses of high-grade glioma predict prognosis, delineate a pattern of disease progression, and resemble stages in neurogenesis. Cancer Cell 2006;9:157–73.

76. Chen R, Nishimura MC, Bumbaca SM, et al. A hierarchy of self-renewing tumor-initiating cell types in glioblastoma. Cancer Cell 2010;17:362–75.

77. Dai C, Celestino JC, Okada Y, et al. PDGF autocrine stimulation dedifferentiates cultured astrocytes and induces oligodendrogliomas and oligoastrocytomas from neural progenitors and astrocytes in vivo. Genes Dev 2001;15:1913–25.

78. Read TA, Fogarty MP, Markant SL, et al. Identification of CD15 as a marker for tumor-propagating cells in a mouse model of medulloblastoma. Cancer Cell 2009;15:135–47.

79. Schuller U, Heine VM, Mao J, et al. Acquisition of granule neuron precursor identity is a critical determinant of progenitor cell competence to form Shh-induced medulloblastoma. Cancer Cell 2008;14: 123–34.

80. Uhrbom L, Dai C, Celestino JC, et al. Ink4a-Arf loss cooperates with KRas activation in astrocytes and neural progenitors to generate glioblastomas of various morphologies depending on activated Akt. Cancer Res 2002;62:5551–8.

81. Yang ZJ, Ellis T, Markant SL, et al. Medulloblastoma can be initiated by deletion of Patched in lineage-restricted progenitors or stem cells. Cancer Cell 2008;14:135–45.

82. Engebraaten O, Hjortland GO, Hirschberg H, et al. Growth of precultured human glioma specimens in nude rat brain. J Neurosurg 1999;90:125–32.

83. Kaloshi G, Mokhtari K, Carpentier C, et al. FABP7 expression in glioblastomas: relation to prognosis,

invasion and EGFR status. J Neurooncol 2007;84: 245–8.

84. Liang Y, Bollen AW, Aldape KD, et al. Nuclear FABP7 immunoreactivity is preferentially expressed in infiltrative glioma and is associated with poor prognosis in EGFR-overexpressing glioblastoma. BMC Cancer 2006;6:97.

85. Arai Y, Funatsu N, Numayama-Tsuruta K, et al. Role of Fabp7, a downstream gene of Pax6, in the maintenance of neuroepithelial cells during early embryonic development of the rat cortex. J Neurosci 2005;25:9752–61.

86. McCord AM, Jamal M, Shankavaram UT, et al. Physiologic oxygen concentration enhances the stem-like properties of CD133+ human glioblastoma cells in vitro. Mol Cancer Res 2009;7: 489–97.

87. Pouyssegur J, Dayan F, Mazure NM. Hypoxia signalling in cancer and approaches to enforce tumour regression. Nature 2006;441:437–43.

88. Keith B, Simon MC. Hypoxia-inducible factors, stem cells, and cancer. Cell 2007;129:465–72.

89. Evans SM, Judy KD, Dunphy I, et al. Hypoxia is important in the biology and aggression of human glial brain tumors. Clin Cancer Res 2004;10: 8177–84.

90. Dings J, Meixensberger J, Jager A, et al. Clinical experience with 118 brain tissue oxygen partial pressure catheter probes. Neurosurgery 1998;43: 1082–95.

91. Platet N, Liu SY, Atifi ME, et al. Influence of oxygen tension on CD133 phenotype in human glioma cell cultures. Cancer Lett 2007;258:286–90.

92. Griguer CE, Oliva CR, Gobin E, et al. CD133 is a marker of bioenergetic stress in human glioma. PLoS One 2008;3:e3655.

93. Li Z, Wang H, Eyler CE, et al. Turning cancer stem cells inside out: an exploration of glioma stem cell signaling pathways. J Biol Chem 2009;284: 16705–9.

94. Matsumoto K, Arao T, Tanaka K, et al. mTOR signal and hypoxia-inducible factor-1 alpha regulate CD133 expression in cancer cells. Cancer Res 2009;69:7160–4.

95. Forristal CE, Wright KL, Hanley NA, et al. Hypoxia inducible factors regulate pluripotency and proliferation in human embryonic stem cells cultured at reduced oxygen tensions. Reproduction 2010; 139:85–97.

96. Tabu K, Sasai K, Kimura T, et al. Promoter hypomethylation regulates CD133 expression in human gliomas. Cell Res 2008;18:1037–46.

97. Yi JM, Tsai HC, Glockner SC, et al. Abnormal DNA methylation of CD133 in colorectal and glioblastoma tumors. Cancer Res 2008;68:8094–103.

98. Jaksch M, Munera J, Bajpai R, et al. Cell cycle-dependent variation of a CD133 epitope in human embryonic stem cell, colon cancer, and melanoma cell lines. Cancer Res 2008;68:7882–6.

99. Gray D, Jubb AM, Hogue D, et al. Maternal embryonic leucine zipper kinase/murine protein serine-threonine kinase 38 is a promising therapeutic target for multiple cancers. Cancer Res 2005;65: 9751–61.

100. El Hallani S, Boisselier B, Peglion F, et al. A new alternative mechanism in glioblastoma vascularization: tubular vasculogenic mimicry. Brain 2010;133: 973–82.

101. Kreisl TN, Kim L, Moore K, et al. Phase II trial of single-agent bevacizumab followed by bevacizumab plus irinotecan at tumor progression in recurrent glioblastoma. J Clin Oncol 2009;27:740–5.

102. Vredenburgh JJ, Desjardins A, Herndon JE 2nd, et al. Phase II trial of bevacizumab and irinotecan in recurrent malignant glioma. Clin Cancer Res 2007;13:1253–9.

103. Soda Y, Marumoto T, Friedmann-Morvinski D, et al. Transdifferentiation of glioblastoma cells into vascular endothelial cells. Proc Natl Acad Sci U S A 2011;108:4274–80.

104. He H, Niu CS, Li MW. Correlation between glioblastoma stem-like cells and tumor vascularization. Oncol Rep 2012;27:45–50.

105. Wang R, Chadalavada K, Wilshire J, et al. Glioblastoma stem-like cells give rise to tumour endothelium. Nature 2010;468:829–33.

106. Ricci-Vitiani L, Pallini R, Biffoni M, et al. Tumour vascularization via endothelial differentiation of glioblastoma stem-like cells. Nature 2010;468: 824–8.

107. Marumoto T, Tashiro A, Friedmann-Morvinski D, et al. Development of a novel mouse glioma model using lentiviral vectors. Nat Med 2009;15:110–6.

108. Bergers G, Benjamin LE. Tumorigenesis and the angiogenic switch. Nat Rev Cancer 2003;3: 401–10.

109. Bertolini F, Shaked Y, Mancuso P, et al. The multifaceted circulating endothelial cell in cancer: towards marker and target identification. Nat Rev Cancer 2006;6:835–45.

110. Gunsilius E, Duba HC, Petzer AL, et al. Evidence from a leukaemia model for maintenance of vascular endothelium by bone-marrow-derived endothelial cells. Lancet 2000;355:1688–91.

111. Streubel B, Chott A, Huber D, et al. Lymphoma-specific genetic aberrations in microvascular endothelial cells in B-cell lymphomas. N Engl J Med 2004;351:250–9.

112. Rigolin GM, Fraulini C, Ciccone M, et al. Neoplastic circulating endothelial cells in multiple myeloma with 13q14 deletion. Blood 2006;107:2531–5.

113. Calabrese C, Poppleton H, Kocak M, et al. A perivascular niche for brain tumor stem cells. Cancer Cell 2007;11:69–82.

114. Fuchs E, Tumbar T, Guasch G. Socializing with the neighbors: stem cells and their niche. Cell 2004; 116:769–78.

115. Moore KA, Lemischka IR. Stem cells and their niches. Science 2006;311:1880–5.

116. Borovski T, De Sousa EMF, Vermeulen L, et al. Cancer stem cell niche: the place to be. Cancer Res 2011;71:634–9.

117. Shen Q, Goderie SK, Jin L, et al. Endothelial cells stimulate self-renewal and expand neurogenesis of neural stem cells. Science 2004;304:1338–40.

118. Ramirez-Castillejo C, Sanchez-Sanchez F, Andreu-Agullo C, et al. Pigment epithelium-derived factor is a niche signal for neural stem cell renewal. Nat Neurosci 2006;9:331–9.

119. Leventhal C, Rafii S, Rafii D, et al. Endothelial trophic support of neuronal production and recruitment from the adult mammalian subependyma. Mol Cell Neurosci 1999;13:450–64.

120. Louissaint A Jr, Rao S, Leventhal C, et al. Coordinated interaction of neurogenesis and angiogenesis in the adult songbird brain. Neuron 2002;34: 945–60.

121. He H, Li MW, Niu CS. The pathological characteristics of glioma stem cell niches. J Clin Neurosci 2012;19(1):121–7.

122. Charles N, Holland EC. The perivascular niche microenvironment in brain tumor progression. Cell Cycle 2010;9:3012–21.

123. Pallini R, Ricci-Vitiani L, Banna GL, et al. Cancer stem cell analysis and clinical outcome in patients with glioblastoma multiforme. Clin Cancer Res 2008;14:8205–12.

124. Beier D, Wischhusen J, Dietmaier W, et al. CD133 expression and cancer stem cells predict prognosis in high-grade oligodendroglial tumors. Brain Pathol 2008;18:370–7.

125. Kong DS, Kim MH, Park WY, et al. The progression of gliomas is associated with cancer stem cell phenotype. Oncology Reports 2008;19:639–43.

126. Bao S, Wu Q, McLendon RE, et al. Glioma stem cells promote radioresistance by preferential activation of the DNA damage response. Nature 2006;444:756–60.

127. Angelastro JM, Lame MW. Overexpression of CD133 promotes drug resistance in C6 glioma cells. Mol Cancer Res 2010;8:1105–15.

128. Salmaggi A, Boiardi A, Gelati M, et al. Glioblastoma-derived tumorospheres identify a population of tumor stem-like cells with angiogenic potential and enhanced multidrug resistance phenotype. Glia 2006;54:850–60.

129. Liu G, Yuan X, Zeng Z, et al. Analysis of gene expression and chemoresistance of CD133+ cancer stem cells in glioblastoma. Mol Cancer 2006;5:67.

130. Das S, Srikanth M, Kessler JA. Cancer stem cells and glioma. Nat Clin Pract Neurol 2008;4: 427–35.

Clinical Trials of Small Molecule Inhibitors in High-Grade Glioma

Samuel E. Day, PhD[a], Allen Waziri, MD[b],*

KEYWORDS

- Glioblastoma • Small molecule inhibitor • Clinical trial

KEY POINTS

- Small molecule inhibitors (SMIs) are highly selective compounds that are generally water soluble with high oral bioavailability. These agents are designed to produce targeted inhibition at the active site of proteins involved with critical pathways in tumor biology.
- Several SMIs, including sunitinib (renal cell carcinoma) and imatinib (chronic myelogenous leukemia), have shown significant therapeutic benefit in clinical trials and are now considered standard of care.
- Several clinical trials of SMIs have been performed in patients with glioblastoma, including drugs targeting epidermal-derived growth factor receptor, platelet-derived growth factor receptor, and vascular endothelial growth factor receptor. To date, there has been no reported clinical benefit associated with the use of currently available agents.
- Increasing insight into the heterogeneous nature of glioblastoma may allow future tailoring of targeted agents for individual patients.

CHEMOTHERAPY: OPPORTUNITIES FOR OPTIMIZATION IN HIGH-GRADE GLIOMA

Modern chemotherapy can be traced to the discovery of the antitumoral properties of nitrogen mustard, a DNA alkylating agent used in chemical warfare.[1] The first trial of nitrogen mustard derivatives, used to treat Hodgkin lymphoma in the 1940s, followed observations of lymphosuppressive and myelosuppressive effects in soldiers exposed to mustard gas. Most historical approaches to treating cancers have incorporated agents that derive a degree of disease specificity by inducing DNA damage in rapidly dividing cells. Chemotherapeutics have traditionally been derived from broadly toxic substances that trigger cascades of programmed cell death in actively dividing tumor cells. However, the sequelae of this strategy are the many nonspecific effects in normal cells with high rates of turnover, such as those in the bone marrow, digestive tract, and hair follicles. Examples of 2 cytotoxic drugs that remain standard of care in primary and recurrent glioblastoma multiforme (GBM) are carmustine (BCNU, Gliadel) and temozolomide (TMZ; Temodar, Temodal).[2–4] These 2 drugs alkylate many cellular functional groups, including sites on guanine and cytosine nucleotides, thereby triggering the DNA damage–detecting checkpoint mechanisms of mitosis that subsequently promote cellular apoptotic cascades.

DNA-damaging approaches are limited in many aggressive tumors, because of mutations resulting in prosurvival traits including defective apoptotic signaling cascades, upregulation of rates of DNA repair, and increased rates of mutation leading to drug resistance. GBM is known to be inherently

[a] Medical Scientist Training Program, University of Colorado School of Medicine; [b] Department of Neurosurgery, University of Colorado, Academic Office Building One, Room 5001, 12631 East, 17th Avenue, Aurora, CO 80045, USA
* Corresponding author.
E-mail address: allen.waziri@ucdenver.edu

Neurosurg Clin N Am 23 (2012) 407–416
doi:10.1016/j.nec.2012.04.004
1042-3680/12/$ – see front matter © 2012 Elsevier Inc. All rights reserved.

resistant to nearly every standard DNA-damaging chemotherapeutic agent. The lack of significant progress with traditional cytotoxic agents has provided the impetus for a new strategy of targeting specific alterations in signaling pathways responsible for the development and maintenance of GBM. Recent genome-wide analyses of human GBM tumor samples have amassed data regarding the commonly altered, mutated, or amplified genes implicated in GBM development,[5] many of which involve receptor tyrosine kinase (RTK) signaling pathways. Several these overactive signaling pathways, which include upstream receptors as well as downstream targets of activation, are the specific focus of many small molecule inhibitor (SMI) drugs.

WHAT IS AN SMI?

A small molecule drug is a nonpolymeric organic compound, generally fewer than 800 to 1000 Da. SMIs are designed to specifically inhibit the activity of a cellular constituent for therapeutic benefit. In practice, SMIs should be soluble in aqueous solution, lipophilic enough to cross the cellular membrane, and bind specifically to a target of interest to effect some change in cellular function. A particular advantage of these compounds is their potential for high selectivity for an active region of a given target, thus minimizing potential side effects. Major additional benefits inherent to small molecule compounds include the potential for oral bioavailability and, in the specific case of brain tumors, potentially superior passage across the blood-brain barrier relative to larger compounds (such as antibodies). These properties, combined with an ability to screen both new and modified compounds in high-throughput fashion, have led to the role of SMIs as a large proportion of drugs under current clinical study for cancer.

Most SMIs find efficacy via inhibition of function; as a result, most of these drugs are targeted toward reducing flux through overactive oncogenic pathways. Many of the SMIs in current clinical use have been identified either serendipitously or through in vitro screens focusing on a desired biologic activity. Several SMIs, designed to inhibit specific kinases that are upregulated in many cancers, have recently changed standard clinical practice for several solid tumors. Examples include lapatinib (Tykerb) for metastatic breast cancer,[6] sunitinib (Sutent) for metastatic renal cell carcinoma (RCC),[7] and sorafenib (Nexavar), which has proved efficacious in both advanced hepatocellular carcinoma[8] and advanced RCC.[9] Perhaps the best-known example of a targeted agent is the tyrosine kinase inhibitor imatinib mesylate (Gleevec). This

small molecule was designed to inhibit a mutated RTK fusion protein, Bcr-Abl, the constitutive activation of which has long been known to cause chronic myelogenous leukemia (CML). In what is considered to be the proof-of-principle success story for SMIs in cancer, patients with chronic-phase CML treated with imatinib generally experience dramatic remission with few side effects.[10]

The remainder of this article focuses on specific SMIs designed to target signaling pathways previously associated with malignant glioma (reviewed in **Fig. 1**) and reviews preliminary results of clinical trials using these drugs.

EPIDERMAL-DERIVED GROWTH FACTOR RECEPTOR

Perhaps the best example of increased RTK signaling in GBM is that of the epidermal-derived growth factor receptor (EGFR), which increases activation of the downstream RAS and PI3K intracellular signaling cascades. Early studies suggested that around 40% of GBM show EGFR amplification and protein overexpression leading to increased pathway flux.[11] Furthermore, approximately 40% of GBM with EGFR amplification also harbor activating EGFR mutations.[12] These findings have been recently supported through integrated genome analysis from The Cancer Genome Atlas (TCGA) Research Network study, which found that 41 of 91 (45%) sequenced tumors harbored EGFR alterations.[13]

Several SMIs designed to inhibit EGFR and its mutant variants have been or are currently under investigation in GBM, including erlotinib (Tarceva), gefitinib (Iressa), lapatinib, and AEE788, as well as a host of monoclonal antibodies outside the scope of this article. Although the drugs seem to be well tolerated, most early single-agent trials of EGFR inhibitors have failed to show significant therapeutic benefit in GBM. In one phase II study, 13% of patients remained progression free for 6 months in response to gefitinib monotherapy.[14] However, results from trials in lung cancer, in which improved clinical and radiographic responses to gefitinib have correlated with documented mutations in the EGFR kinase regions,[15] have not been similarly recapitulated in patients with GBM.[16] Preliminary data from trials focusing on erlotinib[17,18] were slightly more encouraging than the results from gefitinib trials,[14,19] suggesting potentially greater activity of this compound against the constitutively active EGFRvIII mutant receptor[20] frequently found in GBM,[21,22] but limited overall efficacy was seen. Despite disappointing early trials comparing single-agent administration of erlotinib versus temozolomide or BCNU to treat GBMbeing,[23,24]

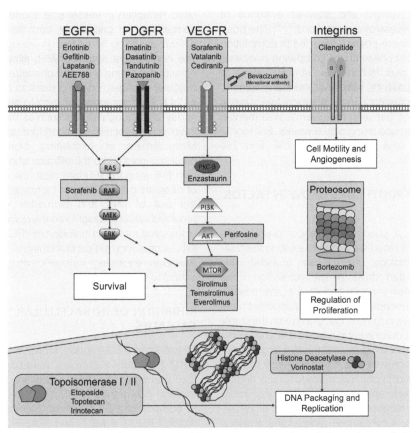

Fig. 1. Molecular targets of interest for SMIs in glioblastoma. EGFR, epidermal-derived growth factor receptor; PDGFR, platelet-derived growth factor receptor, VEGFR, vascular endothelial growth factor receptor.

further study to understand the potential cytostatic effects of EGFR inhibitors on GBM is warranted. To this end, EGFR inhibitors have been incorporated into multidrug trials including standard therapies (radiation therapy [RT] and TMZ) to determine any synergistic effect. One recent phase I/II trial showed no benefit of adding erlotinib to standard RT/TMZ protocols,[25] whereas another phase II trial combining erlotinib with TMZ before and after RT showed increased median survival (19.1 months) relative to historical controls (14.1 months).[26] It is likely that the variety of alterations observed in the RTK signaling axis of GBM means that some patients will find benefit from EGFR inhibition, whereas many will not, and also that combination therapies might be designed to address the most common alterations. Further studies using erlotinib as a component of first-line therapy may continue to elucidate this concept.

PLATELET-DERIVED GROWTH FACTOR RECEPTOR

Platelet-derived growth factor receptor (PDGFR) is another RTK signaling molecule with documented

upregulation of expression in a subset of GBM.[27] Inhibitors of PDGFR include the drugs imatinib, dasatinib (Sprycel), tandutinib, and pazopanib (Votrient). Imatinib, an inhibitor of PDGFR as well as other selected RTKs (including KIT and ABL), is indicated for the treatment of CML and gastrointestinal stromal cell tumors. As mentioned earlier, response to imatinib in these previously untreatable tumors is often dramatic. However, imatinib has generally failed to show similar efficacy as a single-agent therapeutic drug in GBM[28–30] despite studies that detected intact imatinib within the GBM tissue.[31] A recent European Organization for Research and Treatment of Cancer (EORTC) study using imatinib monotherapy in 112 patients with recurrent gliomas showed evidence of radiological response in the form of a reduction of postcontrast T1 gadolinium enhancement but did not show a concomitant improvement in clinical outcomes. It was concluded that, in the range of 600 to 1000 mg/d, imatinib shows a good safety profile but lacks antitumor activity in most patients with recurrent glioma.[32] Two phase II studies of recurrent GBM, using a combination of hydroxyurea (HU) plus imatinib, suggested that this combination strategy was well tolerated by patients and showed evidence of response in excess of expectations.[33,34] The positive results in these phase II trials led to completion of a randomized phase III trial comparing combination imatinib plus HU therapy with HU alone in progressive patients with TMZ-resistant tumors. However, no difference in progression-free survival (PFS) was seen between the 2 arms, with median PFS in both groups being only 6 weeks. Six-month PFS (PFS-6) was also similar at 5% and 7% respectively.[35]

VASCULAR ENDOTHELIAL GROWTH FACTOR RECEPTOR

Angiogenesis, a phenomenon encompassing the creation of new blood vessels from existing vasculature, is a pathologic characteristic of GBM. This process is, in part, driven by the expression of the regulatory protein vascular endothelial growth factor (VEGF) and its receptor (VEGFR). The apparent need for angiogenesis in tumors, compared with the stable vascular networks present in other tissues, has implicated VEGFR signaling as an attractive target for inhibiting tumor growth, which is particularly relevant for GBM, a tumor in which increased vascular density and VEGF levels are associated with poor prognosis.[36] Given recent clinical success with bevacizumab (Avastin), a humanized monoclonal antibody against VEGF, there has been increasing focus on exploring SMIs targeting VEGF/VEGFR in GBM.

SMIs developed to inhibit VEGFR include the drugs vatalanib and cediranib (tentative trade name Recentin), both of which have shown promise in early clinical trials. Vatalanib inhibits both the VEGFR and platelet-derived growth factor receptor (PDGFR), and has shown moderate effect when used alone or in combination with TMZ or lomustine to treat recurrent GBM in phase I/II multicenter trials.[37,38]

A recent study designed to target both EGFR and VEGFR using a combination of erlotinib and bevacizumab (a monoclonal antibody) was well tolerated in patients, but showed no benefit in increasing PFS compared with that of historical regimens containing bevacizumab.[39,40]

A phase II trial of cedirinib, which inhibits many forms of VEGFR, recently showed evidence of activity with a PFS-6 of 27.6%, normalization of vasculature, and reduction of edema in patients with GBM.[41] Because serial sampling of GBM tissue is generally not possible, this study used multiple MRI-based methods to measure functional tissue response to cedirinib over time. These methods included measurements of vessel size, permeability, gadolinium enhancement, and diffusion-weighted imaging (DWI) characteristics. The results showed rapid reduction in vessel size, blood volume, and permeability to gadolinium contrast agents, with a corresponding reduction in vasogenic edema. The noninvasive nature of MRI allowed repeated measurement and temporal characterization of the vascular changes, showing them to begin as early as 24 hours after treatment, and to begin to reverse at day 28, although effects such as the reduction in vascular permeability persisted for up to 4 months. Measurement of circulating biomarkers also provided insight into the efficacy of cedirinib in this trial: following VEGFR inhibition, the concentration of circulating VEGF ligand increased. In addition, the use of MRI and biomarker measurement provided valuable insight into the duration of effects of the small molecule inhibition of VEGFR with cedirinib, suggesting that careful timing of combinatorial therapies (including cytotoxic drugs) might be critical to their success.

INHIBITION OF INTRACELLULAR SIGNALING CASCADES

Overall, the TCGA study found that 88% of all GBM harbored 1 or more mutations increasing the activity of the RTK signaling axis and flux through downstream RAS and PI3K pathways.[13] In addition to EGFR activity, increased signaling of the ERBB2, c-MET, and PDGFR RTKs can all result in activation of RAS and PI3K; whereas signaling through VEGF activates both pathways via PKC-β. However, increased activity of RTKs are not the only drivers of RAS and PI3K signaling. RAS and PI3K are themselves upregulated in many GBM, whereas their endogenous inhibitors NF1 and PTEN (phosphatidylinositol phosphate 3'-phosphatase) are often mutated or lost.[13,42] Loss of PTEN inhibition has been shown to remove sensitivity to EGFR inhibition by erlotinib and gefitinib[43] and is a powerful negative prognostic factor.[44] Subsequent signaling molecules in the 2 pathways have been identified and are also deregulated and mutated, resulting in increased flux through the pathways. The characterization of these downstream alterations gives rise to approaches other than simply targeting more or different cell surface RTKs.

RAS/RAF

RAS signaling ultimately activates the transcription factor extracellular signal-regulated kinase (ERK) by way of the intermediate proteins RAF and MEK. Tipifarnib (Zarnestra) is a farnesyl transferase–inhibiting drug shown to reduce signaling through the RAS pathway. Although early phase I trials determined that tipifarnib is well tolerated by patients with GBM, early phase II trials failed to show a benefit of tipifarnib when added to TMZ and RT. The RAF protein is among those inhibited by the drug sorafenib, currently being studied in GBM. In addition to its effects on RAF, sorafenib also shows inhibitory effects on VEGFR and PDGFR.[45] However, despite potentially complimentary antitumor effects, trials combining sorafenib with TMZ and RT have thus far failed to show benefit, although the drug combination was well tolerated in patients.[46] Similarly, studies of recurrent GBM treated concurrently with sorafenib and TMZ have been unsuccessful in improving outcomes.[47] There are several additional active trials of sorafenib that may provide important information about the effect of combining sorafenib with other agents including erlotinib, the RAS inhibitor tipifarnib, and the mTOR inhibitor temsirolimus (Torisel). A study proposing treatment of recurrent GBM with sorafenib plus the mTOR inhibitor evirolimus (Afinitor, Zortress) has recently been approved, but is not yet recruiting patients.

PI3K

It has been suggested that aberrant activation of the PI3K pathway is universal in human cancer. PI3K pathways regulate several malignant phenotypes including resistance to apoptosis, cell growth, proliferation, and invasion, and PI3K activation is associated with poor prognosis in GBM.[48,49] PI3K signaling activates AKT and subsequently mTOR via phosphorylation of phosphatidylinositol-4,5-bisphosphate (PIP2) to produce phosphatidylinositol-3,4,5-trisphosphate (PIP3). Perifosine is an AKT inhibitor that has shown promise in preclinical studies and is currently being tested in phase II trials.[50] mTOR can also be activated downstream of RAS and is therefore an example of a confluence of the RAS and PI3K pathways. The mTOR-inhibiting drugs sirolimus (Rapamycin, Rapamune) and temsirolimus have been studied in human GBM, though dramatic growth inhibition has not been seen.[51–53] Two single-agent phase II trials of temsirolimus showed altered radiological response after monotherapy, but failed to show a prolongation of survival.[52,53] These trials suggest that mTOR inhibition alone is likely to be insufficient for effective GBM therapy, although these agents continue to have potential as components of multimodal approaches.

β-PROTEIN KINASE C

The β-protein kinase C (PKC-β) signaling molecule is implicated in promoting activity of both the RAS and PI3K pathways after activation through VEGFR. Expression of this receptor, and its subsequent activation of PKC-β, leads to downstream promotion of the prosurvival and progrowth pathways described earlier. The drug enzastaurin, which inhibits PKC-β activity,[54] has been shown to affect total flux through the PI3K and RAS pathways and was determined in preclinical studies to be a good candidate drug for trials in GBM. A recent phase II trial showed a strong radiological response in 26% of patients treated with enzastaurin for recurrent glioma.[55,56] This success was used as rationale to begin a phase III clinical trial comparing enzastaurin with the alkylating drug lomustine (CCNU, CeeNU) for the treatment of recurrent GBM. Although this study was terminated early because of the lack of an increase in median overall survival (OS) or median PFS compared with lomustine, the enzastaurin was better tolerated, suggesting the potential for inclusion of enzastaurin into combination therapies.[57–60] To this end, a study combining enzastaurin with RT and TMZ for the treatment of primary GBM is ongoing (clinicaltrials.gov), and enzastaurin is also being combined with the antiangiogenic antibody bevacizumab and the alkylating agent carboplatin (Paraplatin) in a study for the treatment of recurrent GBM.

OTHER AGENTS

Several SMIs have been developed to target intracellular proteins that are not implicated in the RTK-RAS-PI3K signaling axis. These SMIs include inhibitors of topoisomerase I and II, histone deacetylase, integrins, and the proteasome.

Topoisomerase inhibitors include the drugs etoposide, topotecan, irinotecan, edotecarin, rubitecan, pyrazoloacridine, karenitecin, and gimatecan, many of which have shown efficacy in various types of cancer. Topoisomerase-inhibiting drugs block function of the cellular enzymes topoisomerase I and II, which bind to DNA and result in breakage and ligation of the phosphodiester backbone during the S phase of the cell cycle, allowing unwinding (and, thus, unpackaging) of supercoiled DNA. It is thought that topoisomerase-inhibiting drugs block the ligation step, and thereby produce single-stranded and double-stranded DNA breaks that compromise integrity and result in checkpoint arrest and cellular apoptosis. Several single-agent studies of irinotecan have shown discouraging results in patients with recurrent malignant gliomas.[61–65] Despite this, the unique cytotoxic action of these drugs has made them an attractive potential component of multimodal therapy, especially in patients who have recurrent disease or those whose methylguanine methyltransferase (MGMT) status suggests that they will be resistant to TMZ therapy. Trials combining topoisomerase inhibitors with other therapies have shown some benefit to the addition of these drugs, and the combination of irinotecan and bevacizumab has been shown to have some effect in treating recurrent GBM in a phase II study.[66,67] Another study using etoposide in place of irinotecan showed similar results,[68] supporting the case for combinatorial approaches to using topoisomerase inhibitors in GBM.

Histone deacetylase enzymes (HDAC) remove acetyl groups from histones, allowing for the unpackaging of supercoiled DNA, which is normally stored condensed and wound around the histone proteins. This process is important in DNA replication as well as DNA repair; inhibition of HDAC results in cell cycle arrest and apoptosis in cancer cells. Pretreatment of patients with cancer with HDAC inhibitors has been shown to sensitize GBM cells to RT and DNA-damaging chemotherapeutics.[69–71] In phase II trials of recurrent GBM, vorinostat induced inhibition of HDAC and showed modest single-agent activity. As a result of this finding, and considering the method of action of HDAC, various clinical trials of vorinostat combined with RT, TMZ, erlotinib, bevacizumab, or irinotecan are underway.

Integrins are a class of cell adhesion proteins that are important regulators of motility and angiogenesis in glioma cells.[72] The recent development of cilgenitide, an inhibitor of the a_vb_3 and a_vb_5 integrins has shown some promise in recently completed trials in recurrent[73] as well as newly diagnosed GBM.[74] However, it has been suggested that the improvements seen in these 2 trials were possible artifacts of the progressively improved care common to all add-on TMZ therapies, rather than a result of cilengitide itself.[75] Accrual of patients for an international phase III trial to test the effects of addition of cilengitide to the standard therapy for TMZ and RT in newly diagnosed GBM has just been completed. This CENTRIC study should answer many of the questions regarding the benefit of adding cilengitide to standard therapy when treating GBM.[74]

The ubiquitin-proteasome complex is a critical regulatory element in the scheduled degradation of cell cycle proteins involved in balancing proliferation and apoptosis.[76] Inhibition of the proteasome disrupts the cyclic degradation of these regulatory proteins, and can induce cell growth arrest leading to the induction of apoptosis. The proteasome-inhibiting drug bortezomib (Velcade) showed growth arrest in glioma cells in vitro, and

is currently being tested in several phase II trials in combination with TMZ or other targeted agents. However, one such phase II trial showed no significant benefit from the combination of the HDAC inhibitor vorinostat (Zolinza) with bortezomib.[77]

FUTURE DIRECTIONS

An ever-increasing armamentarium of SMI drugs has resulted from increasing understanding of the altered signaling inherent to many cancers, and many of these agents are dramatically changing care in previously untreatable diseases such as CML and gastrointestinal stromal tumors. Given the dismal prognosis of high-grade glioma, there has been considerable hope that newer drugs would improve outcomes in this aggressive cancer. However, as outlined earlier, few of these new targeted agents have shown significant or prolonged survival benefits in initial studies of patients with GBM.

There are several potential explanations for current failures with the use of SMIs for GBM. Because of the diverse genetic bases of these tumors, a variety of mutations involving oncogene and tumor suppressor pathways may drive tumor progression in individual patients and likely require multiple agents (targeting both antigrowth and proapoptotic functionality) for clinically relevant antitumor effects. Given coactivation and downstream overlap of multiple oncogenic RTK within GBM, it is likely that inhibition of any RTK can be compensated by increased activation of another. For example, PDGFR and c-MET receptors are engaged after EGFR inhibition and maintain downstream pathway activation.[78] Taken together, these findings suggest that multiple targeted agents used in combination might be required to effectively attenuate RTK signal transmission in GBM.[79]

In addition, although increasing OS is the most pertinent goal of any treatment strategy for cancer, this is only 1 of several relevant clinical endpoints to evaluate drug efficacy. Given that many SMIs are cytostatic in nature, it is likely that their effects on tumor cells could be overlooked when using traditional metrics of prolonged survival and radiological response. To this end, the development of biomarkers and molecular imaging tools to report on drug concentration and activity at the site of interest are important goals that would provide valuable information aiding the design of future studies.

In addition, large-scale studies to better characterize the genetic changes associated with GBM will be critically important for integrating the understanding of common molecular alterations and subsequently tailoring specific therapy. In an example of such an approach, recent data from TCGA Research Network has reclassified GBM into 4 distinct subtypes based on abnormalities in commonly altered signaling pathways.[80] The differentiators include upregulation of EGFR and PDGFR-, loss of NF1, and activation of IDH1. This identification of GBM subtypes seems to predict those patients who will respond best to aggressive conventional therapies, versus those who respond only poorly or not at all. This example of a clinically relevant stratification approach, based on commonly altered pathways in GBM, provides researchers with a strong foundation on which to design pathway-targeted combination regimens. This information also serves to identify the patient subtypes most likely to derive benefit from aggressive traditional therapies, versus those who will not and should therefore be encouraged to enroll in trials of experimental therapeutics as first-line agents.

Regarding overall approach, integration of the known effects of targeted agents to provide redundancy in signaling inhibition should be a major focus of future trial design. It may be shown that slowing overactive oncogenic cascades through small molecule inhibition may not provide enough antitumor benefit to improve overall outcomes, emphasizing that this approach may be best applied in conjunction with current cytotoxic treatments such as the current standard therapies TMZ and RT. In other cases, certain SMI drugs such as the topoisomerase inhibitors can induce cytotoxicity through novel mechanisms and could feasibly provide alternative treatment options for recurrent patients or those with inherent resistance to TMZ caused by MGMT status.

REFERENCES

1. Papac RJ. Origins of cancer therapy. Yale J Biol Med 2001;74(6):391–8.

2. Westphal M, Hilt DC, Bortey E, et al. A phase 3 trial of local chemotherapy with biodegradable carmustine (BCNU) wafers (Gliadel wafers) in patients with primary malignant glioma. Neuro Oncol 2003; 5(2):79–88.

3. Brem H, Piantadosi S, Burger PC, et al. Placebo-controlled trial of safety and efficacy of intraoperative controlled delivery by biodegradable polymers of chemotherapy for recurrent gliomas. The Polymer-brain Tumor Treatment Group. Lancet 1995;345(8956):1008–12.

4. Stupp R, Mason WP, van den Bent MJ, et al. Radiotherapy plus concomitant and adjuvant temozolomide for glioblastoma. N Engl J Med 2005;352(10): 987–96.

5. Parsons DW, Jones S, Zhang X, et al. An integrated genomic analysis of human glioblastoma multiforme. Science 2008;321(5897):1807–12.

6. Geyer CE, Forster J, Lindquist D, et al. Lapatinib plus capecitabine for HER2-positive advanced breast cancer. N Engl J Med 2006;355(26):2733–43.

7. Motzer RJ, Michaelson MD, Rosenberg J, et al. Sunitinib efficacy against advanced renal cell carcinoma. J Urol 2007;178(5):1883–7.

8. Llovet JM, Ricci S, Mazzaferro V, et al. Sorafenib in advanced hepatocellular carcinoma. N Engl J Med 2008;359(4):378–90.

9. Escudier B, Eisen T, Stadler WM, et al. Sorafenib for treatment of renal cell carcinoma: final efficacy and safety results of the phase III treatment approaches in renal cancer global evaluation trial. J Clin Oncol 2009;27(20):3312–8.

10. Kantarjian H, Sawyers C, Hochhaus A, et al. Hematologic and cytogenetic responses to imatinib mesylate in chronic myelogenous leukemia. N Engl J Med 2002;346(9):645–52.

11. Wong AJ, Bigner SH, Bigner DD, et al. Increased expression of the epidermal growth factor receptor gene in malignant gliomas is invariably associated with gene amplification. Proc Natl Acad Sci U S A 1987;84(19):6899–903.

12. Frederick L, Wang XY, Eley G, et al. Diversity and frequency of epidermal growth factor receptor mutations in human glioblastomas. Cancer Res 2000; 60(5):1383–7.

13. The Cancer Genome Atlas Research Network. Comprehensive genomic characterization defines human glioblastoma genes and core pathways. Nature 2008;455(7216):1061–8.

14. Rich JN, Reardon DA, Peery T, et al. Phase II trial of gefitinib in recurrent glioblastoma. J Clin Oncol 2004;22(1):133–42.

15. Lynch TJ, Bell DW, Sordella R, et al. Activating mutations in the epidermal growth factor receptor underlying responsiveness of non-small-cell lung cancer to gefitinib. N Engl J Med 2004;350(21):2129–39.

16. Rich JN, Rasheed BK, Yan H. EGFR mutations and sensitivity to gefitinib. N Engl J Med 2004;351(12): 1260–1 [author reply: 1260–1].

17. Cloughesy T, Yung A, Vrendenberg J, et al. Phase II study of erlotinib in recurrent GBM: Molecular predictors of outcome. J Clin Oncol. 2005 ASCO Annual Meeting Proceedings. 2005.

18. Vogelbaum MA, DP, Stevens G, Barnett G, et al. Phase II trial of the EGFR tyrosine kinase inhibitor erlotinib for single agent therapy of recurrent glioblastoma multiforme: interim results. J Clin Oncol. 2004 ASCO Annual Meeting Proceedings (Post-Meeting Edition). vol. 22, No 14S (July 15 Supplement), 2004:1558.

19. Franceschi E, Cavallo G, Lonardi S, et al. Gefitinib in patients with progressive high-grade gliomas:

a multicentre phase II study by Gruppo Italiano Co-
operativo di Neuro-Oncologia (GICNO). Br J Cancer
2007;96(7):1047–51.

20. Iwata KK, Provoncha K, Gibson N. Inhibition of
mutant EGFRvIII transformed cells by tyrosine
kinase inhibitor OSI-774 (Tarceva). Proc Am Soc
Clin Oncol 2002;21:[abstract: 79].

21. Moscatello DK, Holgado-Madruga M, Godwin AK,
et al. Frequent expression of a mutant epidermal
growth factor receptor in multiple human tumors.
Cancer Res 1995;55(23):5536–9.

22. Wikstrand CJ, Hale LP, Batra SK, et al. Monoclonal
antibodies against EGFRvIII are tumor specific and
react with breast and lung carcinomas and malignant gliomas. Cancer Res 1995;55(14):3140–8.

23. van den Bent MJ, Brandes AA, Rampling R, et al.
Randomized phase II trial of erlotinib versus temozo-
lomide or carmustine in recurrent glioblastoma:
EORTC Brain Tumor Group study 26034. J Clin
Oncol 2009;27(8):1268–74.

24. Van den Bent MJ, Brandes AA, Rampling R, et al.
Randomized phase II trial of erlotinib versus temozolomide (TMZ) or BCNU in recurrent glioblastoma
multiforme (GBM): EORTC 26034. Neuro Oncol
2007;9:[abstract: MA-27].

25. Brown PD, Krishnan S, Sarkaria JN, et al. Phase I/II
trial of erlotinib and temozolomide with radiation
therapy in the treatment of newly diagnosed glioblastoma multiforme: North Central Cancer Treatment Group Study N0177. J Clin Oncol 2008;
26(34):5603–9.

26. Prados MD, Chang SM, Butowski N, et al. Phase II
study of erlotinib plus temozolomide during and
after radiation therapy in patients with newly diagnosed glioblastoma multiforme or gliosarcoma.
J Clin Oncol 2009;27(4):579–84.

27. Jendrossek V, Belka C, Bamberg M. Novel chemotherapeutic agents for the treatment of glioblastoma
multiforme. Expert Opin Investig Drugs 2003;12(12):
1899–924.

28. Raymond E, Brandes AA, Dittrich C, et al. Phase II
study of imatinib in patients with recurrent gliomas
of various histologies: a European Organisation for
Research and Treatment of Cancer Brain Tumor
Group Study. J Clin Oncol 2008;26(28):4659–65.

29. Wen PY, Yung WK, Lamborn KR, et al. Phase I/II
study of imatinib mesylate for recurrent malignant gliomas: North American Brain Tumor Consortium Study 99-08. Clin Cancer Res 2006;
12(16):4899–907.

30. Viola FS, Katz A, Arantes A, et al. Barrios phase II
trial of high dose imatinib in recurrent glioblastoma
multiforme (GBM) with platelet derived growth factor receptor (PDGFR) expression. J Clin Oncol
2007;25(Suppl 18). ASCO Annual Meeting Proceedings Part I J Clin Oncol (Meeting Abstracts) 2007;
25(18 Suppl):2056.

31. Razis E, Selviaridis P, Labropoulos S, et al. Phase
II study of neoadjuvant imatinib in glioblastoma:
evaluation of clinical and molecular effects of
the treatment. Clin Cancer Res 2009;15(19):
6258–66.

32. Raymond E, Brandes Alba A, Dittrich Ch, et al.
Phase II study of imatinib in patients with recurrent
gliomas of various histologies: a European Organisation for Research and Treatment of Cancer
Brain Tumor Group study. J Clin Oncol 2008;26:
4659–65.

33. Dresemann G. Imatinib and hydroxyurea in pretreated progressive glioblastoma multiforme:
a patient series. Ann Oncol 2005;16(10):1702–8.

34. Reardon DA, Egorin MJ, Quinn JA, et al. Phase II
study of imatinib mesylate plus hydroxyurea in
adults with recurrent glioblastoma multiforme. J
Clin Oncol 2005;23(36):9359–68.

35. Dresemann G, Weller M, Rosenthal MA, et al. Imatinib in combination with hydroxyurea versus hydroxyurea alone as oral therapy in patients with
progressive pretreated glioblastoma resistant to
standard dose temozolomide. J Neurooncol 2010;
96(3):393–402.

36. Oehring RD, Miletic M, Valter MM, et al. Vascular
endothelial growth factor (VEGF) in astrocytic
gliomas–a prognostic factor? J Neurooncol 1999;
45(2):117–25.

37. Conrad C, Friedman H, Reardon D, et al. A phase I/
II trial of single-agent PTK 787/ZK 222584 (PTK/
ZK), a novel, oral angiogenesis inhibitor, in patients
with recurrent glioblastoma multiforme (GBM). Proc
Am Soc Clin Oncol 2004;22.

38. Reardon D, Friedman H, Yung WKA, et al. A phase
I/II trial of PTK787/ZK 222584 (PTK/ZK), a novel,
oral angiogenesis inhibitor, in combination with
either temozolomide or lomustine for patients with
recurrent glioblastoma multiforme (GBM). Proc Am
Soc Clin Oncol 2004;22.

39. Sathornsumetee S, Desjardins A, Vredenburgh JJ,
et al. Phase II trial of bevacizumab and erlotinib in
patients with recurrent malignant glioma. Neuro Oncol 2010;12(12):1300–10.

40. Sathornsumetee S, Desjardins A, Vredenburgh JJ,
et al. Phase II trial of bevacizumab plus erlotinib
for patients with recurrent malignant gliomas: final
results. J Clin Oncol 2010;28(Suppl 15):[Suppl;
abstract: 2055].

41. Batchelor TT, Sorensen AG, di Tomaso E, et al.
AZD2171, a pan-VEGF receptor tyrosine kinase
inhibitor, normalizes tumor vasculature and alleviates edema in glioblastoma patients. Cancer Cell
2007;11(1):83–95.

42. Maehama T, Dixon JE. The tumor suppressor, PTEN/
MMAC1, dephosphorylates the lipid second mes-
senger, phosphatidylinositol 3,4,5-trisphosphate.
J Biol Chem 1998;273(22):13375–8.

43. Mellinghoff IK, Wang MY, Vivanco I, et al. Molecular determinants of the response of glioblastomas to EGFR kinase inhibitors. N Engl J Med 2005; 353(19):2012–24.

44. Smith JS, Tachibana I, Passe SM, et al. PTEN mutation, EGFR amplification, and outcome in patients with anaplastic astrocytoma and glioblastoma multiforme. J Natl Cancer Inst 2001;93(16): 1246–56.

45. Wilhelm SM, Carter C, Tang L, et al. BAY 43-9006 exhibits broad spectrum oral antitumor activity and targets the RAF/MEK/ERK pathway and receptor tyrosine kinases involved in tumor progression and angiogenesis. Cancer Res 2004;64(19): 7099–109.

46. Hainsworth JD, Ervin T, Friedman E, et al. Concurrent radiotherapy and temozolomide followed by temozolomide and sorafenib in the first-line treatment of patients with glioblastoma multiforme. Cancer 2010;116(15):3663–9.

47. Reardon DA, Vredenburgh JJ, Desjardins A, et al. Effect of CYP3A-inducing anti-epileptics on sorafenib exposure: results of a phase II study of sorafenib plus daily temozolomide in adults with recurrent glioblastoma. J Neurooncol 2011;101(1):57–66.

48. Kleber S, Sancho-Martinez I, Wiestler B, et al. Yes and PI3K bind CD95 to signal invasion of glioblastoma. Cancer Cell 2008;13(3):235–48.

49. Chakravarti A, Zhai G, Suzuki Y, et al. The prognostic significance of phosphatidylinositol 3-kinase pathway activation in human gliomas. J Clin Oncol 2004;22(10):1926–33.

50. Momota H, Nerio E, Holland EC. Perifosine inhibits multiple signaling pathways in glial progenitors and cooperates with temozolomide to arrest cell proliferation in gliomas in vivo. Cancer Res 2005; 65(16):7429–35.

51. Cloughesy TF, Yoshimoto K, Nghiemphu P, et al. Antitumor activity of rapamycin in a phase I trial for patients with recurrent PTEN-deficient glioblastoma. PLoS Med 2008;5(1):e8.

52. Galanis E, Buckner JC, Maurer MJ, et al. Phase II trial of temsirolimus (CCI-779) in recurrent glioblastoma multiforme: a North Central Cancer Treatment Group Study. J Clin Oncol 2005;23(23):5294–304.

53. Chang SM, Wen P, Cloughesy T, et al. Phase II study of CCI-779 in patients with recurrent glioblastoma multiforme. Invest New Drugs 2005;23(4):357–61.

54. Carducci MA, Musib L, Kies MS, et al. Phase I dose escalation and pharmacokinetic study of enzastaurin, an oral protein kinase C beta inhibitor, in patients with advanced cancer. J Clin Oncol 2006;24(25):4092–9.

55. Fine HA, Kim L, Royce C. Results from phase II trial of enzastaurin (LY317615) in patients with recurrent high grade gliomas. J Clin Oncol 2005; 23(Suppl 115):[abstract: 1504].

56. Fine HA, Kim L, Royce C, et al. A phase II trial of LY317615 in patients with recurrent high grade gliomas. J Clin Oncol 2004;22:[abstract: 1511].

57. Fine HA, PV, Chamberlain MC, et al. Enzastaurin (ENZ) versus lomustine (CCNU) in the treatment of recurrent, intracranial glioblastoma multiforme (GBM): a phase III study. J Clin Oncol 2005;26: [abstract: 2005].

58. Puduvalli VK, Wick W, Chamberlain MC, et al. Enzastaurin versus lomustine in the treatment of recurrent, intracranial glioblastoma: a phase III study. Neuro Oncol 2008;10:[abstract: MA-35].

59. Thornton D, Graff J. Enzastaurin: an introduction to a new, targeted agent for the treatment of glioblastoma multiforme. Neuro Oncol 2006;8:[abstract: P142].

60. Wick W, Puduvalli VK, Chamberlain MC, et al. Phase III study of enzastaurin compared with lomustine in the treatment of recurrent intracranial glioblastoma. J Clin Oncol 2010;28(7):1168–74.

61. Friedman HS, Petros WP, Friedman AH, et al. Irinotecan therapy in adults with recurrent or progressive malignant glioma. J Clin Oncol 1999;17(5):1516–25.

62. Chamberlain MC. Salvage chemotherapy with CPT-11 for recurrent glioblastoma multiforme. J Neurooncol 2002;56(2):183–8.

63. Prados MD, Lamborn K, Yung WK, et al. A phase 2 trial of irinotecan (CPT-11) in patients with recurrent malignant glioma: a North American Brain Tumor Consortium study. Neuro Oncol 2006;8(2):189–93.

64. Buckner JC, Reid JM, Wright K, et al. Irinotecan in the treatment of glioma patients: current and future studies of the North Central Cancer Treatment Group. Cancer 2003;97(Suppl 9):2352–8.

65. Batchelor TT, Gilbert MR, Supko JG, et al. Phase 2 study of weekly irinotecan in adults with recurrent malignant glioma: final report of NABTT 97-11. Neuro Oncol 2004;6(1):21–7.

66. Vredenburgh JJ, Desjardins A, Herndon JE, et al. Phase II trial of bevacizumab and irinotecan in recurrent malignant glioma. Clin Cancer Res 2007;13(4): 1253–9.

67. Vredenburgh JJ, Desjardins A, Herndon JE, et al. Bevacizumab plus irinotecan in recurrent glioblastoma multiforme. J Clin Oncol 2007;25(30): 4722–9.

68. Reardon DA, Desjardins A, Vredenburgh JJ. Bevacizumab plus etoposide among recurrent malignant glioma patients: phase II study final results. J Clin Oncol 2009;27(Suppl 15):[abstract: 2046].

69. Conley BA, Wright JJ, Kummar S. Targeting epigenetic abnormalities with histone deacetylase inhibitors. Cancer 2006;107(4):832–40.

70. Chinnaiyan P, Vallabhaneni G, Armstrong E, et al. Modulation of radiation response by histone deacetylase inhibition. Int J Radiat Oncol Biol Phys 2005; 62(1):223–9.

71. Sawa H, Murakami H, Kumagai M, et al. Histone deacetylase inhibitor, FK228, induces apoptosis and suppresses cell proliferation of human glioblastoma cells in vitro and in vivo. Acta Neuropathol 2004; 107(6):523–31.

72. MacDonald TJ, Taga T, Shimada H, et al. Preferential susceptibility of brain tumors to the antiangiogenic effects of an alpha(v) integrin antagonist. Neurosurgery 2001;48(1):151–7.

73. Nabors LB, Mikkelsen T, Rosenfeld SS, et al. Phase I and correlative biology study of cilengitide in patients with recurrent malignant glioma. J Clin Oncol 2007;25(13):1651–7.

74. Stupp R, Hegi ME, Neyns B, et al. Phase I/IIa study of cilengitide and temozolomide with concomitant radiotherapy followed by cilengitide and temozolomide maintenance therapy in patients with newly diagnosed glioblastoma. J Clin Oncol 2010;28(16):2712–8.

75. Chamberlain MC. What role should cilengitide have in the treatment of glioblastoma? J Clin Oncol 2010; 28(33):e695.

76. Mani A, Gelmann EP. The ubiquitin-proteasome pathway and its role in cancer. J Clin Oncol 2005; 23(21):4776–89.

77. Friday BB, Anderson SK, Buckner J, et al. Phase II trial of vorinostat in combination with bortezomib in recurrent glioblastoma multiforme: a north central cancer treatment group study. Neuro Oncol 2010; 12(4):iv69–78.

78. Stommel JM, Kimmelman AC, Ying H, et al. Coactivation of receptor tyrosine kinases affects the response of tumor cells to targeted therapies. Science 2007;318(5848):287–90.

79. Huang TT, Sarkaria SM, Cloughesy TF, et al. Targeted therapy for malignant glioma patients: lessons learned and the road ahead. Neurotherapeutics 2009;6(3):500–12.

80. Verhaak RG, Hoadley KA, Purdom E, et al. Integrated genomic analysis identifies clinically relevant subtypes of glioblastoma characterized by abnormalities in PDGFRA, IDH1, EGFR, and NF1. Cancer Cell 2010;17(1):98–110.

Molecular Characteristics and Pathways of Avastin for the Treatment of Glioblastoma Multiforme

Marko Spasic, BA[a], Frances Chow, BA[a], Claire Tu, BS[a],
Daniel T. Nagasawa, MD[a], Isaac Yang, MD[a,b],*

KEYWORDS

- Avastin • Bevacizumab • VEGF • Chemotherapy • Glioblastoma

KEY POINTS

- The overall benefit of bevacizumab remains controversial.
- Although bevacizumab has been shown to extend progression-free survival, it has not been shown to improve overall survival and may facilitate glioma transformation to a more invasive phenotype.
- The mechanism of bevacizumab is still not sufficiently understood and future studies may need to use novel methods of evaluating and visualizing tumor progression to determine the effectiveness of bevacizumab.

INTRODUCTION

Glioblastoma multiforme (GBM) is one of the most common and aggressive primary brain tumors. Despite surgical resection, radiotherapy, and chemotherapy, prognosis for GBM remains poor. The median progression-free survival (PFS) and overall survival (OS) for patients with GBM who undergo surgical resection followed by radiation therapy and temozolomide chemotherapy are 6.9 and 14.7 months, respectively.[1]

GBM is a highly invasive and one of the most angiogenic and vascularized cancer. Altered pathways in GBM include the loss of function of tumor suppressor genes and the activation of oncogenes.[2] GBM is believed to be characterized by tumor progression through the induction of angiogenesis to form new blood vessels via endothelial cell migration and proliferation.[3] GBM is capable of exhibiting endothelial proliferation and rapid formation of tortuous vessels to supply its increasing metabolic needs; as a result, its poor-quality blood vessels are highly permeable and disorganized. Angiogenesis may play a pivotal role beginning in the earliest phase of tumor development and perhaps represents a critical event in the progression of malignant gliomas.[4] Hence, angiogenesis has been targeted in the treatment of recurrent GBM.

Disclosure of interests: Marko Spasic (first author) was partially supported by an American Association of Neurologic Surgeons Fellowship. Daniel Nagasawa (fourth author) was supported by an American Brain Tumor Association Medical Student Summer Fellowship in Honor of Connie Finc. Isaac Yang (senior author) was partially supported by a Visionary Fund Grant, an Eli and Edythe Broad Center of Regenerative Medicine and Stem Cell Research UCLA Scholars in Translational Medicine Program Award, the Stein Oppenheimer Endowment Award and the STOP CANCER Jason Dessel Memorial Seed Grant.

[a] UCLA Department of Neurosurgery, University of California, Los Angeles, 695 Charles E Young Drive South, Gonda 3357, Los Angeles, CA 90095-1761, USA; [b] University of California Los Angeles, Jonsson Comprehensive Cancer Center, 8-684 Factor Building, Box 951781, Los Angeles, CA 90095-1781, USA

* Corresponding author. UCLA Department of Neurosurgery, UCLA Jonsson Comprehensive Cancer Center, University of California, Los Angeles, David Geffen School of Medicine at UCLA, 695 Charles East Young Drive South, UCLA Gonda 3357, Los Angeles, CA 90095-1761.
E-mail address: iyang@mednet.ucla.edu

neurosurgery.theclinics.com

Recurrent Glioblastoma

Nearly all GBM recur after initial therapy, and only 20% to 25% of patients survive beyond 1 year after the diagnosis of recurrent disease.[5,6] Median survival for patients with recurrent GBM ranges from 3 to 9 months.[7] Several potential treatments are being evaluated in ongoing clinical trials for recurrent GBM. bevacizumab (Avastin), a humanized anti-vascular endothelial growth factor (VEGF) antibody, has shown promising results in phase II clinical trials for recurrent GBM; as a result, in May 2009, the Food and Drug Administration (FDA) approved the use of bevacizumab for the treatment of patients with recurrent GBM, which made bevacizumab the third FDA-approved chemotherapy for GBM along with implantable Gliadel wafers and temozolomide.[8]

Bevacizumab

Since its inception, bevacizumab has led a successful yet controversial path. Initially indicated for metastatic colorectal cancer in 2004, bevacizumab was shown in a randomized, double-blind, stage III clinical trial to significantly extend both PFS and duration of survival.[9] Median PFS in a colorectal cancer control group receiving IFL (irinotecan, fluorouracil, and leucovorin) treatment was 6.2 months, compared with 10.6 months in a group receiving IFL with bevacizumab. Median duration of survival increased from 15.6 months in the IFL control group to 20.3 months in the group receiving IFL and bevacizumab.[9] Because of its versatility and success in treating colorectal cancer, bevacizumab was considered as the first anti-angiogenic therapy approved in the United States. Bevacizumab later gained approval for use in several other solid tumors, including lung cancer, breast cancer, renal cell cancer, and in 2009, was granted accelerated approval for GBM.[9–12]

However, in 2010, the FDA rescinded its approval of bevacizumab for metastatic breast cancer based on the lack of evidence for improved OS in phase III clinical trials when compared with standard anti-mitotic chemotherapies, such as docetaxel, 5-fluorouracil, epirubicin, and cyclophosphamide.[13,14] An additional point of concern was the severity of the side effects, including wound dehiscence, gastrointestinal perforation, hemorrhage, and high-grade thrombosis.[15,16] However, the other indications remain and bevacizumab continues to be evaluated as a promising treatment in clinical trial for patients with recurrent GBM.[17,18] Based on these results, only in GBM is bevacizumab approved as a single agent.

Although bevacizumab prolongs GBM PFS, decreases tumor vascularization, and reduces permeability of vessels, it does not prolong the OS. Bevacizumab alone gives a median PFS of 4 months and 6-month PFS (PFS6) of 29%.[8] A meta-analysis of 548 patients showed that bevacizumab given in combination with other drugs gives a higher PFS6 rate of 45%, a 6-month OS rate of 76%, and an OS of 9.3 months.[19] Another study comparing bevacizumab with combination bevacizumab and irinotecan therapy showed that PFS6 is higher when bevacizumab is taken with irinotecan (PFS6 of 50.2% for combination vs 35.1% for bevacizumab alone). Despite the clear benefit of irinotecan plus bevacizumab on PFS, OS for bevacizumab plus irinotecan is 8.9 months, although bevacizumab alone only marginally extends OS to 9.7 months.[20] This lack of a clear benefit in OS for one therapy over another adds to the uncertainty of the benefit of anti-angiogenic therapies.

Subsequently, the FDA's approval of bevacizumab for the treatment of recurrent GBM was accelerated with PFS being relied on as a metric for drug efficacy rather than OS. However, the validity of PFS as an accurate measurement of treatment outcome has been questioned. Although statistical analysis shows that PFS and OS are strongly associated, it has been argued that PFS is not a replacement for OS and cannot be predictive of tumor growth after treatment.[21]

Furthermore, several studies suggest that 1 adverse consequence of this pharmacologic treatment includes hijacking of healthy nontumorous vasculature. Vessels from normal tissue are recruited via tumor infiltration to supply the lesion in a process known as co-option.[22] In short, the mechanism of bevacizumab is still not sufficiently understood[23,24] and must be further elucidated to evaluate its far-reaching effects.

MOLECULAR MECHANISM OF BEVACIZUMAB

In theory, the mechanism of bevacizumab is exquisitely simple. As an antibody for angiogenic factors, bevacizumab cuts off a tumor's life supply by inhibiting the factors required to promote and sustain vessel growth. Angiogenesis has been extensively studied for decades. Tumors should theoretically stop growing if vascularization is absent or insufficient.[25] However, this mechanism has proven to be more difficult in clinical practice than expected,[26,27] and nonangiogenic pathways that may be affected by bevacizumab are also under scrutiny.

Angiogenesis, or sprouting of new vessels from parent vessels, first involves vascular endothelial breakdown and then proliferation of existing vasculature. Extensive investigation has revealed several

VEGF-dependent and VEGF-independent pathways that regulate angiogenesis.[28] VEGF is recognized as one of the most potent stimuli for angiogenesis, making it a key pathway of deregulation in GBM development and proliferation.

VEGF

VEGF, also known as VPF (vascular permeability factor), comprises a family of 5 proteins (VEGF-A, VEGF-B, VEGF-C, VEGF-D, and placental-derived growth factor) that regulate vasculogenesis during growth, lymphatic development, wound healing, menstruation, and pregnancy.[29] Hypoxia commonly induces VEGF release, and in particular, VEGF-A is released by GBM as a mitogen that accumulates in nearby blood vessels.[30] After release from hypoxic malignant cells, VEGF binds to both pericytes and vascular endothelial cells.

Pericytes typically wrap around the outside surface of vascular endothelial cells to maintain stability of the blood-brain barrier. In mice without pericytes, extravasation occurs as intravenously administered tracers are found to seep out of vessels and into brain tissue. In fact, the proper functioning of the blood-brain barrier depends on the extent of pericyte coverage of vessels.[31] In the presence of VEGF, pericytes detach from the vessel wall, resulting in a weakened vessel basement membrane[32–34] and contributing to the compromised blood-brain barrier that is often observed in proximity to gliomas.[35]

In addition to binding to pericytes, VEGF-A binds to the surface of vascular endothelial cells through either vascular endothelial growth factor receptor (VEGFR) -1 (also known as Flt-1) or VEGFR-2 (also known as KDR or Flk-1).[36] The binding of VEGF-A to VEGFR-2 produces tyrosine kinase activity that is 10 times more potent than the activity of VEGF-B to VEGFR-1 binding.[28] Not coincidentally, bevacizumab targets VEGF-A and neutralizes its many downstream effects. For endothelial cell proliferation, the VEGFR-2 signal transduces through phospholipase C to C-Raf-MAP kinase.[37] For endothelial cell survival and migration, the VEGFR-2 signal transduces through a tyrosine kinase PI3 K-Akt cascade to activate focal adhesion kinase.[38] One of the first cellular changes observed with VEGF binding is a 4-fold increase in intracellular calcium, which may be used as a marker for VEGF pathway activation.[39]

One of several VEGF downstream pathways leads to the phosphorylation of occludin and zonula occludens-1,[40] key proteins of tight junction function and organization.[41] Phosphorylation ultimately causes the gap junctions between endothelial cells to loosen, resulting in fenestrations, vessel dilation, and additional increase in vascular permeability. Permeability allows proteins to extravasate and extracellular matrix to be laid down as the foundation for new vessels. Endothelial cells recruit to the new extracellular matrix, and the cell at the tip of the growing endothelial cell group (known as the tip cell) is responsible for sensing environmental cues to direct vessel growth. HIF-1α (hypoxia-inducible factor) sensitizes these endothelial cells to angiogenic factors.[42] VEGF-A induces vascular hyper-permeability and sprouting of new vessels from preexisting vasculature. Therefore, the hyperplastic vascularization that is characteristic of GBM may be because of the high levels of VEGF.

Dvorak and colleagues[43–45] argue that movement of fluid between endothelial cell tight junctions and compromised endothelial cells is not sufficient to account for all of the extravasation that occurs in the presence of VEGF. Instead, they report that an intracellular system, the vesicular-vacuolar organelle (VVO), is responsible for VEGF-induced microvascular permeability. More organized than caveolae, VVOs are a system of vesicles or vacuoles that transport fluid and molecules across endothelial cells. Moreover, VVO function upregulates in the presence of VEGF (**Fig. 1**).

Upregulation of VEGF in Glioblastoma

In GBM, VEGF-A is upregulated due to hypoxia and necrosis induced by rapid tumor growth.[46,47] The gene sequence for VEGF shares common elements with erythropoietin, which is also transcribed in an oxygen-level–dependent manner.[48] The stress of unmet perfusion demands (resulting in decreased oxygen, reduced nutrients, and insufficient blood flow) induces the release of VEGF. Cells must always be near nutritional support, otherwise necrosis occurs. Hypoxia stabilizes HIF-1α and HIF-2α, which promote metabolic changes to sustain continued tumor growth. Specifically, HIF-1α and -2α have the following effects: (1) block the proteolysis of VEGF by ubiquitin, therefore allowing VEGF to accumulate[28]; (2) upregulate GLUT-1 receptors to increase uptake of glucose from blood[27]; (3) upregulate carbonic anhydrase IX (CAIX) to stabilize pH in hypoxic conditions, making the environment tolerable for continued proliferation[49,50]; and (4) sensitize endothelial cells to angiogenic signals.[42] One group suggests that different degrees of hypoxia induce different sets of rescue proteins: mild hypoxia induces the production of HIF-1α and VEGF, whereas severe hypoxia induces the production of CAIX.[49,50] Ultimately, this results in growth of additional vessels to supply the malignancy with the nutrients needed to support

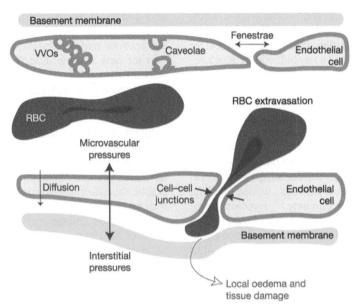

Fig. 1. Mechanisms of VEGF-induced vascular permeability. (*From* Weis SM, Cheresh DA. Pathophysiological consequences of VEGF-induced vascular permeability. Nature 2005;437:497–504; with permission.)

continued growth. All of these adaptive responses make GBM particularly resistant to various treatment modalities.

VEGF AND BEVACIZUMAB

By neutralizing VEGF-A, bevacizumab induces tumor hypoxia and also blocks the mechanism by which new vessels are induced. Although circulating VEGF levels increase after the administration of VEGF antibodies, the compensatory upregulation is not enough to induce substantial angiogenesis. In rats bearing human GBM xenografts, it is observed that the tumor is subjected to hypoxia, resulting in reduced growth, decreased mitochondria, and diminished edema caused by the decreased permeability of vessels.[27]

Tumors treated with bevacizumab do not exhibit the normal histologic characteristics of GBM. Bevacizumab successfully stops proliferation of vessel endothelium and pseudopalisading necrosis. Fewer mitochondria are present within cells, and microareas of cell death, as suggested by the presence of cell lysis, are seen in the core of the tumor. However, the edges of the tumor uniquely comprises loosely connected cells[27] that may suggest increased invasiveness, a potentially harmful consequence of bevacizumab treatment.

Bevacizumab inhibits the VEGF-induced permeability of vessels. Treatment with bevacizumab shows a marked decrease in edema as early as 1 day after treatment according to a phase II trial,[8] therefore replacing the need for corticosteroids given to block transendothelial fluid flow by

regulating endothelial tight junctions.[51] Reduction in edema occurs in 50% of patients, equating to a 59% reduction in corticosteroid doses.[8] As a result, minimized corticosteroid administration allows for a decrease in complications, mortality, and morbidity associated with its chronic use. In a phase II study, bevacizumab significantly decreased abnormal fluid attenuated inversion recovery (FLAIR) signal by more than 5% in 77% of patients; 79% of patients had more than 5% volume reduction on T1-weighted magnetic resonance imaging (MRI) with contrast enhancement.[52] Another study reported that 93.2% of patients showed radiographic response (including complete response, partial response, and minimal response) and 34.1% showed either complete or partial response.[53] T2-weighted MRI taken after bevacizumab treatment shows substantial reduction in contrast enhancement. Similar results are seen in FLAIR signals with bevacizumab treatment.[52] However, this apparent improvement according to MRI does not necessarily correspond to reduction in activity of the tumor[54–56] and may simply be because of the reduction in the vascular permeability of gadolinium, which gives an exaggerated impression of tumor reduction.[57] According to a study comparing changes before and after bevacizumab treatment in T2-weighted MRI and contrast-enhancing volume, there was no significant correlation between tumor volume and PFS or OS (**Table 1**).[56]

However, there is a significant linear correlation between proliferation rate and PFS.[56] In addition, infiltrative GBM after bevacizumab treatment is

Table 1
Prediction of patient survival using traditional magnetic resonance estimates of tumor volume in *n* = 26 patients

Tumor Region of Interest	PFS (*P*-Value)	OS (*P*-Value)
Pretreatment T2 volume	0.2909	0.7226
Posttreatment T2 volume	0.8385	0.6421
Change in T2 volume	0.1624	0.5882
Pretreatment CE volume	0.3142	0.7963
Posttreatment CE volume	0.6914	0.5547
Change in CE volume	0.0760	0.4392

Abbreviation: CE, contrast enhancement.
From Ellingson BM, et al. Cell invasion, motility, and proliferation level estimate (CIMPLE) maps derived from serial diffusion MR images in recurrent glioblastoma treated with bevacizumab. J Neurooncol 2011;105:91–101; with permission.

often nonenhancing, making radiographic evaluation difficult and misleading. Overall, pseudoresponse confounds interpretation of imaging after bevacizumab use and may skew the apparent effectiveness of bevacizumab on tumor size and disease progression.[52] As the glioma response to bevacizumab is difficult to assess with traditional computed tomography and MRI,[58] different imaging methods may be necessary to properly evaluate the benefits of this therapeutic approach.

As the concentration of VEGF correlates with vessel density,[53,59,60] anti-VEGF therapy reduces concentrations of active VEGF and leads to a subsequent decrease in vessel density. Staining of endothelial cells after bevacizumab administration shows that large-sized vessels are reduced by 58%, whereas medium-sized vessels are reduced by 17%. However, there is no change in small-sized vessels,[27] indicating that limits exist in vessel remodeling and destruction. This also suggests the role of other angiogenic pathways in maintaining blood flow to the tumor. In addition, bevacizumab works very rapidly; as visualized by CD34 immunohistochemistry, tumor vessels drop to less than 50% of control density by 1 day after administration, and less than 30% of control vessel density by day 7.[61]

Because of the reduction in vessel density, bevacizumab induces a hypoxic state in tumors, resulting in the accumulation of lactate, alanine, choline, myo-inositol, creatine, taurine, mobile lipids,[62] and HIF-1α.[27,63] Although HIF-1α is involved with critical tumorigenic, survival, and angiogenic pathways in GBM, bevacizumab prevents vascularization associated with HIF-1α. As such, tumor upregulation of HIF-1α is not sufficient to induce substantial angiogenesis, yet the tumor finds other pathways for proliferation and invasion.

Although bevacizumab reduces vascularization of tumors, it also results in glioma transformation from an expansive to an invasive phenotype.[64,65] One group was able to induce invasiveness from a xenograft glioma animal model of previously noninvasive tumor by treating with bevacizumab. The borders of bevacizumab-treated tumors are extremely invasive, spreading far beyond landmark vessels, in comparison with untreated controls.[66] In addition, distant recurrences were common in patients treated with bevacizumab, even if they had reduced radiographic enhancement.[53] It is possible that the physiologic stress of hypoxia and reduction in vascularization after anti-VEGF treatment leads to the highly invasive properties of the xenografts. Several other groups[22,46,63] observed that when angiogenesis is inhibited, the tumor activates an alternate pathway that uses preexisting vessels. This bevacizumab-induced vessel co-option occurs with highly invasive tumors, resulting in a significant increase in satellite tumor area when compared with controls.[22] However, primary tumor size does not change with anti-VEGF antibody, and growth rate slows.[22] Therefore, despite slowed primary tumor progression, bevacizumab treatment may activate a separate highly invasive quality in satellite tumors that infiltrate healthy tissue to take over preexisting blood vessels.[22] Co-option provides a VEGF-independent method of vascularization of tumors and therefore serves as a method of escape from anti-VEGF treatment.

Analysis of gene expression after bevacizumab therapy demonstrates an upregulation of the Wnt pathway indicating a potential mechanism for the differentiation and infiltrative nature of these gliomas after treatment.[67] Similarly, bevacizumab induces more than half of the genes related to the PI3 K/Akt pathway to increase,[27] resulting in pathway activation and reduction in apoptosis. In combination, these factors seem to promote tumor proliferation and invasion, despite anti-angiogenic treatment effects.

THE EFFECT OF BEVACIZUMAB ON OTHER TREATMENTS
Anti-VEGF Effect on Surgery

During tumor resection, the high vascularization and abnormal state of vessels from VEGF-induced angiogenesis increases the risk of bleeding. Therefore, debates exist on the optimal method of approach in the surgical removal of highly vascularized gliomas. Some claim that first finding the edge of the tumor, then progressively moving inwards toward the center (in an "outside-in" en bloc fashion) to remove the mass is more effective than beginning in the center of the tumor and moving outward ("inside-out"). The outside-in method avoids damaging the highly vascular infiltration often found in the center of the growth, thereby minimizing the risk of bleeding from the delicate hyperplastic blood vessels that are characteristic of GBM pathogenesis.[68] The use of anti-angiogenic factors before surgery may be beneficial in normalizing vasculature or promoting the stabilization and return of vasculature to normal healthy states, thereby minimizing the presence of poor-quality vessels and reducing the risk of bleeding. However, a side effect of bevacizumab is altered wound healing, which may complicate surgical recovery.

Anti-VEGF Effect on Radiotherapy and Chemotherapy

Because oxygen sensitizes tissue to radiotherapy, hypoxic tumors such as gliomas have characteristically been less responsive to radiotherapy. Anti-VEGF therapy halts the rapid growth of weak and poorly constructed vessels, sensitizing gliomas to radiation.[69] However, anti-VEGF-induced normalization also attenuates hyperpermeability, therefore decreasing total chemotherapeutic delivery of drugs to the tumor. Vessels seal up and restore the blood-brain barrier, effectively reducing drug movement out of vessels and into tumor tissue. A small window of time exists before further loss of vessels through anti-VEGF treatment will lead again to hypoxia, making delivery of chemotherapy to tumors more difficult.[70] It is believed that hypoxia may select for more aggressive and infiltrative malignant cell types,[71] resulting in recurrence with more invasive and aggressive tumors after bevacizumab therapy.

Dickson and colleagues[61] described phenotypic normalization of GBM vessels after bevacizumab therapy in mice xenografts. Bevacizumab-treated mice had vasculature similar to that of normal skin, whereas control mice had chaotic, dilated, irregular, and unorganized vessels. More importantly, improvement in chemotherapy delivery and efficacy transiently follows bevacizumab treatment. Topotecan penetration into tumor tissue is greater when given 1 day after bevacizumab (51%) than when given after saline control (43%). Topotecan is even more penetrant when given 3 days after bevacizumab (57%) than when given 3 days after saline control (34%). After 7 days; however, drug penetration power is lost (bevacizumab 39% vs saline control 40%) due to either loss in single-dose activity of bevacizumab or treatment-induced normalization of vessels.

Evasive Resistance

Although phase II clinical trials of bevacizumab may seem promising, anti-angiogenic therapies often demonstrate brief intervals of efficacy and are followed by the development of increased tumor growth. This loss of response may be caused by evasion.[72] There are 2 subtypes of bevacizumab evasion: infiltrative bevacizumab evasive gliomas (IBEGs) and nodular enhancing bevacizumab evasive gliomas (NEBEGs).

IBEGs maintain hypoxia but show reduced vascularity, suggesting that the glioma may have relied on invasion to reduce vascular dependence. Through transcription upregulation, IBEGs may be able to overcome the effects of bevacizumab treatment by promoting tumor cell invasion from devascularized areas into those in closer proximity to blood vessels, which results in a subset of bevacizumab-resistant GBM that exhibit an infiltrative radiographic appearance.

NEBEGs result in upregulation of VEGF-A and VEGF-C, but down-regulation of VEGF-B. VEGF-C binds to VEGFR-2 to stimulate angiogenesis.[73,74] The upregulation of VEGF-A and VEGF-C allows NEBEGs to exceed capacity and cross the bevacizumab-mediated VEGF blockade. Subsequently, NEBEGs are capable of reacquiring an increased vascularity and decreased hypoxia status comparable to pretreatment levels. It is therefore possible that VEGF-targeted treatments such as bevacizumab may cause hyperinvasive IBEG or hyperangiogenic NEBEG resulting in bevacizumab evasion.

Other Angiogenic Pathways May Contribute to Unresponsiveness or Adverse Reactions to Bevacizumab

Because GBM is not always responsive to bevacizumab treatment, other angiogenic pathways may be upregulating when VEGF is neutralized. Although VEGF has been shown to be responsible for direct initiation of angiogenesis, other growth factors such as angiopoietin 1 (Ang1), angiopoietin 2 (Ang2), and Delta are responsible for vessel remodeling and maturation.[36] VEGF-independent angiogenesis is regulated by the Angiopoietin-Tie and Delta-Notch pathways. These alternate pathways may be upregulated or adjusted when using anti-VEGF antibodies, resulting in unanticipated side effects or unresponsiveness to bevacizumab treatment.

Although VEGF increases vessel quantity,[36,75–77] Ang1 increases vessel size.[36,77,78] Ang2 is a growth factor released from host vessels during co-option that binds to the tyrosine kinase receptor Tie to destabilize endothelial cell layers. Ang2 is regulated in part by VEGF; in the presence of high VEGF-A, Ang2 will destabilize endothelial cells, with additional subsequent increases in VEGF promoting angiogenesis. However, in the presence of little or no VEGF-A, Ang2 will simply destabilize vessels through apoptosis of endothelial cells.[28,79] This leads to hypoxia and apoptosis of tumor cells, which then induces the release of VEGF to form new vessels.

A ligand for the Delta-Notch pathway, Dll4 (Delta-like ligand 4), is upregulated in endothelial cells of GBM[80–83] because of the induction by VEGF.[84,85] Dll4 stabilizes vessels, thereby inhibiting sprouting and angiogenesis,[86] while also improving the quality of existing vessels and promoting tumor growth.[84] Dll4 is a negative regulator of angiogenesis even though it is a positive regulator of tumor progression.[81] Dll4 provides a pathway for GBM to grow, despite anti-VEGF therapy.

In addition to VEGFR-2, tumor endothelial cell specimens are often found by immunohistochemistry to have elevated levels of platelet-derived growth factor receptors (PDGFR) α and PDGFRβ.[87] The platelet-derived growth factor (PDGF) pathway is yet to be fully elucidated, but sources report that although PDGFRα is present in all astrocytic malignancies, PDGFRβ is found in tumor vasculature and is involved in angiogenesis. PDGF can stimulate and induce the proliferation of tumors.[88,89] In addition, VEGF and PDGF contain some structural similarities and sequence homology—both are transcribed as monomers, contain cysteine knots, and dimerize to facilitate activity[90] In addition, PDGF is believed to complement angiogenesis via PDGFRβ-mediated synthesis and release of VEGF.[91] One study showed that tumors are able to escape from radiation and anti-VEGF therapy by upregulating PDGF in endothelial cells.[92] This may help explain some of the resistance to bevacizumab therapy.

Side Effects

Several clinical studies have shown a higher toxicity profile in patients with GBM compared with other cancer populations. Patients with recurrent GBM who received single-agent bevacizumab showed several adverse effects including complications in wound healing, intracranial hemorrhage, and venous thromboembolic events.[15,16]

Wound healing

Studies show an increased rate of wound-healing complications in patients treated preoperatively with bevacizumab compared with those without VEGF-targeted chemotherapy.[93] Typically, surgical wounds result in increased expression of VEGF and VEGFR-2 for approximately 24 weeks postoperatively[94] to promote angiogenesis essential for normal wound healing. Thus, when bevacizumab reduces angiogenesis by inhibiting VEGF-A from activating VEGFR-1 and VEGFR-2, patients become predisposed to wound-healing complications as reported by Clark and colleagues[93,95] in their study of craniotomy wound-healing. Bevacizumab's relatively long half-life of approximately 20 days[96] represents a fairly sustained interval until complete elimination from the body. Thus, the timing of VEGF-targeted therapy for both preoperative and postoperative therapy is critical. Sugrue and colleagues[97] reported that 78% of postoperative complications occur when therapy starts within 60 days of surgery. However, postoperative complications still remain low. In fact, the 4% to 6% of wound healing complication rate at the craniotomy site was one of the reasons for the accelerated FDA approval of bevacizumab for GBM.[17,98]

Intracranial hemorrhage

Fatal intracranial hemorrhage is one of the most serious complications of anti-angiogenic treatment of GBM. Clinical trial results show that bevacizumab-administered patients have a risk of severe (grade 3) intracranial hemorrhage of 2% to 5%.[17,99,100] Bevacizumab's inhibition of VEGF causes changes in vascular endothelium, which may play a pivotal role in the mechanism of this complication.[101] Thus, an increased risk of intracranial hemorrhage may be caused by the inability to regenerate the endothelium.

Venous thromboembolic events

Bevacizumab causes abnormal endothelial cell apoptosis, which may result in venous thromboembolic events by exposing subendothelial molecules. A possible mechanism for thrombosis could be the loss of VEGF-dependent production of the platelet inhibitors, such as prostaglandin I-2 and nitric oxide.[102] Risk of venous thrombosis is historically increased with the use of angiogenic inhibitors, such as thalidomide and lenalidomide. As another angiogenic inhibitor, bevacizumab has also been suggested by Nalluri and colleagues[103] to be capable of increasing the risk for venous thromboembolic events in an already susceptible population, with relatively high rates in patients with GBM ranging from 7% to 32%.[8,99]

SUMMARY

The overall benefit of bevacizumab remains controversial. Although it inhibits angiogenesis and sensitizes gliomas to radiotherapy and chemotherapy, these treatment advantages and the extended PFS come at a significant price—tumor expansion may be substituted for tumor invasion into adjacent healthy tissue, and OS is not significantly extended. Future studies may need to assess novel methods of evaluating and visualizing tumor progression to determine the effectiveness of bevacizumab. Phase III clinical trials are currently investigating bevacizumab's potential as a therapeutic option for primary GBM.

REFERENCES

1. Stupp R, Mason WP, van den Bent MJ, et al. Radiotherapy plus concomitant and adjuvant temozolomide for glioblastoma. N Engl J Med 2005; 352(10):987–96.

2. Shibuya M. Brain angiogenesis in developmental and pathological processes: therapeutic aspects of vascular endothelial growth factor. FEBS J 2009;276(17):4636–43.

3. Brem S, Cotran R, Folkman J. Tumor angiogenesis: a quantitative method for histologic grading. J Natl Cancer Inst 1972;48(2):347–56.

4. Bello L, Giussani C, Carrabba G, et al. Angiogenesis and invasion in gliomas. Cancer Treat Res 2004;117:263–84.

5. Ballman KV, Buckner JC, Brown PD, et al. The relationship between six-month progression-free survival and 12-month overall survival end points for phase II trials in patients with glioblastoma multiforme. Neuro Oncol 2007;9(1):29–38.

6. Lamborn KR, Yung WK, Chang SM, et al. Progression-free survival: an important end point in evaluating therapy for recurrent high-grade gliomas. Neuro Oncol 2008;10(2):162–70.

7. Vredenburgh JJ, Desjardins A, Herndon JE 2nd, et al. Phase II trial of bevacizumab and irinotecan in recurrent malignant glioma. Clin Cancer Res 2007;13(4):1253–9.

8. Kreisl TN, Kim L, Moore K, et al. Phase II trial of single-agent bevacizumab followed by bevacizumab plus irinotecan at tumor progression in recurrent glioblastoma. J Clin Oncol 2009;27(5):740–5.

9. Hurwitz H, Fehrenbacher L, Novotny W, et al. Bevacizumab plus irinotecan, fluorouracil, and leucovorin for metastatic colorectal cancer. N Engl J Med 2004;350(23):2335–42.

10. Giantonio BJ, Catalano PJ, Meropol NJ, et al. Bevacizumab in combination with oxaliplatin, fluorouracil, and leucovorin (FOLFOX4) for previously treated metastatic colorectal cancer: results from the Eastern Cooperative Oncology Group Study E3200. J Clin Oncol 2007;25(12):1539–44.

11. Sandler A, Gray R, Perry MC, et al. Paclitaxel-carboplatin alone or with bevacizumab for non-small-cell lung cancer. N Engl J Med 2006;355(24): 2542–50.

12. Miller K, Wang M, Gralow J, et al. Paclitaxel plus bevacizumab versus paclitaxel alone for metastatic breast cancer. N Engl J Med 2007;357(26): 2666–76.

13. Miles DW, Chan A, Dirix LY, et al. Phase III study of bevacizumab plus docetaxel compared with placebo plus docetaxel for the first-line treatment of human epidermal growth factor receptor 2-negative metastatic breast cancer. J Clin Oncol 2010; 28(20):3239–47.

14. O'Shaughnessy JA, Brufsky AM. RiBBON 1 and RiBBON 2: phase III trials of bevacizumab with standard chemotherapy for metastatic breast cancer. Clin Breast Cancer 2008;8(4):370–3.

15. Reardon DA, Desjardins A, Rich JN, et al. The emerging role of anti-angiogenic therapy for malignant glioma. Curr Treat Options Oncol 2008;9(1):1–22.

16. Desjardins A, Reardon DA, Herndon JE 2nd, et al. Bevacizumab plus irinotecan in recurrent WHO grade 3 malignant gliomas. Clin Cancer Res 2008;14(21):7068–73.

17. Friedman HS, Prados MD, Wen PY, et al. Bevacizumab alone and in combination with irinotecan in recurrent glioblastoma. J Clin Oncol 2009;27(28): 4733–40.

18. Vredenburgh JJ, Desjardins A, JE Herndon JE 2nd, et al. Bevacizumab plus irinotecan in recurrent glioblastoma multiforme. J Clin Oncol 2007;25(30): 4722–9.

19. Wong ET, Gautam S, Malchow C, et al. Bevacizumab for recurrent glioblastoma multiforme: a meta-analysis. J Natl Compr Canc Netw 2011; 9(4):403–7.

20. Cloughesy T, Prados MD, Wen PY, et al. A phase II, randomized, non-comparative clinical trial of the effect of bevacizumab (BV) alone or in combination with irinotecan (CPT) on a 6-month progression free survival (PFS6) in recurrent, treatment-refractory glioblastoma (GBM). ASCO Annual Meeting 2010. J Clin Oncol 2008;26.

21. Wilkerson J, Fojo T. Progression-free survival is simply a measure of a drug's effect while administered and is not a surrogate for overall survival. Cancer J 2009;15(5):379–85.

22. Rubenstein JL, Kim J, Ozawa T, et al. Anti-VEGF antibody treatment of glioblastoma prolongs survival but results in increased vascular cooption. Neoplasia 2000;2(4):306–14.

23. Grothey A, Galanis E. Targeting angiogenesis: progress with anti-VEGF treatment with large molecules. Nat Rev Clin Oncol 2009;6(9):507–18.

24. Rapisarda A, Hollingshead M, Uranchimeg B, et al. Increased antitumor activity of bevacizumab in combination with hypoxia inducible factor-1 inhibition. Mol Cancer Ther 2009;8(7):1867–77.

25. Folkman J. Tumor angiogenesis: therapeutic implications. N Engl J Med 1971;285(21):1182–6.

26. Ellis LM, Hicklin DJ. Pathways mediating resistance to vascular endothelial growth factor-targeted therapy. Clin Cancer Res 2008;14(20):6371–5.

27. Keunen O, Johansson M, Oudin A, et al. Anti-VEGF treatment reduces blood supply and increases tumor cell invasion in glioblastoma. Proc Natl Acad Sci U S A 2011;108(9):3749–54.

28. Shibuya M. Vascular endothelial growth factor-dependent and -independent regulation of angiogenesis. BMB Rep 2008;41(4):278–86.

29. Brown LF, Yeo KT, Berse B, et al. Expression of vascular permeability factor (vascular endothelial growth factor) by epidermal keratinocytes during wound healing. J Exp Med 1992;176(5):1375–9.

30. Dvorak HF, Sioussat TM, Brown LF, et al. Distribution of vascular permeability factor (vascular endothelial growth factor) in tumors: concentration in tumor blood vessels. J Exp Med 1991;174(5):1275–8.

31. Armulik A, Genove G, Mae M, et al. Pericytes regulate the blood-brain barrier. Nature 2010;468(7323):557–61.

32. Inai T, Mancuso M, Hashizume H, et al. Inhibition of vascular endothelial growth factor (VEGF) signaling in cancer causes loss of endothelial fenestrations, regression of tumor vessels, and appearance of basement membrane ghosts. Am J Pathol 2004;165(1):35–52.

33. Abramsson A, Berlin O, Papayan H, et al. Analysis of mural cell recruitment to tumor vessels. Circulation 2002;105(1):112–7.

34. Morikawa S, Baluk P, Kaidoh T, et al. Abnormalities in pericytes on blood vessels and endothelial sprouts in tumors. Am J Pathol 2002;160(3):985–1000.

35. Rosso L, Brock CS, Gallo JM, et al. A new model for prediction of drug distribution in tumor and normal tissues: pharmacokinetics of temozolomide in glioma patients. Cancer Res 2009;69(1):120–7.

36. Yancopoulos GD, Davis S, Gale NW, et al. Vascular-specific growth factors and blood vessel formation. Nature 2000;407(6801):242–8.

37. Pajusola K, Aprelikova O, Armstrong E, et al. Two human FLT4 receptor tyrosine kinase isoforms with distinct carboxy terminal tails are produced by alternative processing of primary transcripts. Oncogene 1993;8(11):2931–7.

38. Hicklin DJ, Ellis LM. Role of the vascular endothelial growth factor pathway in tumor growth and angiogenesis. J Clin Oncol 2005;23(5):1011–27.

39. Brock TA, Dvorak HF, Senger DR. Tumor-secreted vascular permeability factor increases cytosolic Ca2+ and von Willebrand factor release in human endothelial cells. Am J Pathol 1991;138(1):213–21.

40. Antonetti DA, Barber AJ, Hollinger LA, et al. Vascular endothelial growth factor induces rapid phosphorylation of tight junction proteins occludin and zonula occluden 1. A potential mechanism for vascular permeability in diabetic retinopathy and tumors. J Biol Chem 1999;274(33):23463–7.

41. Papadopoulos MC, Saadoun S, Davies DC, et al. Emerging molecular mechanisms of brain tumour oedema. Br J Neurosurg 2001;15(2):101–8.

42. Carmeliet P, Jain RK. Molecular mechanisms and clinical applications of angiogenesis. Nature 2011;473(7347):298–307.

43. Dvorak HF, Brown LF, Detmar M, et al. Vascular permeability factor/vascular endothelial growth factor, microvascular hyperpermeability, and angiogenesis. Am J Pathol 1995;146(5):1029–39.

44. Kohn S, Nagy JA, Dvorak HF, et al. Pathways of macromolecular tracer transport across venules and small veins. Structural basis for the hyperpermeability of tumor blood vessels. Lab Invest 1992;67(5):596–607.

45. Qu H, Nagy JA, Senger DR, et al. Ultrastructural localization of vascular permeability factor/vascular endothelial growth factor (VPF/VEGF) to the abluminal plasma membrane and vesiculovacuolar organelles of tumor microvascular endothelium. J Histochem Cytochem 1995;43(4):381–9.

46. Kunkel P, Ulbricht U, Bohlen P, et al. Inhibition of glioma angiogenesis and growth in vivo by systemic treatment with a monoclonal antibody against vascular endothelial growth factor receptor-2. Cancer Res 2001;61(18):6624–8.

47. Plate KH, Breier G, Weich HA, et al. Vascular endothelial growth factor is a potential tumour angiogenesis factor in human gliomas in vivo. Nature 1992;359(6398):845–8.

48. Goldberg MA, Schneider TJ. Similarities between the oxygen-sensing mechanisms regulating the expression of vascular endothelial growth factor and erythropoietin. J Biol Chem 1994;269(6):4355–9.

49. Korkolopoulou P, Perdiki M, Thymara I, et al. Expression of hypoxia-related tissue factors in astrocytic gliomas. A multivariate survival study with emphasis upon carbonic anhydrase IX. Hum Pathol 2007;38(4):629–38.

50. Giatromanolaki A, Koukourakis MI, Sivridis E, et al. Expression of hypoxia-inducible carbonic anhydrase-9 relates to angiogenic pathways and independently to poor outcome in non-small cell lung cancer. Cancer Res 2001;61(21):7992–8.

51. Underwood JL, Murphy CG, Chen J, et al. Glucocorticoids regulate transendothelial fluid flow

resistance and formation of intercellular junctions. Am J Physiol 1999;277(2 Pt 1):C330–42.

52. Ellingson BM, Cloughesy TF, Lai A, et al. Quantitative volumetric analysis of conventional MRI response in recurrent glioblastoma treated with bevacizumab. Neuro Oncol 2011;13(4):401–9.

53. Chamberlain MC. Bevacizumab for recurrent malignant gliomas: efficacy, toxicity, and patterns of recurrence. Neurology 2009;72(8):772–3 [author reply: 773–4].

54. Pope WB, Lai A, Nghiemphu P, et al. MRI in patients with high-grade gliomas treated with bevacizumab and chemotherapy. Neurology 2006; 66(8):1258–60.

55. Ananthnarayan S, Bahng J, Roring J, et al. Time course of imaging changes of GBM during extended bevacizumab treatment. J Neurooncol 2008;88(3):339–47.

56. Ellingson BM, Cloughesy TF, Lai A, et al. Cell invasion, motility, and proliferation level estimate (CIMPLE) maps derived from serial diffusion MR images in recurrent glioblastoma treated with bevacizumab. J Neurooncol 2011;105:91–101.

57. Macdonald DR, Cascino TL, Schold SC Jr, et al. Response criteria for phase II studies of supratentorial malignant glioma. J Clin Oncol 1990;8(7): 1277–80.

58. Vos MJ, Uitdehaag BM, Barkhof F, et al. Interobserver variability in the radiological assessment of response to chemotherapy in glioma. Neurology 2003;60(5):826–30.

59. Zhou YH, Tan F, Hess KR, et al. The expression of PAX6, PTEN, vascular endothelial growth factor, and epidermal growth factor receptor in gliomas: relationship to tumor grade and survival. Clin Cancer Res 2003;9(9):3369–75.

60. Chaudhry IH, O'Donovan DG, Brenchley PE, et al. Vascular endothelial growth factor expression correlates with tumour grade and vascularity in gliomas. Histopathology 2001;39(4):409–15.

61. Dickson PV, Hamner JB, Sims TL, et al. Bevacizumab-induced transient remodeling of the vasculature in neuroblastoma xenografts results in improved delivery and efficacy of systemically administered chemotherapy. Clin Cancer Res 2007;13(13):3942–50.

62. Howe FA, Barton SJ, Cudlip SA, et al. Metabolic profiles of human brain tumors using quantitative in vivo 1H magnetic resonance spectroscopy. Magn Reson Med 2003;49(2):223–32.

63. Holash J, Maisonpierre PC, Compton D, et al. Vessel cooption, regression, and growth in tumors mediated by angiopoietins and VEGF. Science 1999;284(5422):1994–8.

64. Leenders WP, Kusters B, Verrijp K, et al. Antiangiogenic therapy of cerebral melanoma metastases results in sustained tumor progression via vessel co-option. Clin Cancer Res 2004;10(18 Pt 1): 6222–30.

65. Claes A, Gambarota G, Hamans B, et al. Magnetic resonance imaging-based detection of glial brain tumors in mice after antiangiogenic treatment. Int J Cancer 2008;122(9):1981–6.

66. de Groot JF, Fuller G, Kumar AJ, et al. Tumor invasion after treatment of glioblastoma with bevacizumab: radiographic and pathologic correlation in humans and mice. Neuro Oncol 2010;12(3):233–42.

67. Sakariassen PO, Prestegarden L, Wang J, et al. Angiogenesis-independent tumor growth mediated by stem-like cancer cells. Proc Natl Acad Sci U S A 2006;103(44):16466–71.

68. Hentschel SJ, Lang FF. Current surgical management of glioblastoma. Cancer J 2003;9(2): 113–25.

69. Jain RK. Normalization of tumor vasculature: an emerging concept in antiangiogenic therapy. Science 2005;307(5706):58–62.

70. Stark-Vance V. Bevacizumab and CPT-11 in the treatment of relapsed malignant glioma. In: World Federation of Neuro-Oncology Meeting. 2005 May 5-8; Edinburgh, United Kingdom; 2005. p. 91.

71. Hockel M, Schlenger K, Aral B, et al. Association between tumor hypoxia and malignant progression in advanced cancer of the uterine cervix. Cancer Res 1996;56(19):4509–15.

72. Rose SD, Aghi MK. Mechanisms of evasion to antiangiogenic therapy in glioblastoma. Clin Neurosurg 2010;57:123–8.

73. Tille JC, Wang X, Lipson KE, et al. Vascular endothelial growth factor (VEGF) receptor-2 signaling mediates VEGF-C(deltaNdeltaC)- and VEGF-A-induced angiogenesis in vitro. Exp Cell Res 2003; 285(2):286–98.

74. Kadambi A, Mouta Carreira C, Yun CO, et al. Vascular endothelial growth factor (VEGF)-C differentially affects tumor vascular function and leukocyte recruitment: role of VEGF-receptor 2 and host VEGF-A. Cancer Res 2001;61(6):2404–8.

75. Detmar M, Brown LF, Schon MP, et al. Increased microvascular density and enhanced leukocyte rolling and adhesion in the skin of VEGF transgenic mice. J Invest Dermatol 1998;111(1):1–6.

76. Larcher F, Murillas R, Bolontrade M, et al. VEGF/VPF overexpression in skin of transgenic mice induces angiogenesis, vascular hyperpermeability and accelerated tumor development. Oncogene 1998;17(3):303–11.

77. Thurston G, Suri C, Smith K, et al. Leakage-resistant blood vessels in mice transgenically overexpressing angiopoietin-1. Science 1999;286(5449): 2511–4.

78. Suri C, McClain J, Thurston G, et al. Increased vascularization in mice overexpressing angiopoietin-1. Science 1998;282(5388):468–71.

79. Scharpfenecker M, Fiedler U, Reiss Y, et al. The Tie-2 ligand angiopoietin-2 destabilizes quiescent endothelium through an internal autocrine loop mechanism. J Cell Sci 2005;118(Pt 4):771–80.

80. Gale NW, Dominguez MG, Noguera I, et al. Haploinsufficiency of delta-like 4 ligand results in embryonic lethality due to major defects in arterial and vascular development. Proc Natl Acad Sci U S A 2004;101(45):15949–54.

81. Li JL, Sainson RC, Shi W, et al. Delta-like 4 Notch ligand regulates tumor angiogenesis, improves tumor vascular function, and promotes tumor growth in vivo. Cancer Res 2007;67(23):11244–53.

82. Mailhos C, Modlich U, Lewis J, et al. Delta4, an endothelial specific notch ligand expressed at sites of physiological and tumor angiogenesis. Differentiation 2001;69(2–3):135–44.

83. Patel NS, Li JL, Generali D, et al. Up-regulation of delta-like 4 ligand in human tumor vasculature and the role of basal expression in endothelial cell function. Cancer Res 2005;65(19):8690–7.

84. Noguera-Troise I, Daly C, Papadopoulos NJ, et al. Blockade of Dll4 inhibits tumour growth by promoting non-productive angiogenesis. Nature 2006;444(7122):1032–7.

85. Liu ZJ, Shirakawa T, Li Y, et al. Regulation of Notch1 and Dll4 by vascular endothelial growth factor in arterial endothelial cells: implications for modulating arteriogenesis and angiogenesis. Mol Cell Biol 2003;23(1):14–25.

86. Real C, Remedio L, Caiado F, et al. Bone marrow-derived endothelial progenitors expressing Delta-like 4 (Dll4) regu-late tumor angiogenesis. PLoS One 2011;6(4):e18323.

87. Batchelor TT, Sorensen AG, di Tomaso E, et al. AZD2171, a pan-VEGF receptor tyrosine kinase inhibitor, normalizes tumor vasculature and alleviates edema in glioblastoma patients. Cancer Cell 2007;11(1):83–95.

88. Uhrbom L, Hesselager G, Nister M, et al. Induction of brain tumors in mice using a recombinant platelet-derived growth factor B-chain retrovirus. Cancer Res 1998;58(23):5275–9.

89. Dai C, Celestino JC, Okada Y, et al. PDGF autocrine stimulation dedifferentiates cultured astrocytes and induces oligodendrogliomas and oligoastrocytomas from neural progenitors and astrocytes in vivo. Genes Dev 2001;15(15):1913–25.

90. Muller YA, Li B, Christinger HW, et al. Vascular endothelial growth factor: crystal structure and functional mapping of the kinase domain receptor binding site. Proc Natl Acad Sci U S A 1997; 94(14):7192–7.

91. Homsi J, Daud AI. Spectrum of activity and mechanism of action of VEGF/PDGF inhibitors. Cancer Control 2007;14(3):285–94.

92. Timke C, Zieher H, Roth A, et al. Combination of vascular endothelial growth factor receptor/platelet-derived growth factor receptor inhibition markedly improves radiation tumor therapy. Clin Cancer Res 2008;14(7):2210–9.

93. Clark AJ, Butowski NA, Chang SM, et al. Impact of bevacizumab chemotherapy on craniotomy wound healing. J Neurosurg 2011;114(6):1609–16.

94. Kumar I, Staton CA, Cross SS, et al. Angiogenesis, vascular endothelial growth factor and its receptors in human surgical wounds. Br J Surg 2009;96(12): 1484–91.

95. Bose D, Meric-Bernstam F, Hofstetter W, et al. Vascular endothelial growth factor targeted therapy in the perioperative setting: implications for patient care. Lancet Oncol 2010;11(4):373–82.

96. Lu JF, Bruno R, Eppler S, et al. Clinical pharmacokinetics of bevacizumab in patients with solid tumors. Cancer Chemother Pharmacol 2008; 62(5):779–86.

97. Sugrue M, Bauman A, Jones F, et al. Clinical examination is an inaccurate predictor of intraabdominal pressure. World J Surg 2002;26(12):1428–31.

98. Gutin PH, Iwamoto FM, Beal K, et al. Safety and efficacy of bevacizumab with hypofractionated stereotactic irradiation for recurrent malignant gliomas. Int J Radiat Oncol Biol Phys 2009;75(1): 156–63.

99. Lai A, Tran A, Nghiemphu PL, et al. Phase II study of bevacizumab plus temozolomide during and after radiation therapy for patients with newly diagnosed glioblastoma multiforme. J Clin Oncol 2011; 29(2):142–8.

100. Raizer JJ, Grimm S, Chamberlain MC, et al. A phase 2 trial of single-agent bevacizumab given in an every-3-week schedule for patients with recurrent high-grade gliomas. Cancer 2010; 116(22):5297–305.

101. Khasraw M, Holodny A, Goldlust SA, et al. Intracranial hemorrhage in patients with cancer treated with bevacizumab: the Memorial Sloan-Kettering experience. Ann Oncol 2012;23(2):458–63.

102. Yang R, Thomas GR, Bunting S, et al. Effects of vascular endothelial growth factor on hemodynamics and cardiac performance. J Cardiovasc Pharmacol 1996;27(6):838–44.

103. Nalluri SR, Chu D, Keresztes R, et al. Risk of venous thromboembolism with the angiogenesis inhibitor bevacizumab in cancer patients: a meta-analysis. JAMA 2008;300(19):2277–85.

Potential Usefulness of Radiosensitizers in Glioblastoma

Yasuaki Harasaki, MD, Allen Waziri, MD*

KEYWORDS

- Radiosensitizers • Glioblastoma • Cancer • Chemotherapy

KEY POINTS

- Concurrent use of radiation with a range of sensitizing agents, including various chemotherapeutic drugs, can augment treatment efficacy through several well-defined biologic pathways.
- Mechanisms of radiosensitization include spatial cooperation, cytotoxic enhancement, biologic cooperation, temporal modulation, and protection of normal tissues.
- Temozolamide is the only chemotherapeutic agent that has been shown to provide a survival advantage when included with standard radiation therapy as an initial adjuvant approach for glioblastoma, an effect that has been associated with radiosensitization.
- Several agents, including angiogenesis inhibitors, are currently being studied for potential use in radiosensitization.

INTRODUCTION

In spite of recent success in the treatment of various forms of systemic cancer, glioblastoma multiforme (GBM) remains resistant to most current therapies. Various tumor characteristics have contributed to this resistance, including diffuse infiltration at the time of diagnosis, significant cellular heterogeneity (both intratumor and intertumor), and the role of tumor stem/progenitor cells in reestablishment of resistant disease following cytotoxic treatments. Current standard treatment of GBM consists of the regimen established by the European Organization for Research and Treatment of Cancer (EORTC) and the National Cancer Institute of Canada Clinical Trials Group (NCIC) in a landmark phase III trial published in 2005. Following maximal surgical resection, patients are treated with 60 Gy involved-field radiation therapy (IFRT), in which the involved field is defined as the radiographically evident tumor along with a margin of 2 to 3 cm. Treatment is administered in 30 fractions of 2 Gy each over 6 weeks with concurrent daily doses of the alkylating chemotherapeutic agent temozolomide (TMZ) at 75 mg/m^2. This standardized chemoradiation therapy is followed by TMZ alone at 200 mg/m^2 for 5 days every 4 weeks for a total of 6 months.[1]

The development of this combined adjuvant approach stemmed from several decades of clinical effort to improve outcomes for patients with GBM. Early studies in the 1970s had shown median survival for patients with malignant glioma, treated with surgical resection alone, to be less than 4 months.[2,3] A growing experience with postoperative radiation therapy to the brain was initiated in the late 1960s and early 1970s. The survival benefit of whole brain radiation (WBR) to greater than 50 Gy was shown through a large trial performed at the Montreal Neurology Institute in 1966 and confirmed by studies from the Brain Tumor Study Group within the National Institutes of Health in the 1970s.[4] Higher dosing strategies were explored by Salazar and colleagues in the 1970s, who concluded that doses of 70 to 80 Gy

Department of Neurosurgery, University of Colorado School of Medicine, 12631 East 17th Avenue, C307, Aurora, CO 80045, USA
* Corresponding author.
E-mail address: allen.waziri@ucdenver.edu

Neurosurg Clin N Am 23 (2012) 429–437
doi:10.1016/j.nec.2012.04.005
1042-3680/12/$ – see front matter © 2012 Elsevier Inc. All rights reserved.

were well tolerated by patients but did not eradicate tumor and did not significantly improve survival compared with the 60-Gy dose. Based on histologic changes seen in autopsy specimens of the patients receiving 70 to 80 Gy, they cautioned that higher doses than this would likely involve significant risk for extensive tissue necrosis.[5]

By the mid-1970s, there was increasing interest in application of IFRT to high-grade glioma, based on increasing understanding from clinical experience that most tumors are localized and that focal treatment allows minimization of the complications of radiation.[6] It was also during this time that early reports of successful stereotactic radiosurgery suggested that precise localization of radiation was both technically possible and could be of clinical benefit. The rationale for IFRT was validated by Hochberg and Pruitt,[7] who reviewed autopsy and imaging data for patients with GBM. They concluded that microscopic disease was limited to a 2-cm margin of the primary tumor in 29 out of 35 patients examined, and that 90% of recurrences also occurred in this margin. Further, multifocal disease occurred in only 4% of untreated patients, and was always identified on imaging.[7] Ramsey and Brand[6] in 1973 randomized 34 patients to WBR versus limited-field radiation, and showed that there was a survival benefit to higher dose (60 Gy) IFRT versus lower dose (40 Gy) WBR. These results have been validated in numerous subsequent studies and, in conjunction with technical improvements such as the introduction of multileaf collimators and associated planning algorithms for linear accelerators, have become the standard of care.[4]

There has similarly been a long history of correlative adjuvant therapy in GBM through the addition of chemotherapeutic agents. Temozolomide, a second-generation DNA alkylating agent, has been the only chemotherapeutic agent to show a clear survival benefit in combination with radiotherapy (RT). The recent EORTC/NCIC study, which established the current standard of treatment, compared surgical resection plus RT versus surgical resection plus RT plus temozolomide. Median survival for patients aged 18 to 70 years was 12.1 months for surgery and RT alone to 14.6 months for surgery and RT combined with temozolomide. In a 5-year follow-up to this initial study, the benefit of the addition of temozolomide durable throughout the period of follow-up.[8] A recent review of all patients with GBM in the United States in the SEER (Surveillance, Epidemiology and End Results) database comparing 2 years before the institution of the EORTC/NCIC regimen as standard care (2002–2004) with 2 years after (2005–2007) shows a gain in median survival from 11.5 to 12.5 months in the same age group,[9]

confirming that the additive effects of TMZ are mild in terms of clinical efficacy.

New therapeutic approaches are needed to provide a significant survival advantage for patients with GBM. The potential usefulness of radiosensitizing agents has been an intriguing possibility for these purposes and is the topic of this article.

RADIOSENSITIZATION: A CONCEPTUAL BASIS

Radiosensitizers are agents that are broadly defined as those that enhance the efficacy of radiation. In response to the increasing combination of radiation and chemotherapeutic agents available for the treatment of cancer in the late 1970s, Steel and Peckham[10] described 4 exploitable mechanisms of radiosensitization derived from the interaction of various therapeutic modalities. Their system was recently updated by Bentzen and colleagues[11] to provide further clinical relevance and take into account the effects of newer chemotherapeutic agents that are not directly cytotoxic. This more recent system of classification consists of 5 mechanisms of radiosensitization, which are summarized in this article.

Spatial Cooperation

The purpose of radiation therapy is locoregional control of disease, whereas chemotherapeutic agents target systemic disease that may or may not be clinically apparent. This approach allows for intensification of treatment via radiation in tissues with the greatest disease burden. Because this effect is spatial, it does not require concurrent administration of the 2 modes of therapy, and sequential treatment is generally preferred to minimize toxicity. This strategy has been effectively used in the context of various types of metastatic disease.

Cytotoxic Enhancement

The primary mechanism through which cytotoxicity is induced by ionizing radiation is the formation of free radicals within target tissues, which subsequently lead to DNA damage. Cytotoxic enhancement refers to the ability of a chemotherapeutic agent, given concurrently with radiation, to enhance DNA damage in the irradiated tissue by facilitating damage or by inhibiting repair. This approach may include inhibition of DNA replication, inhibition of mitosis, or induction of redox stress.

Biologic Cooperation

Although cytotoxic enhancement includes targeted effects of radiation and a chemotherapeutic agent on a common cell population, biologic cooperation refers to the presence of synergistic effects exerted by the chemotherapeutic agent through either different effector mechanisms and/or the activity of different cell populations. Commonly cited examples of agents showing biologic cooperation are antiangiogenic agents (eg, bevacizumab [BEV]) and bioreductive agents.

Temporal Modulation

Temporal modulation is the enhancement of the so-called 4 R effects of radiation dose fractionation through concurrent administration of a chemotherapeutic agent. The Rs consist of (1) preferential repair of DNA in normal tissues, reducing the toxicity of radiation if administered in a single fraction; (2) reoxygenation of previously hypoxic, and therefore radioresistant, central portions of tumor following the killing of the well-vascularized peripheral portions of tumor; (3) treatment by successive fractions of tumor repopulation following cytotoxic insult; and (4) redistribution of surviving tumor cells through the cell cycle to the more radiosensitive G2 and M phases. Agents targeting DNA repair mechanisms may be involved in both temporal modulation and cytotoxic enhancement.

Protection of Normal Tissue

This mechanism refers to minimization of acute or late radiation toxicity through the administration of a systemic agent. An example is a free radical scavenger with preferential cytoprotective effects in normal tissues.

Through the aforementioned mechanisms, a variety of agents have been proposed to have radiosensitizing properties in clinical use for malignant glioma (outlined in **Table 1**). The remainder of this article provides a brief overview of several of these agents, focusing on proposed mechanism of action as well as initial clinical experience with their use.

INHIBITION OF DNA REPLICATION
Temozolomide

Temozolomide (TMZ) is currently the only radiosensitizing agent used for GBM with class I evidence of benefit. TMZ was developed in the 1980s under the sponsorship of the Cancer Research Campaign in the United Kingdom (now Cancer Research UK) and entered clinical use in the late 1990s, with accelerated US Food and Drug Administration (FDA) approval for use in anaplastic astrocytoma granted in 1999.[29] It is a second-generation alkylating agent that is provided as a prodrug. Following administration through the enteral route, it undergoes hydrolysis in physiologic pH to its active form methyltraizeno-imidazoleoarboxamid (MTIC).

The main mechanism of action of MTIC, as with other alkylating agents, is to transfer a methyl group to the middle guanine in a GGG sequence to convert it to O6-methylguanine. Chakravarti and colleagues[30] showed that, in combination with radiation, TMZ exhibits cytotoxic enhancement by increasing the number of double-strand breaks and subsequently causes a greater number of the treated cells to undergo apoptosis. Hirose and colleagues[12] showed that there is also a temporal modulation effect, increasing radiosensitivity in the tumor by causing G2/M cycle arrest.

Based on the EORTC/NCIC data, Hegi and colleagues[31] showed that patient response to TMZ, as with other alkylating agents, was dependent on O6-methylguanine-DNA methyltransferase (MGMT) activity. MGMT is a DNA repair protein that reverses the O6-guanine methylation and therefore directly counteracts the action of alkylating agents. Hegi and colleagues[31] showed prolonged survival in patients in whom MGMT had been epigenetically silenced via hypermethylation of the MGMT promoter. Because MGMT is consumed in the process of performing this function, some approaches to depleting MGMT have been attempted. These approaches have included manipulation of dosing schedules of TMZ,[32] locally increased TMZ delivery to the tumor resection bed in biodegradable polymer wafers,[33] and administration of competing MGMT substrate O6-benzylguanine before TMZ administration.[34,35] A difficulty with these approaches has been the rapid de novo synthesis of MGMT and restoration of function within hours of depletion.[36]

Nitrogen Mustards

Carmustine or bis-chloroethylnitrosourea (BCNU) is a nitrogen mustard that, like temozolomide, is an alkylating agent and therefore similarly susceptible to reversal of its effect by MGMT. A recent retrospective study suggests that BCNU in biodegradable polymer wafers placed at the resection site before the current EORTC/NCIC protocol confers survival benefit compared with BCNU and radiation alone.[13]

Topoisomerase I Inhibitors

Camptothecin was first isolated from the deciduous tree *Camptotheca acuminata* in the screening program for cytotoxic plant-based substances at the Cancer Chemotherapy National Service Center (CCNSC) under the National Cancer Institute. Its discovery and antitumor activity were first described in 1966. However, it was not until 1985 that its mechanism of action via inhibition of topoisomerase I was elucidated.[14]

Table 1
Agents that have been proposed to have radiosensitizing properties in clinical use for malignant glioma

Class	Agent	Mechanism
Inhibition of DNA replication		
Alkylating agents	Temozolomide	Covalent transfer of alkyl group to guanine, increased apoptosis, and G2/M cell cycle arrest[12]
	Carmustine	Covalent transfer of alkyl group to guanine, increased apoptosis[13]
Topoisomerase I inhibitors	Camptothecin	Stabilization of topoisomerase I–DNA complex, inhibition of DNA religation[14,15]
	Topotecan	Stabilization of topoisomerase I–DNA complex, inhibition of DNA religation[15]
	Irinotecan	Stabilization of topoisomerase I–DNA complex, inhibition of DNA religation[15]
Topoisomerase II inhibitors	Doxorubicin	Stabilization of topoisomerase II–DNA complex, inhibition of DNA religation[15]
Inhibition of mitosis		
Microtubule stabilizers	Paclitaxel	Disruption of microtubule organization during mitosis
Microtubule destabilizers	Vinca alkaloids	Disruption of microtubule organization during mitosis
	Verubulin	Disruption of microtubule organization during mitosis
Augmentation of redox stress		
Nitroimidazoles	Metronidazole	Depletion of free radical scavengers
	Misonidazole	Depletion of free radical scavengers
Novel agents	Tirapazamine	Depletion of free radical scavengers
	Motexafin gadolinium	Depletion of free radical scavengers
Inhibition of angiogenesis		
Thalidomide derivatives	Lenalidomide	Inhibition of migration of endothelial cells[16]
Novel VEGF Inhibitors	Bevacizumab	Monoclonal antibody against VEGF-A[17]
	Aflibercept	VEGFR mimic, competes with VEGFR-1 and VEGFR-2[18]
Receptor tyrosine kinase inhibitors	Cediranib	Inhibits PDGFR, c-kit, all subtypes of VEGFR[19,20]
	Vandetanib	Inhibits EGFR, RET kinases, VEGFR-1, VEGFR-2[21,22]
	Sorafenib	Inhibits BRAF, PDGFR-β, c-Kit, RAS, p38 α, VEGFR-1, VEGFR-2[23]
	Cabozantinib	Inhibits VEGFR-2 and MET[24]
	Dasatinib	Inhibits BCR-Abl and Src family tyrosine kinases[25]
Adnectins	CT-322	Inhibits VEGFR-2[26]
Integrin inhibitors	Cilengitide	Inhibits signaling initiated by contact of cell with extracellular matrix[27]
Alternate signal pathway inhibition		
Receptor tyrosine kinase inhibitors	Erlotinib	Inhibition of EGFR[28]

Abbreviations: EGFR, epidermal growth factor receptor; PDGFR, platelet-derived growth factor receptor; RET; receptor tyrosine; VEGF, vascular endothelial growth factor; VEGFR, VEGF receptor.

Topoisomerase I binds covalently to 1 strand of the double-stranded DNA, cuts the other strand to relax supercoils, then religates the strand before disengaging the DNA. The primary action of camptothecin and its derivatives are S-phase specific, by reversibly binding the topoisomerase I–DNA complex and stabilizing it, specifically inhibiting the religation step. A collision of the camptothecin–topo-I-DNA complex with the replication fork during DNA replication leads to irreversible arrest of the replication fork followed by RNA polymerase during transcription. This collision is thought to result in a DNA double-strand break that, if unrepaired, leads to cell death.[14] Clinical trials with camptothecin in the 1970s were not pursued beyond a small phase 2 study because of toxicity. Since that time, 2 derivatives, topotecan and irinotecan, have been developed and are in clinical use.

As radiosensitizing agents, topoisomerase I inhibitors exhibit cytotoxic enhancement by targeting S-phase cells, which are radioresistant. There are currently multiple studies in progress examining the effectiveness of these agents as adjuncts to the EORTC/NCIC protocol.

Topoisomerase II Inhibitors

Doxorubicin, an anthracycline antibiotic, acts by intercalating DNA. Its main mode of action is in inhibition of the religation action of topoisomerase II, leading to double-strand breaks. Topoisomerase II, in contrast with topoisomerase I, forms double-strand breaks before religation, allowing it to not only relax supercoils but also to perform catenation-decatenation as well as knotting-deknotting. Doxorubicin not only exhibits cytotoxicity during replication but also during transcription.[15] Although doxorubicin was known to have activity against GBM cells in vitro, it had not seen clinical use because of its poor penetration of the blood brain barrier (BBB). Following recent availability of pegylated liposomal doxorubicin (PLD), there have been trials to assess its usefulness in GBM. A recent phase II study of postradiation administration of PLD within the EORTC/NCIC protocol has shown no clear benefit.[37]

MICROTUBULE STABILIZERS/DESTABILIZERS

Microtubule stabilizers and destabilizers cause mitotic arrest in dividing cells. Both the microtubule stabilizer paclitaxel and microtubule destabilizing vinca alkaloids have previously been susceptible to development of resistance through upregulation of efflux pumps. Verubulin (MPC-6827) is a recently introduced microtubule destabilizer binding the same site on β-tubulin as colchicine. In contrast with vinca alkaloids, verubulin is not susceptible to multidrug resistance efflux pumps. A phase I dose escalation trial has been completed,[38] and phase II trials of verubulin in conjunction with standard therapy are under way. Similarly, there has been renewed interest in paclitaxel, a first-generation microtubule stabilizing agent, which is being studied with new delivery methods that are less susceptible to cellular efflux. However, there are no current studies examining paclitaxel with radiation.

AUGMENTATION OF REDOX STRESS
Trans-Sodium Crocetinate

Radiation causes DNA damage in target tissues through the action of reactive oxygen species (ROS) with unpaired, highly chemically reactive electrons in their outer shells, such as superoxide, hydrogen peroxide, hydroxyl radical, and singlet oxygen. In the presence of molecular oxygen, this leads to formation of DNA organic peroxides that cannot be reversed, thereby fixing the damage. In the absence of oxygen, it forms DNA free radicals that can be reversed by the action of antioxidants, typically through reaction with an -SH group.[39]

Early attempts at radiosensitization of hypoxic tissues with nitroimidazoles such as metronidazole and misonidazole seemed promising in vitro but failed to show any clinical effect,[4] and have largely been abandoned with recent interest focused on their use in imaging of hypoxia.

More recently, tirapazamine, a bioreductive prodrug shown to significantly enhance radiation response in an animal model,[40] was studied as a radiosensitizing agent. In hypoxic tissues, it is reduced to reactive radical forms by intracellular reductases, leading to DNA single-strand and double-strand breaks. In the presence of oxygen, it is rapidly oxidized back to its inactive prodrug form, limiting its effect to tissues with low oxygen tension.[41] A phase II trial of tirapazamine given at 2 dose levels in conjunction with radiation showed no benefit compared with historical controls.

Motaxefin Gadolinium

Motexafin gadolinium (MGd) is a redox-active compound consisting of a porphyrinlike aromatic macromolecule complexed with gadolinium (III). In vivo in the presence of oxygen, it first accepts an electron from compounds with sufficient reduction potentials to form a radical, then subsequently transfers that electron to molecular oxygen to form a superoxide in a process known as redox cycling. The reducing agents are substances such as nicotinamide adenine dinucleotide (NADH)/nicotinamide adenine dinucleotide phosphate hydrogen (NADPH), glutathione, and ascorbic acid that act as antioxidant agents.[42] By depleting these cellular free radical scavenging mechanisms, MGd confers radiosensitization through cytotoxic enhancement. Recent literature suggests that reduction of MGd by NADPH may be catalyzed by thioredoxin reductase, which participates in various cellular functions via its protein disulfide reductase activity. In addition, MGd may have a direct inhibitory effect on ribonucleotide reductase, which is necessary for the reduction of all ribonucleotides to deoxyribonucleotides.[43]

A phase I dose escalation study of MGd with radiation in newly diagnosed GBM showed promising results, with median survival of 16.1 months in the treatment group versus 11.8 months in case-matched historical controls receiving radiation only.[44] A separate phase I dose escalation study of MGd with radiation in newly diagnosed pediatric pontine glioma has been completed,[45] and a phase II study of MGd plus TMZ and radiation is ongoing.

INHIBITION OF ANGIOGENESIS

Microvascular proliferation has long been known to be one of the histologic hallmarks of GBM, in large part because of increased expression of vascular endothelial growth factor (VEGF) in response to the hypoxic and acidotic tumor microenvironment. VEGF binds to a tyrosine kinase receptor (VEGF receptor [VEGFR]) that then initiates various signaling cascades. Of the VEGF subtypes, VEGF-A, in particular, is known to stimulate both angiogenesis and vasculogenesis as well as increase endothelial permeability and breakdown of the BBB.[46]

Inhibition of angiogenesis is thought to exert radiosensitizing effects on 2 levels. Prevention of the development of new capillaries between radiation fractions is thought to prevent the repopulation and tissue invasion response of the tumor to a cytotoxic insult, an example of biologic cooperation. Second, Jain and colleagues[46] introduced the concept of vascular normalization that may occur in neoadjuvant administration of antiangiogenic agents. The abundant vasculature in GBM is known to have various structural abnormalities, including poor organization, excessive tortuosity, and lack of an intact BBB. Flow through this abnormal vasculature has been noted in animal models to be heterogeneous with areas of poor or static flow. The increased VEGF levels constitute one possible mechanism, and anti-VEGF agents are thought to correct this abnormality and restore structurally and functionally more normal vasculature, providing cytotoxic enhancement via the reduction of hypoxic radioresistant regions within the tumor.[46]

Thalidomide Derivatives

Thalidomide was among the first-generation agents known to inhibit angiogenesis. Because of toxicity, various derivatives with improved tolerance have been developed, among them lenalidomide. The mechanism of the antiangiogenic effects of these agents is not clearly understood. A phase II study of thalidomide and topoisomerase I inhibitor irinotecan (CPT) in both newly diagnosed and recurrent GBM was performed before the establishment of the EORTC/NCIC standard. Six-month progression-free survival (PFS-6) was 40% and 19% in the newly diagnosed and recurrent groups, respectively.[47] A phase II trial of thalidomide administered during and following radiation in pediatric GBM and brainstem gliomas in a small cohort showed no clear benefit.[48] A phase II study of lenalidomide and radiation in newly diagnosed GBM has been published.[49] The corresponding phase II study has been completed and is awaiting publication of results.

VEGF Inhibitors

An antiangiogenic agent currently of interest is BEV, a humanized monoclonal antibody against VEGF-A. Because of previous success in treating colorectal cancer with the combination of BEV and CPT, this combination has been used in many phase II studies of high-grade glioma. In a recent prospective randomized trial comparing BEV with BEV plus CPT in recurrent GBM, PFS-6 was 42.6% in the BEV group and 50.3% in the BEV plus CPT group, compared with 15% for salvage chemotherapy and CPT alone.[17] There are currently multiple studies examining the use of BEV in a neoadjuvant or concurrent dosing with the radiation in the EORTC/NCIC protocol.

A second strategy for inhibition of VEGF has been the use of a VEGF receptor (VEGFR) mimic that reversibly competes with VEGFR for binding of VEGF, effectively reducing the concentration of available VEGF. Aflibercept (VEGF-Trap), a fusion protein consisting of extracellular domains of both VEGFR-1 and VEGFR-2 bound to the Fc region of human immunoglobulin G. In contrast with the VEGF-A–specific BEV, VEGF-Trap binds VEGF-A, VEGF-B, and placental growth factor (PlGF), also implicated in GBM angiogenesis, with high affinity. A recently published phase II trial showed no clear benefit and moderate toxicity of aflibercept monotherapy in recurrent GBM.[18] There is an ongoing study examining aflibercept with TMZ and radiation in both newly diagnosed and recurrent BM.

Another approach targets VEGF signaling. Small molecule receptor tyrosine kinase inhibitors (RTKI) compete for adenosine triphosphate (ATP) binding sites and subsequently prevent phosphorylation of the tyrosine kinase. This approach, as with VEGF-Trap, has the benefit of having multiple targets of activity. Cediranib has pan-VEGFR activity, as well as activity against platelet-derived growth factor (PDGF) and c-kit.[19,20] A phase II trial of cediranib monotherapy in recurrent GBM showed promising results with a median PFS-6 of 25.8% versus historical controls of 15%, and overall survival of 227 days versus 175 days in controls. Vandetanib has activity against VEGFR-1, VEGFR-2, epidermal growth factor receptor (EGFR), and receptor tyrosine (RET) kinases. Phase I trials in recurrent GBM have shown good tolerance of vandetanib in combination with radiation.[21,22] Sorafenib is active against VEGFR-2 and VEGFR-3, as well as BRAF, PDGF receptor-β (PDGFR-β), c-Kit, RAS, and p38-α. A recent trial examining administration of sorafenib after radiation within the EORTC/NCIC protocol showed no clear benefit, but there was a large drop-out rate before the initiation of sorafenib because of early disease progression.[23] There are also 2 newer tyrosine kinase inhibitors with few previous data in GBM: cabozontinib targeting VEGFR-2 and MET,[24] and dasatinib, targeting BCR-Abl and Src family tyrosine kinases.[25] There are ongoing trials examining all of these agents administered concurrently with radiation within the EORTC/NCIC protocol for newly diagnosed GBM.

A recently introduced class of target-binding proteins, adnectins, are currently being studied in GBM. These are proteins based on the 10th type III domain of fibronectin with its binding redirected to various targets. CT-322, an adnectin active against VEGFR-2, has been shown to be well tolerated in a phase I trial,[26] and is currently undergoing phase II evaluation.

SIGNAL PATHWAY INHIBITION
Epidermal Growth Factor Signaling

EGFR amplification is a hallmark in the pathogenesis of primary GBMs. EGFR is a tyrosine kinase receptor belonging to the human endothelial growth factor receptor (HER) family and is known to be involved in differentiation, proliferation, and migration of cells in the central nervous system during development.[50] In primary GBM, it is amplified in approximately 40% and overexpressed in greater than 60% of tumors.[51] Inhibition of the EGFR pathway may confer temporal modulation by inhibiting repopulation of the tumor between radiation fractions.

Tyrosine Kinase Inhibitors

One of the signaling pathways activated by EGFR and other receptor tyrosine kinases is the PI3 K/AKT/mTOR pathway, which is involved in cell growth, survival, and proliferation.[52] Agents targeting various points along this pathway are currently under investigation, and could potentially act as radiosensitizers in the same ways as the EGFR inhibitors. Simultaneously targeting multiple levels of a single pathway may yield synergistic effects. Clinical trials of these agents administered with radiation are pending.

FUTURE DIRECTIONS

In spite of improved understanding of the biology of many tumors in recent decades, there has been only modest improvement in prognosis for GBM associated with treatment. The combination of surgical resection, radiation, and temozolomide has been shown to provide a survival benefit. However, as understanding of the role of MGMT in therapeutic response shows, the era of 1-size-fits-all therapy is ending. As understanding of the signaling pathways involved in tumorigenesis continues to improve, a shift toward rationally tailored treatment based on tumor biomarkers can be expected to maximize the additive and synergistic effects of chemotherapy with radiation.

REFERENCES

1. Stupp R, Mason WP, van den Bent MJ, et al. Radiotherapy plus concomitant and adjuvant temozolomide for glioblastoma. N Engl J Med 2005;352(10): 987–96.

2. Walker MD, Alexander E Jr, Hunt WE, et al. Evaluation of mithramycin in the treatment of anaplastic gliomas. J Neurosurg 1976;44(6):655–67.

3. Walker MD, Alexander E Jr, Hunt WE, et al. Evaluation of BCNU and/or radiotherapy in the treatment of anaplastic gliomas. A cooperative clinical trial. J Neurosurg 1978;49(3):333–43.

4. Chang JE, Khuntia D, Robins HI, et al. Radiotherapy and radiosensitizers in the treatment of glioblastoma multiforme. Clin Adv Hematol Oncol 2007;5(11): 894–902, 907–15.

5. Salazar OM, Rubin P, Feldstein ML, et al. High dose radiation therapy in the treatment of malignant gliomas: final report. Int J Radiat Oncol Biol Phys 1979;5(10):1733–40.

6. Ramsey RG, Brand WN. Radiotherapy of glioblastoma multiforme. J Neurosurg 1973;39(2): 197–202.

7. Hochberg FH, Pruitt A. Assumptions in the radiotherapy of glioblastoma. Neurology 1980;30(9): 907–11.

8. Stupp R, Hegi ME, Mason WP, et al. Effects of radiotherapy with concomitant and adjuvant temozolomide versus radiotherapy alone on survival in

glioblastoma in a randomized phase III study: 5-year analysis of the EORTC-NCIC trial. Lancet Oncol 2009;10(5):459–66.

9. Darefsky AS, King JT, Dubrow R. Adult glioblastoma multiforme survival in the temozolomide era: a population-based analysis of surveillance, epidemiology, and end results registries. Cancer 2012;118(8): 2163–72.

10. Steel GG, Peckham MJ. Exploitable mechanisms in combined radiotherapy-chemotherapy: the concept of additivity. Int J Radiat Oncol Biol Phys 1979;5(1): 85–91.

11. Bentzen SM, Harari PM, Bernier J. Exploitable mechanisms for combining drugs with radiation: concepts, achievements and future directions. Nat Clin Pract Oncol 2007;4(3):172–80.

12. Hirose Y, Berger MS, Pieper RO. p53 effects both the duration of G2/M arrest and the fate of temozolomide-treated human glioblastoma cells. Cancer Res 2001;61(5):1957–63.

13. McGirt MJ, Than KD, Weingart JD, et al. Gliadel (BCNU) wafer plus concomitant temozolomide therapy after primary resection of glioblastoma multiforme. J Neurosurg 2009;110(3):583–8.

14. Wall ME. Campothecin and taxol: discovery to clinic. Med Res Rev 1998;18(5):299–314.

15. Pommier Y, Leo E, Zang H, et al. DNA topoisomerases and their poisoning by anticancer and antibacterial drugs. Chem Biol 2010;17(5):421–33.

16. Teo SK. Properties of thalidomide and its analogues: implications for anticancer therapy. AAPS J 2005; 7(1):E14–9.

17. Friedman HS, Prados MD, Wen PY, et al. Bevacizumab alone and in combination with irinotecan in recurrent glioblastoma. J Clin Oncol 2009;27(28): 4733–40.

18. de Groot JF, Lamborn KR, Chang SM, et al. Phase II study of aflibercept in recurrent malignant glioma: a North American Brain Tumor Consortium study. J Clin Oncol 2011;29(19):2689–95.

19. Chi AS, Sorensen AG, Jain RK, et al. Angiogenesis as a therapeutic target in malignant gliomas. Oncologist 2009;14(6):621–36.

20. Gerstner ER, Sorensen AG, Jain RK, et al. Antivascular endothelial growth factor therapy for malignant glioma. Curr Neurol Neurosci Rep 2009;9(3): 254–62.

21. Drappatz J, Norden AD, Wong ET, et al. Phase I study of vandetanib with radiotherapy and temozolomide for newly diagnosed glioblastoma. Int J Radiat Oncol Biol Phys 2010;78(1):85–90.

22. Fields EC, Damek D, Gaspar LE, et al. Phase I dose escalation trial of vandetanib with fractionated radiosurgery in patients with recurrent malignant gliomas. Int J Radiat Oncol Biol Phys 2012;82(1):51–7.

23. Hainsworth JD, Ervin T, Friedman E, et al. Concurrent radiotherapy and temozolomide followed by

temozolomide and sorafenib in the first-line treatment of patients with glioblastoma multiforme. Cancer 2010;116(15):3663–9.

24. Yakes FM, Chen J, Tan J, et al. Cabozantinib (XL184), a novel MET and VEGFR2 inhibitor, simultaneously suppresses metastasis, angiogenesis, and tumor growth. Mol Cancer Ther 2011;10(21):2298–308.

25. Wick W, Weller M, Weiler M, et al. Pathway inhibition: emerging molecular targets for treating glioblastoma. Neuro Oncol 2011;13(6):566–79.

26. Tolcher AW, Sweeney CJ, Papadopoulos K, et al. Phase I and pharmacokinetic study of CT-322 (BMS-844203), a targeted Adnectin inhibitor of VEGFR-2 based on a domain of human fibronectin. Clin Cancer Res 2011;17(2):363–71.

27. Tabatabai G, Weller M, Nabors B, et al. Targeting integrins in malignant glioma. Target Oncol 2010;5(3): 175–81.

28. Peereboom DM, Shepard DR, Ahluwalia MS, et al. Phase II trial of erlotinib with temozolomide and radiation in patients with newly diagnosed glioblastoma multiforme. Neuro Oncol 2011;13(12):1331–8.

29. Newlands ES, Stevens MF, Wedge SR, et al. Temozolomide: a review of its discovery, chemical properties, pre-clinical development and clinical trials. Cancer Treat Rev 1997;23(1):35–61.

30. Chakravarti A, Erkkinen MG, Nestler U, et al. Temozolomide-mediated radiation enhancement in glioblastoma: a report on underlying mechanisms. Clin Cancer Res 2006;12(15):4738–46.

31. Hegi ME, Diserens AC, Gorlia T, et al. MGMT gene silencing and benefit from temozolomide in glioblastoma. N Engl J Med 2005;352(10):997–1003.

32. Clarke JL, Iwamoto FM, Sul J, et al. Randomized phase II trial of chemoradiotherapy followed by either dose-dense or metronomic temozolomide for newly diagnosed glioblastoma. J Clin Oncol 2009; 27(23):3861–7.

33. Brem S, Tyler B, Li K, et al. Local delivery of temozolomide by biodegradable polymers is superior to oral administration in a rodent glioma model. Cancer Chemother Pharmacol 2007;60(5):643–50.

34. Quinn JA, Desjardins A, Weingart J, et al. Phase I trial of temozolomide plus O6-benzylguanine for patients with recurrent or progressive malignant glioma. J Clin Oncol 2005;23(28):7178–87.

35. Quinn JA, Jiang SX, Reardon DA, et al. Phase I trial of temozolomide plus O6-benzylguanine 5-day regimen with recurrent malignant glioma. Neuro Oncol 2009;11(5):556–61.

36. Tolcher AW, Gerson SL, Denis L, et al. Marked inactivation of O6-alkylguanine-DNA alkyltransferase activity with protracted temozolomide schedules. Br J Cancer 2003;88(7):1004–11.

37. Ananda S, Nowak AK, Cher L, et al. Phase 2 trial of temozolomide and pegylated liposomal doxorubicin

in the treatment of patients with glioblastoma multiforme following concurrent radiotherapy and chemotherapy. J Clin Neurosci 2011;18(11):1444–8.

38. Tsimberidou AM, Akerley W, Schabel MC, et al. Phase I clinical trial of MPC-6827 (Azixa), a microtubule destabilizing agent, in patients with advanced cancer. Mol Cancer Ther 2010;9(12):3410–9.

39. Halliwell B. Free radicals, antioxidants, and human disease: curiosity, cause, or consequence? Lancet 1994;344(8924):721–4.

40. Brown JM, Lemmon MJ. Tumor hypoxia can be exploited to preferentially sensitize tumors to fractionated irradiation. Int J Radiat Oncol Biol Phys 1991;20(3):457–61.

41. Reddy SB, Williamson SK. Tirapazamine: a novel agent targeting hypoxic tumor cells. Expert Opin Investig Drugs 2009;18(1):77–87.

42. Magda D, Miller RA. Motexafin gadolinium: a novel redox active drug for cancer therapy. Semin Cancer Biol 2006;16(6):466–76.

43. Hashemy SI, Ungerstedt JS, Zahedi Avval F, et al. Motexafin gadolinium, a tumor-selective drug targeting thioredoxin reductase and ribonucleotide reductase. J Biol Chem 2006;281(16):10691–7.

44. Ford JM, Seiferheld W, Alger JR, et al. Results of the phase I dose-escalating study of motexafin gadolinium with standard radiotherapy in patients with glioblastoma multiforme. Int J Radiat Oncol Biol Phys 2007;69(3):831–8.

45. Bradley KA, Pollack IF, Reid JM, et al. Motexafin gadolinium and involved field radiation therapy for intrinsic pontine glioma of childhood: a Children's Oncology Group phase I study. Neuro Oncol 2008; 10(5):752–8.

46. Jain RK, di Tomaso E, Duda DG, et al. Angiogenesis in brain tumours. Nat Rev Neurosci 2007;8(8):610–22.

47. Fadul CE, Kingman LS, Meyer LP, et al. A phase II study of thalidomide and irinotecan for treatment of glioblastoma multiforme. J Neurooncol 2008;90(2): 229–35.

48. Turner CD, Chi S, Marcus KJ, et al. Phase II study of thalidomide and radiation in children with newly diagnosed brain stem gliomas and glioblastoma multiforme. J Neurooncol 2007;82(1):95–101.

49. Drappatz J, Wong ET, Schiff D, et al. A pilot safety study of lenalidomide and radiotherapy for patients with newly diagnosed glioblastoma multiforme. Int J Radiat Oncol Biol Phys 2009;73(1):222–7.

50. Nicholas MK, Lukas RV, Jafri NF, et al. Epidermal growth factor receptor - mediated signal transduction in the development and therapy of gliomas. Clin Cancer Res 2006;12(24):7261–70.

51. Ohgaki H, Kleihues P. Genetic pathways to primary and secondary glioblastoma. Am J Pathol 2007; 170(5):1445–53.

52. Cheng CK, Fan QW, Weiss WA. PI3K signaling in glioma-animal models and therapeutic challenges. Brain Pathol 2009;19(1):112–20.

Nanotechnology Applications for Glioblastoma

Edjah K. Nduom, MD, Alexandros Bouras, MD,
Milota Kaluzova, PhD, Costas G. Hadjipanayis, MD, PhD*

KEYWORDS

- Malignant brain tumors • Glioblastoma • Magnetic nanoparticles • Nanoparticles
- Convection-enhanced delivery • MRI • EGFR • Thermotherapy

KEY POINTS

- GBM remains a difficult tumor to treat due to its infiltrative nature.
- Nanoparticles present a new way to target infiltrating cells.
- Magnetic nanoparticles (MNPs) can be used as MRI contrast agents as well as therapeutic agents by the use of thermotherapy.
- In a nanoparticle formulation chemotherapeutics can be more efficacious than conventional chemotherapeutic agents due to their ability to target GBM cells and release drug.
- Gene delivery through the use of nanoparticles may be a safe option to deliver therapeutic genes to tumor cells.
- Brachytherapy delivered by radioactive nanoparticles can provide long-term focused radiation therapy to these lesions.
- Gold nanoparticles can be used to treat tumors through phototherapy, where deep penetrating near-infrared light can be used to inhibit tumor growth.
- Nanoparticles can be delivered safely systemically or by bulk flow using convection-enhanced delivery (CED) directly to the tumor.
- Magnetic targeting can be used to enhance the delivery of MNPs by directing the delivered particles to the area of interest.

INTRODUCTION

Glioblastoma (GBM) is the most common primary malignancy of the brain as well as its most malignant.[1] The median survival after radiation and chemotherapy ranges from 12 to 15 months, despite advances in surgery, radiation, and chemotherapy.[2] GBM tumors are nearly uniformly fatal due to local recurrence.[3–5] Even for lesions amenable to gross surgical resection, infiltrating cancer cells beyond the boundaries of the enhancing lesion are responsible for tumor recurrence as well as radiation and chemotherapy resistance.[6,7]

Cancer nanotechnology has recently emerged as a field that may provide answers to some of the difficulties encountered in treating GBM. Nanoparticles, defined as particles less than 100 nm in hydrodynamic size, have been used in the

Disclosures: Financial support—EN, no funding to disclose; AB, American Association of Neurological Surgeons/Congress of Neurological Surgeons Section on Tumors/Brainlab International Fellowship; MK, no funding to disclose; and CGH, National Institutes of Health (NS053454), Georgia Cancer Coalition, Distinguished Cancer Clinicians and Scientists Program, Robbins Scholar Award, and Dana Foundation.
Conflicts of interest—No conflicts to report.
Brain Tumor Nanotechnology Laboratory, Department of Neurosurgery, Emory University School of Medicine, 1365C Clifton Road NE, Winship Cancer Institute of Emory University, Atlanta, GA 30322, USA
* Corresponding author. Department of Neurosurgery, Emory University School of Medicine, 1365B Clifton Road Northeast, Suite 6200, Atlanta, GA 30322.
E-mail address: chadjip@emory.edu

treatment of various cancers.[8] The use of biocompatible nanomaterials has permitted the fabrication of nanoparticles with capabilities that surpass those of conventional agents. Chemotherapy-loaded nanoparticles have resulted in sustained-release formulations that can lower systemic toxicity and produce greater antitumor effects. Recently developed nanoparticles can cross the blood-brain barrier (BBB) after systemic administration or be distributed in the brain by CED to target GBM cells therapeutically while harboring elements that may enable imaging of the particle and the target. The field has been moving at a rapid pace, enabling nanoparticles to be used in recent clinical trials.[9] Although not exhaustive, the list of nanoparticles used in the treatment of experimental GBM includes polymeric particles, micelles,[10] nanoshells,[11] quantum dots,[12] and magnetic iron oxide nanoparticles (IONPs).[13] Nanotubes are another formulation of nanoparticle, used to create structures that can trap diagnostic or therapeutic modalities within a cage. This article discusses the use of different nanoparticle formulations in strategies to image and treat GBM, including delivery schemes.

MAGNETIC NANOPARTICLES
MRI Contrast Properties of MNPs

The base of the promise for theranostic nanoparticles with both therapeutic and diagnostic ability hinges on the idea that such nanoparticles will be able to image where the lesion is and treat it. MNPs have attracted particular interest in this respect due to their unique paramagnetic properties that enable their detection by MRI.[14,15] These MNPs have shown great potential as T_1 or T_2 contrast agents in MRI,[16,17] with superparamagnetic iron oxide–based nanoparticles (SPIOs) as the most commonly investigated type of MRI contrast agents.[18] Since 1990, ultrasmall SPIOs (USPIOs), smaller than 50 nm, have been considered an MRI contrast agent,[19] and most of the MRI data regarding nanoparticles references these particles. USPIOs can be visualized in T_2-weighted MRI sequences (T_2 contrast agents) as a hypointense (dark) signal (negative contrast enhancement) or with T_1-weighted MRI sequences (T_1 contrast agents) as a hyperintense (bright) signal (positive contrast enhancement).[20–22]

USPIOs can provide contrast for a longer period of time[23] compared with gadolinium (Gd)-based contrast agents that are rapidly eliminated by the kidney.[24,25] USPIOs are also taken up by tumor cells as well as by reactive phagocytic cells (eg, microglia) found in brain tumors. The USPIOs can reside within brain tumors much longer than Gd-based agents, with a peak enhancement noted at 24 to 28 hours and persisting up to 72 hours after administration.[26,27] These agents may provide a safe alternative for patients at risk for nephrogenic systemic fibrosis, because preliminary studies have shown no adverse renal effects.[27,28]

MNPs for Targeted Brain Tumor Imaging

Targeting of tumor cells can increase the benefits provided by nanoparticles as contrast agents. IONPs are taken up by GBM cells both in vivo and in vitro.[29,30] Surface functionalization further enhances tumor uptake of these particles.[31] Tumor-specific ligands conjugated to MNPs can further enhance the uptake within targeted tumor tissue (**Fig. 1**).[32,33] Antibodies, peptides (including toxins), cytokines, and chemotherapeutic agents have been reported as possible MNP ligands.[34] Amphiphilic triblock copolymer IONPs can be conjugated with a purified antibody that selectively

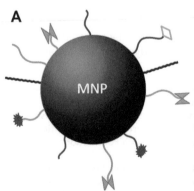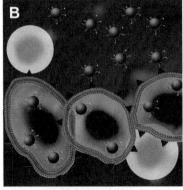

Fig. 1. Theranostic MNPs and tumor targeting. (*A*) Illustration of an MNP with different functional groups on the surface, which permit molecular targeting, imaging, enhanced plasma circulation times, and/or therapy. (*B*) Illustration of MNPs functionalized with tumor cell–specific ligands binding cancer cells (*large irregular cells*) instead of normal cells (*pink*). Internalization of MNPs is shown in cancer cells as well.

binds to the epidermal growth factor receptor (EGFR) deletion mutant, EGFR vIII, which is solely expressed by a population of GBM tumors.[35] Such nanoparticles exhibit MR contrast enhancement of GBM cells and can target these therapy-resistant cancer cells in vitro and in vivo.

Chlorotoxin, derived from scorpion venom, specifically binds to matrix metalloproteinase 2 (MMP-2), which is overexpressed on the surface of GBM cells.[36,37] MMP-2 degrades the extracellular matrix during tumor invasion, and chlorotoxin can be used to bind the MMP-2 and inhibit infiltration.[38,39] Chlorotoxin conjugated to MNPs can act as MRI contrast agents and the addition of a Cy5.5 molecule makes these suitable for use as an intraoperative fluorescent dye as well.[40–42]

F3 is a small peptide that specifically binds to nucleolin overexpressed on proliferating endothelial cells of tumor cells and the associated vasculature.[43] F3-coated IONPs can provide significant MRI contrast enhancement of intracranial rat-implanted tumors, compared with noncoated F3 nanoparticles, when administered intravenously.[44]

A molecular MRI contrast agent, consisting of SPIO coated with dextran, was functionalized with an anti–insulinlike growth factor binding protein 7 (anti-IGFBP7) single-domain antibody and was found by both MRI and in vivo fluorescent imaging to target the vasculature of GBM cells.[45]

Gd has also been incorporated into some therapeutic nanoparticles to enable them to be tracked using MRI. One group has designed nanoparticles containing Gd, which are rapidly taken up by the GL261 tumor cell line and show MRI contrast when these cells are then cultured in a chick embryo host.[46] Gd nanoparticles functionalized with diethylenetriaminepentaacetic acid (DTPA) can also be used as a radiosensitizing agent.[47] Fullerene magnetic nanotubes have been made such that Gd can be trapped within these structures to make them an effective contrast agent, along with whatever therapeutic modality is also associated with the fullerene cage.[48,49] It is also possible to internalize IONPs in these larger nanotube structures so that the magnetic properties of iron oxide can be used, allowing clinicians to localize these particles to a particular area. This, together with surface targeting, can greatly increase the amount of intake and resultant therapeutic effect of these particles.[50]

MNPs for Optical Delineation of Brain Tumors

Although surgical intervention is not curative in GBM, obtaining a maximal resection is important for survival.[51] The use of intraoperative MRI and neuronavigation has increased extent of resection and outcome.[52–54] Recently, fluorescence-guided surgery after oral administration of 5-aminolevulinic acid (5-ALA) has resulted in more complete resection of malignant gliomas.[55,56] Laboratory studies have attempted to find ways to use optical aides to increase the contrast between normal and tumor tissue,[57–59] and these methods have shown improvement in the extent of tumor resection in clinical use.[60,61]

Fluorescent molecules have already been successfully incorporated into several nanoparticles. An IONP-Cy5.5 molecule has been used in many preclinical studies,[40,41,62] giving it the dual benefits of MRI detection and possibly enhanced surgical contrast using the fluorescent properties of the particle. This also could lead to theranostic particles that could be injected preoperatively to outline malignant tissue that would need to be resected at surgery.

MNPs for Stem Cell Tracking

The ability of MNPs to act as MRI contrast agents can be used to track stem cell tropism to malignant brain tumors in vivo. Intracranially administered neural stem cells have tropism for GBM tumors, making them attractive for tumor-targeting gene therapy.[63–65] Mesenchymal stem cells have also been found to migrate to tumor cells.[66] By labeling these cells with IONPs, this migration can be visualized on MRI.[67,68] Magnetically labeled hematopoietic stem cells can also be tracked to gliomas in this fashion.[69]

MNPs for Thermotherapy of GBM

One of the more unique features of MNPs is the ability to induce hyperthermia when exposed to alternating magnetic fields. Temperature elevations in the range of 41°C to 46°C can cause cells to undergo heat stress, resulting in protein denaturation, protein folding, aggregation, and DNA cross-linking.[70] This process can induce apoptosis and heat shock protein expression. At the tissue level, moderate hyperthermia causes changes in pH, perfusion, and oxygenation of the tumor microenvironment.[71–74] These effects, combined with chemotherapy and radiation, can have a synergistic effect.[74–78]

Hyperthermia can be induced in MNPs through the use of an appropriate alternating magnetic field of the right amplitude and frequency to heat up the nanoparticles. A predictable and sufficient amount of heat known as the specific absorption rate is produced. The MNPs use several different mechanisms to convert the magnetic energy into heat energy. Néel relaxation is caused by rapidly occurring changes in the direction of magnetic moments relative to crystal lattice. Brownian relaxation results from the physical rotation of MNPs within the medium in which they are placed. Both internal (Néel) and external (brownian) sources of friction lead to a phase lag between applied magnetic field and the direction of magnetic moment, producing thermal losses (**Fig. 2**).

MNPs can be specifically engineered to maximize their suitability for hyperthermia by producing greater saturation magnetization, optimal anisotropy, and larger size within the constraints of nanoparticle production.[79–81] MNPs suitable for thermotherapy can be made from a combination of various metals, including manganese (Mn), iron (Fe), cobalt (Co), nickel (Ni), zinc (Zn), and magnesium (Mg) and their oxides.[82–89] Ferrites of the various metals are frequently used in these settings, such as cobalt ferrites ($CoFe_2O_4$), manganese ferrites ($MnFe_2O_4$), nickel ferrites ($NiFe_2O_4$), lithium ferrites ($Li_{0.5}Fe_{2.5}O_4$), mixed ferrites of nickel–zinc–copper, and cobalt–nickel ferrites.[85–91] There are also ferromagnetic nanoparticles that are iron based and have greater magnetic properties than IONPs.[79] These cobalt ferrites–based nanoparticles produce greater hyperthermia effects at much lower concentrations than IONPs. FeNPs are comprised of an iron core surrounded by an iron oxide layer to permit stability. Nevertheless, owing to their lack of toxicity, excellent biocompatibility, and their capacity to be metabolized,[92–94] iron oxide–based MNPs are actively being studied for thermotherapy of brain tumors.

MNP-based hyperthermia has been evaluated for feasibility in animal models and in human patients with malignant brain tumors. Dextran-coated or aminosilane-coated IONPs have been used for thermotherapy in a rodent GBM model[95] and in a human clinical trial in patients with recurrent GBM.[9,96] Intratumoral injection of aminosilane-coated IONPs (core size 12 nm) and application of an alternating magnetic field (100 kHz) in several sessions before and after adjuvant fractionated radiation therapy was given. With a high concentration of IONPs (>100 mg/mL), this achieved effective thermotherapy with a median peak temperature within the tumor of 51.2°C. This phase II clinical trial successfully demonstrated safety and efficacy of thermotherapy of malignant brain tumors with MNPs in humans, with a significant increase in overall survival compared with a reference population. Further randomized studies will be required to validate the promise of this treatment modality.

NANOPARTICALIZED CHEMOTHERAPEUTIC AGENTS

Although few conventional chemotherapeutics have been proved effective in GBM, chemotherapeutics in a nanoparticle formulation offer possible advantages. These often can be targeted, evade the reticuloendothelial system for prolonged circulatory time, and potentially cross the BBB better then standard chemotherapy agents. Polyethylene glycol (PEG)-coated paclitaxel (taxol) nanoparticles have been shown to offer superior bioavailability compared with free paclitaxel with a survival advantage shown in a rodent glioma model.[97] Poly(d,l-lactide-co-glycolide) (PLGA) nanoparticles are another form of biocompatible nanoparticles. CED of these nanoparticles, loaded with camptothecin, has been shown efficacious in a rodent glioma model.[98] Although the controlled release offered by nanoparticles can reduce systemic toxicity and allow drug to be slowly released only when it has reached its target, there is also a need to ensure that an adequate dose is delivered to the lesion being treated. Nanoparticles have been developed that are thermosensitive, releasing their drug preferentially when the temperature has been increased.[99] When delivered with gold nanorods, concurrent photothermal hyperthermia can release the drug from the heat sensitive nanoparticle, thus increasing efficacy.

GENE DELIVERY WITH NANOPARTICLES

The Cancer Genome Atlas has revealed the multiple genetic aberrations in GBM tumors that can serve as therapeutic targets provide targets.[100] Cationic solid lipid nanoparticles can be conjugated to PEGylated therapeutic *c-Met* small interfering RNA and reduce human GBM tumor growth in a rodent model without significant toxicity.[101] Another nanoparticle, containing the integrin-binding motif RGD, together with the PEG-polyethylenimine (PEI) nonviral gene carrying

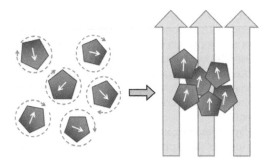

Fig. 2. MNP response to alternating magnetic fields and thermotherapy. Application of applied magnetic fields (*arrows*) orients the MNPs on the right from their random orientation on the left in the absence of magnetic fields. Random orientation on the left produces thermal losses, allowing for hyperthermia generation by the MNPs.

nanoparticle, was able to deliver a plasmid expressing the tumor necrosis factor-related apoptosis-inducing ligand with increased efficiency and increase survival in a rodent glioma model.[102]

NANOPARTICLES FOR BRACHYTHERAPY

Brachytherapy, where localized radiotherapy is delivered directly to a tumor, has been explored as a strategy with nanoparticles. In an orthotopic xenograft brain tumor model, a functionalized fullerene nanoparticle (^{177}Lu-DOTA-f-Gd$_3$N@C$_{80}$), with radiolabeled lutetium 177 (^{177}Lu) and tetraazacyclododecane tetraacetic acid (DOTA), provided an anchor to deliver effective brachytherapy and longitudinal imaging of the tumor.[103] Internal fractionated radiation has also been achieved using a lipid nanoparticle formulation of radionucliides, such as ^{188}Re-SSS in the 9L rat glioma cell line.[75]

GOLD NANOPARTICLE PHOTOTHERAPY

Gold nanoparticles can be designed as nanoshells, consisting of a spherical dielectric core nanoparticle surrounded by thin sheet metal.[76] The size of each layer of the nanoshell can be tailored to enable it to have a peak light absorption at 800 nm, in the near infrared range. Light in this region of the electromagnetic spectrum has minimal absorption by water and biologic chromophores, allowing it to pass deep into tissues without losing much of its energy. This region of the electromagnetic spectrum is notable for minimal absorption by water and biologic chromophores. Thus, light of this wavelength may penetrate deep into tissues with minimal disruption. This has enabled researchers to produce these gold nanoparticles, which can be activated by light and kill GBM cells in vitro.[77] One group has used macrophages loaded with gold nanoshells to deliver these particles to glioma spheroids to then be activated by near infrared light, inhibiting growth.[78]

MALIGNANT BRAIN TUMOR DELIVERY OF NANOPARTICLES

Delivery of therapeutic agents to GBM tumors remains a formidable challenge. Systemic delivery is limited by the BBB, nonspecific uptake, nontargeted distribution, and systemic toxicity. The benefits and drawbacks of the use of systemic delivery, systemic delivery augmented by magnetic targeting, and direct infusion in the brain known as CED are examined.

Systemic Delivery

The reticuloendothelial system can significantly reduce the amount of nanoparticle available to treat the lesion by nonspecific uptake in the liver, kidney, spleen, and circulating macrophages.[104,105] This can be addressed by biocompatible surface coating of nanoparticles, which can increase their circulation time.[106] The BBB further obstructs delivery by preventing the entry of most particles from the circulation into the interstitial space of the brain. It is well known that the vasculature in GBM, however, is not phenotypically normal, due to open endothelial gaps and atypical angiogenesis, allowing more efflux of intravascular material into the tumor mass.[107–109] The enhanced permeability and retention effect is used to describe the selective extravasation of macromolecules into the tumor interstitium through the hyperpermeable tumor vasculature.[110] By attaching tumor-specific targeting ligands, delivery has been shown to be increased in a rodent model, because the extravasated treatment is more likely to be taken up by the lesion.[44,111]

Integrins are overexpressed in GBM at the brain tumor border, and one of the integrin-binding motifs is RGD. Conjugating this peptide to PEG and PEI creates a nanoparticle, which was targeted to GBM and found to prolong survival in rodents implanted with human intracranial GBM xenografts.[102] Meng and colleagues used PEI conjugated to DNA and myristic acid, a hydrophobic molecule, can enhance the ability of the PEI/DNA complexed nanoparticles to cross the BBB, thus showing a treatment effect in GBM tumor models.[112]

PLGA nanoparticles have been shown to cross the BBB. The use of surfactants, such as poloxamer 188 (Pluronic F-68) or polysorbate 80 (Tween 80), can enhance the transport of the particles and increase the delivery of drugs conjugated to them and increase intracellular uptake.[113–115] A recent study demonstrated that conjugating transferrin, a protein known to be actively transported across the BBB, enhances the delivery of these particles to the brain, with an intact BBB as well as a disrupted BBB with an intracranial lesion.[116]

The α-helical amphipathic peptide $_D$[KLAKLAK]$_2$ was originally designed as a synthetic antibacterial peptide that disrupts the bacterial cell membrane but is less toxic to eukaryotic cells. When conjugated to a mitochondrial peptide, CGKRK, IONP-derived nanoworms (due to their elongated shape), these particles localize to the mitochondria of tumor cells and cure tumors in a rodent tumor model. The nanoparticles could be seen to localize to the tumor on MRI.[111]

Magnetic Targeting

The concept of magnetic targeting of malignant brain tumors has also been demonstrated in preclinical rodent models[117,118] as a method to enhance the systemic delivery of MNPs to malignant brain tumors. By using a magnetic field targeted to the region of interest, it has been shown that delivery of MNPs can be increased over the delivery to lesions when a magnetic field is not used.[119] There are concerns in how efficacious the translation of this technique will be to human studies, because the depth of the lesions in the human brain limit the ability to precisely target a lesion with a magnetic field.[118] Nevertheless, this remains an area for increased study.

In an effort to enhance the delivery and deposition of MNPs into malignant brain tumors, many studies have examined using strategies to open the BBB. Focal ultrasound represents a noninvasive technique, which can selectively disrupt the BBB and increase the enhanced permeability and retention effect in a targeted region of the brain.[120–122] Focal ultrasound and magnetic targeting have been used synergistically to enhance the delivery and the deposition of chemotherapy (epirubicin)-loaded MNPs into tumor-bearing animals. Epirubicin delivery and brain tumor accumulation was significantly enhanced by the combined focal ultrasound/magnetic targeting approach of epirubicin-MNPs.[123]

Convection-Enhanced Delivery

CED, where bulk flow is used to distribute infusate throughout the brain with a pressure gradient, is a well-established technique for delivery of molecules to the brain.[124] CED bypasses the BBB, allowing targeted delivery of infusate to the parenchyma of a region of interest through a catheter. A pump is connected to each infusion catheter to ensure a positive pressure gradient during delivery for convection of molecules through the interstitium of the brain. The pressure gradient created by the pump greatly augments the delivery that would be achieved by the use of simple diffusion alone.[125]

The size of nanoparticles makes them optimal to be delivered with CED. Penetration of nanoparticles through the extracellular matrix in the brain is possible due to the larger effective pore size of the extracellular matrix (50 nm).[126] CED of dextran-coated maghemite MNPs have recently been depicted by MRI in a normal rat brain model,[127] showing that these particles could be directly imaged and tracked. They also showed that increased viscosity of the infusate increased efficacy of delivery and reduced leak back.

Imaging the infusate in CED is critical for ensuring adequate drug delivery to regions of interest. Valuable feedback can be gained from tracking infusate delivered into the brain to enable clinicians to properly plan further treatments and avoid pitfalls, such as placement of catheters near sulci or ventricles.[128,129] Trials of conventional chemotherapeutics have failed to show significant benefit with CED, and lack of adequate drug delivery is often cited as the reason for this.[130] Although progress has been made using surrogate tracers, such as Gd-DTPA,[131] directly imaging the therapeutic particle would provide even more accurate information.

The authors have studied the CED of theranostic MNPS in mice (**Fig. 3**).[35] This particle consisted of an IONP core, coated by polymer and conjugated to an EGFR vIII antibody, specific for a subset of GBM tumors. The ability of the nanoparticles to localize to and image the lesion treated and its treatment effect were assessed. CED enabled a broad distribution of the nanoparticles in the region of the tumor and the surrounding brain, and repeat imaging showed that this effect remained for days after the nanoparticle delivery.

FUTURE STUDIES

Although researchers have made great strides in developing nanoparticles that address the difficulties in treating GBM, many challenges remain. In the use of MNPs for thermotherapy and magnetic targeting, clinical equipment needs to be further developed and improved[132] to make these cost effective and freely available for further clinical trials. Phase III studies need to be undertaken to prove their effectiveness. In addition, drug delivery remains an issue with nanoparticles, and as further targeting motifs are studied, delivery of these

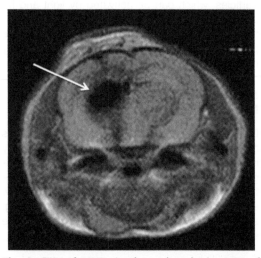

Fig. 3. CED of MNPs in the rodent brain. MRI of a rodent brain depicting the hypointense (*white arrow*) area in the brain that represents distribution of MNPs after CED with no leak back.

particles will be enhanced, further expanding their possible effectiveness.

SUMMARY

Nanotechnology has quickly become a promising tool in the ongoing research to tackle the difficulties in treating GBM. The authors expect translational research to continue to elucidate further uses for this technology as these various particles come into widespread clinical use.

REFERENCES

1. Brat DJ, Prayson RA, Ryken TC, et al. Diagnosis of malignant glioma: role of neuropathology. J Neurooncol 2008;89:287–311.
2. Stupp R, Mason WP, van den Bent MJ, et al. Radiotherapy plus concomitant and adjuvant temozolomide for glioblastoma. N Engl J Med 2005;352: 987–96.
3. Legler JM, Ries LA, Smith MA, et al. Cancer surveillance series [corrected]: brain and other central nervous system cancers: recent trends in incidence and mortality. J Natl Cancer Inst 1999;91:1382–90.
4. Brem H, Piantadosi S, Burger PC, et al. Placebo-controlled trial of safety and efficacy of intraoperative controlled delivery by biodegradable polymers of chemotherapy for recurrent gliomas. The Polymer-brain Tumor Treatment Group. Lancet 1995;345:1008–12.
5. Vredenburgh JJ, Desjardins A, Herndon JE 2nd, et al. Bevacizumab plus irinotecan in recurrent glioblastoma multiforme. J Clin Oncol 2007;25:4722–9.
6. Kelly PJ, Daumas-Duport C, Kispert DB, et al. Imaging-based stereotaxic serial biopsies in untreated intracranial glial neoplasms. J Neurosurg 1987;66:865–74.
7. Demuth T, Berens ME. Molecular mechanisms of glioma cell migration and invasion. J Neurooncol 2004;70:217–28.
8. Hayashi C, Ryozi U, Tasaki A. Ultra-fine particles: exploratory science and technology. Westwood (NJ): Noyes Publications; 1997. p. 2.
9. Maier-Hauff K, Ulrich F, Nestler D, et al. Efficacy and safety of intratumoral thermotherapy using magnetic iron-oxide nanoparticles combined with external beam radiotherapy on patients with recurrent glioblastoma multiforme. J Neurooncol 2011; 103(2):317–24.
10. Liu L, Venkatraman SS, Yang YY, et al. Polymeric micelles anchored with TAT for delivery of antibiotics across the blood-brain barrier. Biopolymers 2008;90:617–23.
11. Loo C, Lin A, Hirsch L, et al. Nanoshell-enabled photonics-based imaging and therapy of cancer. Technol Cancer Res Treat 2004;3:33–40.
12. Xing Y, Chaudry Q, Shen C, et al. Bioconjugated quantum dots for multiplexed and quantitative immunohistochemistry. Nat Protoc 2007;2:1152–65.
13. Provenzale JM, Silva GA. Uses of nanoparticles for central nervous system imaging and therapy. AJNR Am J Neuroradiol 2009;30:1293–301.
14. Jain TK, Richey J, Strand M, et al. Magnetic nanoparticles with dual functional properties: drug delivery and magnetic resonance imaging. Biomaterials 2008;29:4012–21.
15. Sun C, Lee JS, Zhang M. Magnetic nanoparticles in MR imaging and drug delivery. Adv Drug Deliv Rev 2008;60:1252–65.
16. Corot C, Robert P, Idee JM, et al. Recent advances in iron oxide nanocrystal technology for medical imaging. Adv Drug Deliv Rev 2006; 58:1471–504.
17. Lodhia J, Mandarano G, Ferris N, et al. Development and use of iron oxide nanoparticles (Part 1): synthesis of iron oxide nanoparticles for MRI. Biomed Imaging Interv J 2010;6:e12.
18. Thorek DL, Chen AK, Czupryna J, et al. Superparamagnetic iron oxide nanoparticle probes for molecular imaging. Ann Biomed Eng 2006;34:23–38.
19. Weissleder R, Elizondo G, Wittenberg J, et al. Ultrasmall superparamagnetic iron oxide: characterization of a new class of contrast agents for MR imaging. Radiology 1990;175:489–93.
20. Pan D, Caruthers SD, Hu G, et al. Ligand-directed nanobialys as theranostic agent for drug delivery and manganese-based magnetic resonance imaging of vascular targets. J Am Chem Soc 2008; 130:9186–7.
21. Na HB, Lee JH, An K, et al. Development of a T1 contrast agent for magnetic resonance imaging using MnO nanoparticles. Angew Chem Int Ed Engl 2007;46:5397–401.
22. Bridot JL, Faure AC, Laurent S, et al. Hybrid gadolinium oxide nanoparticles: multimodal contrast agents for in vivo imaging. J Am Chem Soc 2007; 129:5076–84.
23. Bourrinet P, Bengele HH, Bonnemain B, et al. Preclinical safety and pharmacokinetic profile of ferumoxtran-10, an ultrasmall superparamagnetic iron oxide magnetic resonance contrast agent. Invest Radiol 2006;41:313–24.
24. Aime S, Caravan P. Biodistribution of gadolinium-based contrast agents, including gadolinium deposition. J Magn Reson Imaging 2009;30:1259–67.
25. Abraham JL, Thakral C. Tissue distribution and kinetics of gadolinium and nephrogenic systemic fibrosis. Eur J Radiol 2008;66:200–7.
26. Varallyay P, Nesbit G, Muldoon LL, et al. Comparison of two superparamagnetic viral-sized iron oxide particles ferumoxides and ferumoxtran-10 with a gadolinium chelate in imaging intracranial tumors. AJNR Am J Neuroradiol 2002;23:510–9.

27. Neuwelt EA, Varallyay CG, Manninger S, et al. The potential of ferumoxytol nanoparticle magnetic resonance imaging, perfusion, and angiography in central nervous system malignancy: a pilot study. Neurosurgery 2007;60:601–11 [discussion: 611–2].

28. Neuwelt EA, Hamilton BE, Varallyay CG, et al. Ultra-small superparamagnetic iron oxides (USPIOs): a future alternative magnetic resonance (MR) contrast agent for patients at risk for nephrogenic systemic fibrosis (NSF)? Kidney Int 2009;75:465–74.

29. Moore A, Marecos E, Bogdanov A Jr, et al. Tumoral distribution of long-circulating dextran-coated iron oxide nanoparticles in a rodent model. Radiology 2000;214:568–74.

30. Zimmer C, Weissleder R, Poss K, et al. MR imaging of phagocytosis in experimental gliomas. Radiology 1995;197:533–8.

31. Villanueva A, Canete M, Roca AG, et al. The influence of surface functionalization on the enhanced internalization of magnetic nanoparticles in cancer cells. Nanotechnology 2009;20:115103.

32. Rhyner MN, Smith AM, Gao X, et al. Quantum dots and multifunctional nanoparticles: new contrast agents for tumor imaging. Nanomedicine (Lond) 2006;1:209–17.

33. Peng XH, Qian X, Mao H, et al. Targeted magnetic iron oxide nanoparticles for tumor imaging and therapy. Int J Nanomedicine 2008;3:311–21.

34. Remsen LG, McCormick CI, Roman-Goldstein S, et al. MR of carcinoma-specific monoclonal antibody conjugated to monocrystalline iron oxide nanoparticles: the potential for noninvasive diagnosis. AJNR Am J Neuroradiol 1996; 17:411–8.

35. Hadjipanayis CG, Machaidze R, Kaluzova M, et al. EGFRvIII antibody-conjugated iron oxide nanoparticles for magnetic resonance imaging-guided convection-enhanced delivery and targeted therapy of glioblastoma. Cancer Res 2010;70:6303–12.

36. Soroceanu L, Gillespie Y, Khazaeli MB, et al. Use of chlorotoxin for targeting of primary brain tumors. Cancer Res 1998;58:4871–9.

37. Lyons SA, O'Neal J, Sontheimer H. Chlorotoxin, a scorpion-derived peptide, specifically binds to gliomas and tumors of neuroectodermal origin. Glia 2002;39:162–73.

38. Deshane J, Garner CC, Sontheimer H. Chlorotoxin inhibits glioma cell invasion via matrix metalloproteinase-2. J Biol Chem 2003;278:4135–44.

39. Veiseh O, Gunn JW, Kievit FM, et al. Inhibition of tumor-cell invasion with chlorotoxin-bound superparamagnetic nanoparticles. Small 2009;5:256–64.

40. Veiseh O, Sun C, Fang C, et al. Specific targeting of brain tumors with an optical/magnetic resonance imaging nanoprobe across the blood-brain barrier. Cancer Res 2009;69:6200–7.

41. Veiseh O, Sun C, Gunn J, et al. Optical and MRI multifunctional nanoprobe for targeting gliomas. Nano Lett 2005;5:1003–8.

42. McFerrin MB, Sontheimer H. A role for ion channels in glioma cell invasion. Neuron Glia Biol 2006;2:39–49.

43. Christian S, Pilch J, Akerman ME, et al. Nucleolin expressed at the cell surface is a marker of endothelial cells in angiogenic blood vessels. J Cell Biol 2003;163:871–8.

44. Reddy GR, Bhojani MS, McConville P, et al. Vascular targeted nanoparticles for imaging and treatment of brain tumors. Clin Cancer Res 2006; 12:6677–86.

45. Tomanek B, Iqbal U, Blasiak B, et al. Evaluation of brain tumor vessels specific contrast agents for glioblastoma imaging. Neuro Oncol 2012;14:53–63.

46. Faucher L, Guay-Begin AA, Lagueux J, et al. Ultra-small gadolinium oxide nanoparticles to image brain cancer cells in vivo with MRI. Contrast Media Mol Imaging 2011;6:209–18.

47. Mowat P, Mignot A, Rima W, et al. In vitro radiosensitizing effects of ultrasmall gadolinium based particles on tumour cells. J Nanosci Nanotechnol 2011;11:7833–9.

48. Fillmore HL, Shultz MD, Henderson SC, et al. Conjugation of functionalized gadolinium metallofullerenes with IL-13 peptides for targeting and imaging glial tumors. Nanomedicine (Lond) 2011;6:449–58.

49. Leung K. TAMRA-IL-13-Conjugated functionalized gadolinium metallofullerene (Gd3N@C80(OH)-26(CH2CH2COOH)-16), Molecular Imaging and Contrast Agent Database (MICAD). Bethesda (MD): National Library of Medicine (US), NCBI; 2004–2009. Available at: http://micad.nih.gov. Accessed April 27, 2012.

50. Lu YJ, Wei KC, Ma CC, et al. Dual targeted delivery of doxorubicin to cancer cells using folate-conjugated magnetic multi-walled carbon nanotubes. Colloids Surf B Biointerfaces 2012;89:1–9.

51. Sanai N, Polley MY, McDermott MW, et al. An extent of resection threshold for newly diagnosed glioblastomas. J Neurosurg 2011;115:3–8.

52. Senft C, Franz K, Blasel S, et al. Influence of iMRI-guidance on the extent of resection and survival of patients with glioblastoma multiforme. Technol Cancer Res Treat 2010;9:339–46.

53. Mehdorn HM, Schwartz F, Dawirs S, et al. High-field iMRI in glioblastoma surgery: improvement of resection radicality and survival for the patient? Acta Neurochir Suppl 2011;109:103–6.

54. Willems PW, Taphoorn MJ, Burger H, et al. Effectiveness of neuronavigation in resecting solitary intracerebral contrast-enhancing tumors: a randomized controlled trial. J Neurosurg 2006;104:360–8.

55. Hadjipanayis CG, Jiang H, Roberts DW, et al. Current and future clinical applications for optical imaging of cancer: from intraoperative surgical

guidance to cancer screening. Semin Oncol 2011; 38:109–18.

56. Van Meir EG, Hadjipanayis CG, Norden AD, et al. Exciting new advances in neuro-oncology: the avenue to a cure for malignant glioma. CA Cancer J Clin 2010;60:166–93.

57. Moore GE, Peyton WT, French LA, et al. The clinical use of fluorescein in neurosurgery; the localization of brain tumors. J Neurosurg 1948;5:392–8.

58. Britz GW, Ghatan S, Spence AM, et al. Intracarotid RMP-7 enhanced indocyanine green staining of tumors in a rat glioma model. J Neurooncol 2002; 56:227–32.

59. Ozawa T, Britz GW, Kinder DH, et al. Bromophenol blue staining of tumors in a rat glioma model. Neurosurgery 2005;57:1041–7 [discussion: 1041–7].

60. Stummer W, Pichlmeier U, Meinel T, et al. Fluorescence-guided surgery with 5-aminolevulinic acid for resection of malignant glioma: a randomised controlled multicentre phase III trial. Lancet Oncol 2006;7:392–401.

61. Eljamel MS, Goodman C, Moseley H. ALA and Photofrin fluorescence-guided resection and repetitive PDT in glioblastoma multiforme: a single centre Phase III randomised controlled trial. Lasers Med Sci 2008;23:361–7.

62. Kircher MF, Mahmood U, King RS, et al. A multimodal nanoparticle for preoperative magnetic resonance imaging and intraoperative optical brain tumor delineation. Cancer Res 2003;63:8122–5.

63. Aboody KS, Brown A, Rainov NG, et al. Neural stem cells display extensive tropism for pathology in adult brain: evidence from intracranial gliomas. Proc Natl Acad Sci U S A 2000;97:12846–51.

64. Yang SY, Liu H, Zhang JN. Gene therapy of rat malignant gliomas using neural stem cells expressing IL-12. DNA Cell Biol 2004;23:381–9.

65. Benedetti S, Pirola B, Pollo B, et al. Gene therapy of experimental brain tumors using neural progenitor cells. Nat Med 2000;6:447–50.

66. Hamada H, Kobune M, Nakamura K, et al. Mesenchymal stem cells (MSC) as therapeutic cytoreagents for gene therapy. Cancer Sci 2005;96: 149–56.

67. Wu X, Hu J, Zhou L, et al. In vivo tracking of superparamagnetic iron oxide nanoparticle-labeled mesenchymal stem cell tropism to malignant gliomas using magnetic resonance imaging. Laboratory investigation. J Neurosurg 2008;108:320–9.

68. Tang C, Russell PJ, Martiniello-Wilks R, et al. Concise review: Nanoparticles and cellular carriers-allies in cancer imaging and cellular gene therapy? Stem Cells 2010;28:1686–702.

69. Arbab AS, Janic B, Knight RA, et al. Detection of migration of locally implanted AC133+ stem cells by cellular magnetic resonance imaging with histological findings. FASEB J 2008;22:3234–46.

70. Goldstein LS, Dewhirst MW, Repacholi M, et al. Summary, conclusions and recommendations: adverse temperature levels in the human body. Int J Hyperthermia 2003;19:373–84.

71. Hildebrandt B, Wust P, Ahlers O, et al. The cellular and molecular basis of hyperthermia. Crit Rev Oncol Hematol 2002;43:33–56.

72. Wust P, Hildebrandt B, Sreenivasa G, et al. Hyperthermia in combined treatment of cancer. Lancet Oncol 2002;3:487–97.

73. Suto R, Srivastava PK. A mechanism for the specific immunogenicity of heat-shock protein-chaperoned peptides. Science 1995;269:1585–8.

74. Santos-Marques MJ, Carvalho F, Sousa C, et al. Cytotoxicity and cell signalling induced by continuous mild hyperthermia in freshly isolated mouse hepatocytes. Toxicology 2006;224:210–8.

75. Vanpouille-Box C, Lacoeuille F, Belloche C, et al. Tumor eradication in rat glioma and bypass of immunosuppressive barriers using internal radiation with (188)Re-lipid nanocapsules. Biomaterials 2011;32:6781–90.

76. Hirsch LR, Gobin AM, Lowery AR, et al. Metal nanoshells. Ann Biomed Eng 2006;34:15–22.

77. Bernardi RJ, Lowery AR, Thompson PA, et al. Immunonanoshells for targeted photothermal ablation in medulloblastoma and glioma: an in vitro evaluation using human cell lines. J Neurooncol 2008;86: 165–72.

78. Baek SK, Makkouk AR, Krasieva T, et al. Photothermal treatment of glioma; an in vitro study of macrophage-mediated delivery of gold nanoshells. J Neurooncol 2011;104:439–48.

79. Hadjipanayis CG, Bonder MJ, Balakrishnan S, et al. Metallic iron nanoparticles for MRI contrast enhancement and local hyperthermia. Small 2008;4:1925–9.

80. Mehdaoui B, Meffre A, Carrey J, et al. Optimal size of nanoparticles for magnetic hyperthermia: a combined theoretical and experimental study. Adv Funct Mater 2011;21:4573–81.

81. Dennis CL, Jackson AJ, Borchers JA, et al. Nearly complete regression of tumors via collective behavior of magnetic nanoparticles in hyperthermia. Nanotechnology 2009;20:395103.

82. Lee JH, Jang JT, Choi JS, et al. Exchange-coupled magnetic nanoparticles for efficient heat induction. Nat Nanotechnol 2011;6:418–22.

83. Wijaya A, Brown KA, Alper JD, et al. Magnetic field heating study of Fe-doped Au nanoparticles. J Magn Magn Mater 2007;309:15–9.

84. Sharma R, Chen CJ. Newer nanoparticles in hyperthermia treatment and thermometry. J Nanopart Res 2009;11:671–89.

85. Pradhan P, Giri J, Samanta G, et al. Comparative evaluation of heating ability and biocompatibility of different ferrite-based magnetic fluids for

hyperthermia application. J Biomed Mater Res B Appl Biomater 2007;81:12–22.

86. Kim DH, Thai YT, Nikles DE, et al. Heating of aqueous dispersions containing MnFe(2)O(4) nanoparticles by radio-frequency magnetic field induction. IEEE Trans Magn 2009;45:64–70.

87. Kaman O, Pollert E, Veverka P, et al. Silica encapsulated manganese perovskite nanoparticles for magnetically induced hyperthermia without the risk of overheating. Nanotechnology 2009;20: 275610.

88. Atsarkin VA, Levkin LV, Posvyanskiy VS, et al. Solution to the bioheat equation for hyperthermia with La1-xAgyMnO3-nanoparticles: the effect of temperature autostabilization. Int J Hyperthermia 2009;25:240–7.

89. Bae S, Lee SW, Takemura Y, et al. Dependence of frequency and magnetic field on self-heating characteristics of NiFe2O4 nanoparticles for hyperthermia. IEEE Trans Magn 2006;42:3566–8.

90. Kim DH, Lee SH, Kim KN, et al. Temperature change of various ferrite particles with alternating magnetic field for hyperthermic application. J Magn Magn Mater 2005;293:320–7.

91. Kim DH, Lee SH, Kim KN, et al. In vitro and in vivo characterization of various ferrites for hyperthermia in cancer-treatment. In: Li P, Zhang K, Colwell CW Jr, editors. Bioceramics, vol. 17. (Key Engineering Materials) Switzerland: Trans Tech Publications; 2005. p. 827–30.

92. Huber DL. Synthesis, properties, and applications of iron nanoparticles. Small 2005;1:482–501.

93. Pradhan P, Giri J, Banerjee R, et al. Cellular interactions of lauric acid and dextran-coated magnetite nanoparticles. J Magn Magn Mater 2007;311:282–7.

94. Luis Corchero J, Villaverde A. Biomedical applications of distally controlled magnetic nanoparticles. Trends Biotechnol 2009;27:468–76.

95. Jordan A, Scholz R, Maier-Hauff K, et al. The effect of thermotherapy using magnetic nanoparticles on rat malignant glioma. J Neurooncol 2006;78:7–14.

96. Maier-Hauff K, Rothe R, Scholz R, et al. Intracranial thermotherapy using magnetic nanoparticles combined with external beam radiotherapy: results of a feasibility study on patients with glioblastoma multiforme. J Neurooncol 2007;81:53–60.

97. Jiang X, Xin H, Sha X, et al. PEGylated poly (trimethylene carbonate) nanoparticles loaded with paclitaxel for the treatment of advanced glioma: in vitro and in vivo evaluation. Int J Pharm 2011; 420:385–94.

98. Sawyer AJ, Saucier-Sawyer JK, Booth CJ, et al. Convection-enhanced delivery of camptothecin-loaded polymer nanoparticles for treatment of intracranial tumors. Drug Deliv Transl Res 2011;1:34–42.

99. Agarwal A, Mackey MA, El-Sayed MA, et al. Remote triggered release of doxorubicin in tumors by synergistic application of thermosensitive liposomes and gold nanorods. ACS Nano 2011;5: 4919–26.

100. Cancer Genome Atlas Research Network. Comprehensive genomic characterization defines human glioblastoma genes and core pathways. Nature 2008;455:1061–8.

101. Jin J, Bae KH, Yang H, et al. In vivo specific delivery of c-Met siRNA to glioblastoma using cationic solid lipid nanoparticles. Bioconjug Chem 2011;22:2568–72.

102. Zhan C, Meng Q, Li Q, et al. Cyclic RGD-polyethylene glycol-polyethylenimine for intracranial glioblastoma-targeted gene delivery. Chem Asian J 2012;7:91–6.

103. Shultz MD, Wilson JD, Fuller CE, et al. Metallofullerene-based nanoplatform for brain tumor brachytherapy and longitudinal imaging in a murine orthotopic xenograft model. Radiology 2011;261:136–43.

104. Nie S, Xing Y, Kim GJ, et al. Nanotechnology applications in cancer. Annu Rev Biomed Eng 2007;9: 257–88.

105. Peer D, Karp JM, Hong S, et al. Nanocarriers as an emerging platform for cancer therapy. Nat Nanotechnol 2007;2:751–60.

106. Gref R, Minamitake Y, Peracchia MT, et al. Biodegradable long-circulating polymeric nanospheres. Science 1994;263:1600–3.

107. van der Sanden BP, Rozijn TH, Rijken PF, et al. Noninvasive assessment of the functional neovasculature in 9L-glioma growing in rat brain by dynamic 1H magnetic resonance imaging of gadolinium uptake. J Cereb Blood Flow Metab 2000;20: 861–70.

108. Vajkoczy P, Menger MD. Vascular microenvironment in gliomas. J Neurooncol 2000;50:99–108.

109. Batchelor TT, Sorensen AG, di Tomaso E, et al. AZD2171, a pan-VEGF receptor tyrosine kinase inhibitor, normalizes tumor vasculature and alleviates edema in glioblastoma patients. Cancer Cell 2007;11:83–95.

110. Son YJ, Jang JS, Cho YW, et al. Biodistribution and anti-tumor efficacy of doxorubicin loaded glycol-chitosan nanoaggregates by EPR effect. J Control Release 2003;91:135–45.

111. Agemy L, Friedmann-Morvinski D, Kotamraju VR, et al. Targeted nanoparticle enhanced proapoptotic peptide as potential therapy for glioblastoma. Proc Natl Acad Sci U S A 2011;108:17450–5.

112. Li J, Gu B, Meng Q, et al. The use of myristic acid as a ligand of polyethylenimine/DNA nanoparticles for targeted gene therapy of glioblastoma. Nanotechnology 2011;22:435101.

113. Tahara K, Kato Y, Yamamoto H, et al. Intracellular drug delivery using polysorbate 80-modified poly(D, L-lactide-co-glycolide) nanospheres to glioblastoma cells. J Microencapsul 2011;28:29–36.

114. Gelperina S, Maksimenko O, Khalansky A, et al. Drug delivery to the brain using surfactant-coated poly(lactide-co-glycolide) nanoparticles: influence of the formulation parameters. Eur J Pharm Biopharm 2010;74:157–63.

115. Wohlfart S, Khalansky AS, Gelperina S, et al. Efficient chemotherapy of rat glioblastoma using doxorubicin-loaded PLGA nanoparticles with different stabilizers. PLoS One 2011;6:e19121.

116. Chang J, Paillard A, Passirani C, et al. Transferrin adsorption onto PLGA nanoparticles governs their interaction with biological systems from blood circulation to brain cancer cells. Pharm Res 2011; 29:1495–505.

117. Chertok B, Moffat BA, David AE, et al. Iron oxide nanoparticles as a drug delivery vehicle for MRI monitored magnetic targeting of brain tumors. Biomaterials 2008;29:487–96.

118. Chertok B, David AE, Huang Y, et al. Glioma selectivity of magnetically targeted nanoparticles: a role of abnormal tumor hydrodynamics. J Control Release 2007;122:315–23.

119. Pulfer SK, Ciccotto SL, Gallo JM. Distribution of small magnetic particles in brain tumor-bearing rats. J Neurooncol 1999;41:99–105.

120. Hynynen K, McDannold N, Vykhodtseva N, et al. Focal disruption of the blood-brain barrier due to 260-kHz ultrasound bursts: a method for molecular imaging and targeted drug delivery. J Neurosurg 2006;105:445–54.

121. Pardridge WM. Drug and gene delivery to the brain: the vascular route. Neuron 2002;36:555–8.

122. Muldoon LL, Soussain C, Jahnke K, et al. Chemotherapy delivery issues in central nervous system malignancy: a reality check. J Clin Oncol 2007; 25:2295–305.

123. Liu HL, Hua MY, Yang HW, et al. Magnetic resonance monitoring of focused ultrasound/magnetic nanoparticle targeting delivery of therapeutic agents to the brain. Proc Natl Acad Sci U S A 2010;107:15205–10.

124. Bobo RH, Laske DW, Akbasak A, et al. Convection-enhanced delivery of macromolecules in the brain. Proc Natl Acad Sci U S A 1994;91:2076–80.

125. Allard E, Passirani C, Benoit JP. Convection-enhanced delivery of nanocarriers for the treatment of brain tumors. Biomaterials 2009;30:2302–18.

126. Thorne RG, Nicholson C. In vivo diffusion analysis with quantum dots and dextrans predicts the width of brain extracellular space. Proc Natl Acad Sci U S A 2006;103:5567–72.

127. Perlstein B, Ram Z, Daniels D, et al. Convection-enhanced delivery of maghemite nanoparticles: increased efficacy and MRI monitoring. Neuro Oncol 2008;10:153–61.

128. Sampson JH, Brady ML, Petry NA, et al. Intracerebral infusate distribution by convection-enhanced delivery in humans with malignant gliomas: descriptive effects of target anatomy and catheter positioning. Neurosurgery 2007;60:ONS89–98 [discussion: ONS98–9].

129. Varenika V, Dickinson P, Bringas J, et al. Detection of infusate leakage in the brain using real-time imaging of convection-enhanced delivery. J Neurosurg 2008;109:874–80.

130. Sampson JH, Archer G, Pedain C, et al. Poor drug distribution as a possible explanation for the results of the PRECISE trial. J Neurosurg 2010;113:301–9.

131. Asthagiri AR, Walbridge S, Heiss JD, et al. Effect of concentration on the accuracy of convective imaging distribution of a gadolinium-based surrogate tracer. J Neurosurg 2011;115:467–73.

132. Silva AC, Oliveira TR, Mamani JB, et al. Application of hyperthermia induced by superparamagnetic iron oxide nanoparticles in glioma treatment. Int J Nanomedicine 2011;6:591–603.

Endogenous Vaults and Bioengineered Vault Nanoparticles for Treatment of Glioblastomas
Implications for Future Targeted Therapies

Jian Yang, PhD[a], Daniel T. Nagasawa, MD[b],
Marko Spasic, BA[b], Misha Amolis, BS[b], Winward Choy, BA[b],
Heather M. Garcia, BS[b], Robert M. Prins, PhD[b,c],
Linda M. Liau, MD, PhD[d], Isaac Yang, MD[b,c,*]

KEYWORDS

- Brain tumor • Immunotherapy • Nanoparticle • Targeted therapy • Vault

KEY POINTS

- Endogenous vaults are ribonucleoproteins expressed throughout various cell types and across numerous species.
- The vault has been hypothesized to play a role in cellular transport implicated in innate immunity, multidrug resistance, and intracellular signaling.
- Gangliogliomas, schwannomas, meningiomas, neurofibromas, astrocytomas, and gliomas have all been reported to exhibit high levels of major vault protein (MVP), which constitutes approximately 70% of the overall mass of endogenous vaults.
- In vitro culture of dendritic cells with antibodies against MVP demonstrates decreased dendritic cell functioning, particularly a reduction in their ability to induce antigen-specific T cell proliferation, indicating that MVP may play a critical role in dendritic cell activation and cellular immunity.
- Bioengineered vault nanoparticles seem to be ideally suited for use as nanocapsules in the delivery of various therapeutic agents and immunogenic proteins, representing a promising prospect for CNS tumor immunotherapy.

Daniel Nagasawa was supported by an American Brain Tumor Association Medical Student Summer Fellowship in Honor of Connie Finc. Isaac Yang (senior author) was partially supported by a Visionary Fund Grant, an Eli and Edythe Broad Center of Regenerative Medicine and Stem Cell Research UCLA Scholars in Translational Medicine Program Award, the Stein Oppenheimer Endowment Award, and the STOP CANCER Jason Dessel Memorial Seed Grant.

[a] Department of Biological Chemistry, David Geffen School of Medicine at University of California, Los Angeles, 310 BSRB, P.O. Box 951737, Los Angeles, CA 90095-1737, USA; [b] Department of Neurosurgery Surgery, University of California, Los Angeles, 695 Charles E Young Drive South, Gonda 3357, Los Angeles, CA 90095-1761, USA; [c] University of California Los Angeles Jonsson Comprehensive Cancer Center, 8-684 Factor Building, Box 951781, Los Angeles, CA 90095-1781, USA; [d] Department of Neurosurgery, UCLA Medical Center, 10833 Le Conte Avenue, CHS 74-145, Los Angeles, CA 90095-6901, USA
* Corresponding author. UCLA Department of Neurosurgery, UCLA Jonsson Comprehensive Cancer Center, University of California, Los Angeles, David Geffen School of Medicine at UCLA, 695 Charles East Young Drive South, UCLA Gonda 3357, Los Angeles, CA 90095-1761.
E-mail address: iyang@mednet.ucla.edu

Neurosurg Clin N Am 23 (2012) 451–458
doi:10.1016/j.nec.2012.04.012

INTRODUCTION

Endogenous vaults are the largest ribonucleoproteins expressed in numerous higher organism species and cell types. Their precise role and function, however, remain largely uncharacterized. The 4 major components of endogenous vaults are major vault protein (MVP), vault poly (ADP) ribose polymerase (vPARP), telomerase-associated protein (TEP1), and untranslated vault RNA (vRNA) molecules. MVP, also described as human lung resistance protein (LRP), has been investigated for its expression in numerous cancers and its possible role in chemoresistance. This article provides an overview of endogenous vaults and the work on bioengineered vault nanoparticles in order to better elucidate the potential role that these complexes may play in a targeted therapy for the central nervous system (CNS). It will focus, in particular, on primary human brain cancers such as malignant gliomas. Lastly, the authors hope to highlight the implications that current research holds in potentially utilizing bioengineered vault nanoparticles for future targeted therapies against human glioblastoma.

VAULT NANOPARTICLES: AN OVERVIEW

Vaults were first characterized by Kedersha and Rome in 1986.[1,2] By using a negative stain for electron microscopy (EM) rather than the positive-staining heavy metal salts that detect nucleic acid and membrane components, Kedersha and Rome were able to visualize the presence of protein-rich nanoparticles with a structural morphology similar to vaulted ceilings in cathedrals.[1,2] Vaults have since been characterized as barrel-like ribonucleoproteins with a mass of approximately 12.9 MDa and dimensions of 420 × 420 × 750 Å. This enormous size classifies vault nanoparticles as among the largest ribonucleoproteins (RNPs) ever characterized.[1,3-7]

The macrostructure of endogenous vaults have been investigated in order to elucidate key insights into their cellular function. The 4 main components of the vault nanoparticle are the structural 100 kDa MVP, the enzymatic 193 kDa ADPvPARP, the RNA-binding 240 kDa TEP1, and vRNA.[8-10] MVP and vRNAs constitute approximately 70% and 5% of the overall mass of endogenous vaults, respectively.[4,11] In each cell, there may be between 10,000 and 10,000,000 of these endogenous barrel-like complexes.[12,13] Vaults localize predominately to the cytoplasm of the cell, but they occasionally can be found in the nucleus, congregating around nucleoli, on the outside of the nuclear envelope, and at the nuclear pore complexes (NPCs), potentially mediating exchange across the nuclear membrane.[14-16] In the cellular cytoplasm, endogenous vaults can be associated with cytoskeletal elements such as actin stress fibers or microtubules.[14,17,18]

Kedersha and colleagues initially utilized quantitative scanning transmission EM to describe bioengineered vault nanoparticles as dimers, with each half resembling a barrel-like structure that consists of 8 rectangular petals that open into a flowerlike structure (**Fig. 1**). Each petal was hypothesized to consist of 6 molecules of MVP.[4] Cryo-EM and single-particle reconstruction indicate that the vault nanoparticle is a hollow, barrel-like structure with an approximate volume of 5×10^7 Å^3.[19] The protein shell of the vault has an invaginated waist with 2 caps protruding on either end of the vault.[6,19-22] Although some evidence has confirmed Kedersha's initial hypothesis of an 8-fold dihedral symmetry, more recent investigations suggest a potential 39-fold dihedral axis or 42-fold rotational symmetry.[20,23,24] In either instance, the bioengineered vault nanoparticle seems to consist of a barrel-like structure with 78 to 96 MVP molecules arranged pole-to-pole, and 39 to 48 copies of MVP forming each half-vault.[6,20,21] For endogenous vaults, each vault has been predicted to contain 1 or more copies of TEP1 and approximately 4 copies of VPARP; additionally, the vRNA also appears to localize to the ends of the vault caps, where it associates with TEP1.[6,10,25]

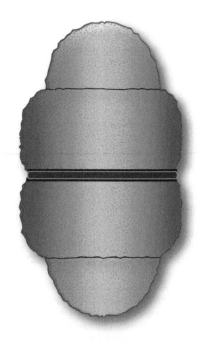

Fig. 1. A schematic rendering of the bioengineered vault nanoparticle, which may encapsulate a therapeutic agent or immunogenic antigen.

One of the most interesting findings of endogenous vault investigations has been their reported upregulation in certain types of cancers. For example, expression upregulation has been reported in breast tumors,[26,27] nonsmall cell lung cancer (NSCLC),[28–30] and other malignancies.[31–49] Several researchers have also reported upregulation of MVP in several brain tumors. Gangliogliomas, schwannomas, meningiomas, neurofibromas, astrocytomas, and gliomas have all been reported to exhibit high levels of the MVP protein.[50–54]

Functionally, the endogenous vault barrel-like structure has been hypothesized to have a possible role in the cellular transport implicated in innate immunity, multidrug resistance (MDR), and intracellular signaling.[55] Most recently, vaults have been studied as possible vectors for therapeutic delivery. Here, the authors will identify and discuss the endogenous vault components and highlight their expression in the CNS and CNS tumors. They will also discuss future implications for targeted therapeutics and the potential role of bioengineered vault nanoparticles for the induction of immune responses and their prospective utilization as a novel method of immunotherapy.

MVP: THE MVP SUBUNIT

The human MVP gene localizes to chromosome 16p11.2.[56–58] The MVP protein also structurally forms the outer shell of the bioengineered vault nanoparticle.[19] Several interesting structural domains have been described within MVP. First, the C-terminus of MVP contains a coiled-coil protein structure that is formed by a long α-helical domain.[59] This C-terminal appears to localize to the vault end cap, and it is hypothesized that these coiled-coil interactions allow MVP particles to interact with one another, providing a likely mechanism for how vaultlike complexes were demonstrated in vault-less Sf9 insect cells after ectopic rat MVP was expressed in these cells.[21,60] When the coiled-coil domain is partially deleted in a yeast 2-hybrid system, this interaction does not appear possible.[59] Secondly, the N terminus of MVP consists of 7 repeats of approximately 55 amino acids. This terminus localizes to the vault's equator, where it forms the sidewalls via noncovalent interactions between particle halves. In addition, part of the N terminus also protrudes interiorly from this equator waistline.[6,20,21,61]

MVP, the major component of bioengineered vault nanoparticles, has also been implicated in innate immunity. While dendritic cell function is still normal in mice that lack MVP,[62] in vitro culture of dendritic cells with antibodies against MVP demonstrate decreased dendritic cell functioning, particularly a reduction in their ability to induce antigen-specific T-cell proliferation.[63] These findings suggest that MVP may play a critical role in innate immunity and dendritic cell activation, providing a key component for the utilization of vault nanoparticles for an immunotherapeutic approach.

vPARP: THE vPARP SUBUNIT

The vPARP gene, located on chromosome 13q11, encodes a protein with 1724 amino acids.[9,64] The enzymatically active PARP domain was first described after an experiment demonstrated that vPARP is able to catalyze the ADP ribosylation of both itself and MVP.[9] ADP ribosylation is most often associated with a post-translational modification of histones and other nuclear proteins that occur principally in response to DNA damage by PARP1. Enzymes with a PARP domain are able to transfer ADP-ribose groups to aspartic and glutamic residues. These altered substrates interact differently with DNA, creating a delay in DNA replication that gives cells enough time to recruit repair enzymes to the site of the DNA damage.[65–67] At least 7 proteins with PARP activity have been described, with PARP1 being the best characterized in this family. These family members, however, are not homologous outside of their catalytic domains.[68,69]

The archetypal PARP1 binds to single- or double-strand DNA breaks in the nucleus and appears to play a role in the base excision pathway.[68,70] Interestingly, vPARP shares a 28% sequence homology with PARP1 but does not appear to be activated in response to DNA damage.[9] This is further suggested by experiments with knockout mice in which a (-/-) vPARP genotype demonstrated neither chromosomal instability nor endogenous vault disturbances.[71] However, a significant increase in carcinogen-induced tumors has been reported in vPARP-deficient mice and may indicate a potential pathway for vPARP in chemically-induced neoplasia.[72]

TEP1: THE TEP1 SUBUNIT

TEP1, the other endogenous vault associated protein, was found to be identical to the previously described mammalian telomerase-associated component TEP1.[10,73] The human TEP1 gene maps to chromosome 14q11.2. The TEP1 protein is comprised of 2629 amino acids and contains a number of interesting domains: an amino–terminal repeat domain, an RNA binding domain, and an adenosine triphosphate (ATP)/guanosine triphosphate binding domain.[73,74] The repeats at the N terminus do not have a known function, but have been hypothesized to serve as binding sites for vPARP.[6] The RNA binding domain appears to be necessary for interaction with both vRNA and telomerase RNA.[75–77]

Endogenous vaults have been isolated from TEP1 knockout mice that appear normal; however, closer examination by 3-dimensional reconstruction demonstrates reduced density in the vault cap, where TEP1 appears to localize. Furthermore, the stable association between vRNA and the vault complex is completely disrupted in these knockouts. Both the half-life of vRNA and its expression in these tissues decrease. Thus, it appears that TEP1 seems to play a key role in vRNA stability and its binding to the vault complex.[25]

UNTRANSLATED RNA

The human vRNA genes are a triple-repeat structure on chromosome 5q33.1.[8,10,12,25,78,79] The vRNAs are transcribed by RNA polymerase 3,[80] but their expression in each cell seems to differ by organ. Data from northern analysis suggests that one of the lowest levels of vRNA expression occurs in the brain.[8]

Concentrated at the ends of vault caps, vRNAs appear to interact with structural endogenous vault proteins, but it does not appear that they are required to maintain the structural integrity of the bioengineered vault nanoparticle. vRNA loss by ribonuclease digestion fails to cause any detectable conformational change of the bioengineered vault nanoparticle complex. This suggests that vRNAs do not play a critical structural role in bioengineering of vault nanoparticles.[4,6,81]

VAULTS AND THE CNS

While endogenous vaults are present in all cell types, they appear to be differentially expressed depending on the cell of origin. The highest levels of MVP/LRP are found in macrophages, keratinocytes, kidney tubules, and epithelial cells of the bronchus and digestive tract.[13,50,64,82] Brain tissue, however, appears to only have low levels of MVP/LRP.[50,52,53] In rat brains, the highest expression of MVP is found in microglia during embryonic development, but in the adult animal, MVP is evident in the amoeboid microglia and choroid plexus. The motile character of these structures may explain their association with endogenous vaults, given the potential of endogenous vaults to interact with cytoskeletal elements.[18,83]

Upregulation of MVP/LRP, however, has been reported in a wide range of brain tumors.[50–54,84]

Conversely, medulloblastomas and neuroblastomas have been reported to demonstrate low levels of MVP.[51] Increased levels of MVP/LRP have also been found in tumor vessels, in dorsal root ganglion tissue after nerve ligation, and in macrophages after brain infarction or acute contusion injury.[52,53,85] Berger and colleagues, utilizing both mRNA and protein assays, have reported high levels of MVP in astrocytomas, meningiomas, and gliomas. With cytotoxicity analysis of astrocytomas, this study also reported that MVP expression was significantly correlated with resistance to adriamycin, daunomycin, etoposide, and cisplatin.[51]

To further characterize the expression of MVP in primary tumors of the CNS, Sasaki and colleagues performed immunohistochemistry on 69 archival CNS tumors and demonstrated that 56 of the samples (81.2%) expressed LRP. Specifically, the protein was found in specimens of neurofibroma, schwannoma, meningioma, oligoastrocytoma, ependymoma, oligodendroglioma, and astrocytoma. Interestingly, neither tumor grade nor invasion appeared to be correlated with the presence of MVP.[84,86]

Focusing on primary and secondary glioblastomas, Tews and colleagues reported consistent upregulation of MVP. Moreover, 78% of World Health Organization (WHO) grade II precursor astrocytomas and all WHO grade III tumors exhibited MVP expression. Because none of these tissues had been subjected to previous chemotherapy, increased MVP expression was likely due to the inherent upregulated expression of MVP in glioma cells, which differs from the low levels of MVP in normal glial cells.[52]

POTENTIAL USES FOR FUTURE THERAPIES

Due to the large internal volume and simple structure of bioengineered vault nanoparticles, they seem to be ideally suited for use as nanocapsules for delivery of therapeutic agents. Several successful encapsulations have been described. In 2005, Kickhoefer and colleagues were able to engineer a vault nanoparticle complex that sequestered 2 proteins and remained viable in living cells.[61] Goldsmith and colleagues were able to demonstrate the capability to load the vault nanoparticle interior,[87] while Ng and colleagues were also able to effectively use the bioengineered vault cage to enclose a semiconducting polymer.[88]

To analyze their potential therapeutic potential, Esfandiary and colleagues investigated the bioengineered vault nanoparticle structural changes in response to various pH and temperature conditions. This analysis found that bioengineered vault nanoparticles remained the most stable below

40°C and that the flowerlike petal structures open at an acidic pH. This opening could serve as a potential mechanism to release therapeutic contents from inside the bioengineered vault nanoparticle.[89] Investigating a different potential mechanism of delivery, Lai and colleagues incorporated the membrane lytic domain of adenovirus protein VI (pVI) into vault interiors, where its activity was maintained. After being ingested by murine macrophages, these novel bioengineered vault nanoparticle complexes aided in the delivery of a soluble ribotoxin and a cDNA plasmid.[90]

Recently, Kickhoefer and colleagues have constructed vault nanoparticles to specifically target the epidermal growth factor receptor (EGFR) by tagging the C terminus of MVP with wither epidermal growth factor or a monoclonal antibody to EGFR.[91] Champion and colleagues recently engineered vault nanoparticles to deliver the major outer membrane protein of *Chlamydia muridarum*. In mice, the application of these bioengineered vault nanoparticles induced mucosal immunity without inducing harmful inflammation. This novel vaccine, utilizing bioengineered vault nanoparticles delivered intranasally, represents a significant advance in the ability to induce an effective cellular immune response utilizing vault nanoparticles.[92]

SUMMARY

Further studies are needed to elucidate the mechanisms of endogenous vault function and gene expression. These advances may enable the development of targeted therapies that may prevent cancer cells from acquiring MVP-related drug resistance. The use of bioengineered vault nanoparticles as delivery vectors for therapeutic agents and immunogenic proteins may be a promising utilization for vault nanoparticles as a potential method of brain tumor therapy.

ACKNOWLEDGMENTS

The authors would like to thank Dr Nancy Huh for the work on **Fig. 1**, and Dr Valerie Kickhoefer and Dr Leonard Rome for their assistance with the manuscript. Marko Spasic was partially supported by an American Association of Neurological Surgeons Fellowship. Daniel Nagasawa was supported by an American Brain Tumor Association Medical Student Summer Fellowship in Honor of Connie Finc. Isaac Yang (senior author) was partially supported by a Visionary Fund Grant, an Eli and Edythe Broad Center of Regenerative Medicine and Stem Cell Research UCLA Scholars in Translational Medicine Program Award, the Stein Oppenheimer Endowment Award and the STOP CANCER Jason Dessel Memorial Seed Grant.

REFERENCES

1. Kedersha N, Rome L. Isolation and characterization of a novel ribonucleoprotein particle: large structures contain a single species of small RNA. J Cell Biol 1986;103:699–709.
2. Rome L, Kedersha N, Chugani D. Unlocking vaults: organelles in search of function. Trends Cell Biol 1991;1:47–50.
3. Kedersha N, Miquel M, Bittner D, et al. Vaults. II. Ribonucleoprotein structures are highly conserved among higher and lower eukaryotes. J Cell Biol 1990;110:895–901.
4. Kedersha N, Heuser J, Chugani D, et al. Vaults. III. Vault ribonucleoprotein particles open into flowerlike structures with octagonal symmetry. J Cell Biol 1991;112:225–35.
5. Batey R, Rambo R, Lucast L, et al. Crystal structure of the ribonucleoprotein core of the signal recognition particle. Science 2000;287:1232–9.
6. Kong L, Siva A, Kickhoefer V, et al. RNA location and modeling of a WD40 repeat domain within the vault. RNA 2000;6:890–900.
7. Suprenant K. Vault ribonucleoprotein particles: sarcophagi, gondolas, or safety deposit boxes? Biochemistry 2002;41:14447–54.
8. Kickhoefer V, Seales R, Kedersha N, et al. Vault ribonucleoprotein particles from rat and bullfrog contain a related small RNA that is transcribed by RNA polymerase III. J Biol Chem 1993;268:7868–73.
9. Kickhoefer V, Siva A, Kedersha N, et al. The 193-kD vault protein, VPARP, is a novel poly(ADP-ribose) polymerase. J Cell Biol 1999;146:917–28.
10. Kickhoefer V, Stephen A, Harrington L, et al. Vaults and telomerase share a common subunit, TEP1. J Biol Chem 1999;274:32712–7.
11. Kickhoefer V, Poderycki M, Chan E, et al. The La RNA-binding protein interacts with the vault RNA and is a vault-associated Protein. J Biol Chem 2002;277:41282–6.
12. Kickhoefer V, Rajavel K, Scheffer G, et al. Vaults are up-regulated in multidrug-resistant cancer cell lines. J Biol Chem 1998;273:8971–4.
13. Hamill D, Suprenant K. Characterization of the sea urchin major vault protein: a possible role for vault ribonucleoprotein particles in nucleocytoplasmic transport. Dev Biol 1997;190:117–28.
14. Chugani D, Rome L, Kedersha N. Evidence that vault ribonucleoprotein particles localize to the nuclear pore complex. J Cell Sci 1993;106:23–9.
15. Rout M, Wente S. Pores for thought: nuclear pore complex proteins. Trends Cell Biol 1994;4:357–65.

16. Vollmar F, Hacker C, Zahedi R, et al. Assembly of nuclear pore complexes mediated by major vault protein. J Cell Sci 2009;122:780–6.

17. Kedersha N, Rome L. Vaults: large cytoplasmic RNPs that associate with cytoskeletal elements. Mol Biol Rep 1990;14:121–2.

18. Herrmann C, Golkaramnay E, Inman E, et al. Recombinant major vault protein is targeted to neuritic tips of PC12 cells. J Cell Biol 1999;144:1163–72.

19. Kong L, Siva A, Rome L, et al. Structure of the vault, a ubiquitous cellular component. Structure 1999;7: 371–9.

20. Mikyas Y, Makabi M, Raval-Fernandes S, et al. Cryoelectron microscopy imaging of recombinant and tissue derived vaults: localization of the MVP N termini and VPARP. J Mol Biol 2004;344: 91–105.

21. Kozlov G, Vavelyuk O, Minailiuc O, et al. Solution structure of a two-repeat fragment of major vault protein. J Mol Biol 2006;356:444–52.

22. Anderson D, Kickhoefer V, Sievers S, et al. Draft crystal structure of the vault shell at 9-Å resolution. PLoS Biol 2007;5:2661–70.

23. Kato K, Tanaka H, Sumizawa T, et al. A vault ribonucleoprotein particle exhibiting 39-fold dihedral symmetry. Acta Crystallogr D Biol Crystallogr 2008; 64:525–31.

24. Tanaka H, Kato K, Yamashita E, et al. The structure of rat liver vault at 3.5 vault angstrom resolution. Science 2009;323:384–8.

25. Kickhoefer V, Liu Y, Kong L, et al. The telomerase/vault-associated protein TEP1 is required for vault RNA stability and its association with the vault particle. J Cell Biol 2001;152:157–64.

26. Beck J, Bohnet B, Brugger D, et al. Multiple gene expression analysis reveals distinct differences between G2 and G3 stage breast cancers, and correlations of PKC eta with MDR1, MRP and LRP gene expression. Br J Cancer 1998;77:87–91.

27. Burger H, Foekens J, Look M, et al. RNA expression of breast cancer resistance protein, lung resistance-related protein, multidrug resistance-associated proteins 1 and 2, and multidrug resistance gene 1 in breast cancer: correlation with chemotherapeutic response. Clin Cancer Res 2003;9:827–36.

28. Bouhamyia L, Chantot-Bastaraud S, Zaidi S, et al. Immunolocalization and cell expression of lung resistance-related protein (LRP) in normal and tumoral human respiratory cells. J Histochem Cytochem 2007;55:773–82.

29. Dingemans A, van Ark-Otte J, van der Valk P, et al. Expression of the human major vault protein LRP in human lung cancer samples and normal lung tissues. Ann Oncol 1996;7:625–30.

30. Volm M, Koomagi R, Mattern J, et al. Protein expression profiles indicative for drug resistance of nonsmall cell lung cancer. Br J Cancer 2002; 87:251–7.

31. Damiani D, Michieli M, Ermacora A, et al. P-glycoprotein (PGP), and not lung resistance-related protein (LRP), is a negative prognostic factor in secondary leukemias. Haematologica 1998;83:290–7.

32. de Figueiredo-Pontes L, Pintão M, Oliveira L, et al. Determination of P-glycoprotein, MDR-related protein 1, breast cancer resistance protein, and lung-resistance protein expression in leukemic stem cells of acute myeloid leukemia. Cytometry B Clin Cytom 2008;74:163–8.

33. Huh H, Park C, Jang S, et al. Prognostic significance of multidrug resistance gene 1 (MDR1), multidrug resistance-related protein (MRP) and lung resistance protein (LRP) mRNA expression in acute leukemia. J Korean Med Sci 2006;21:253–8.

34. Valera E, Scrideli C, de Paula Queiroz R, et al. Multiple drug resistance protein (MDR-1), multidrug resistance-related protein (MRP) and lung resistance protein (LRP) gene expression in childhood acute lymphoblastic leukemia. Sao Paulo Med J 2004;122:166–71.

35. Ohno N, Tani A, Uozumi K, et al. Expression of functional lung resistance–related protein predicts poor outcome in adult T-cell leukemia. Blood 2001;98: 1160–5.

36. Filipits M, Drach J, Pohl G, et al. Expression of the lung resistance protein predicts poor outcome in patients with multiple myeloma. Clin Cancer Res 1999;5:2426–30.

37. Filipits M, Jaeger U, Simonitsch I, et al. Clinical relevance of the lung resistance protein in diffuse large B-cell lymphomas. Clin Cancer Res 2000;6:3417–23.

38. Hodorova I, Rybarova S, Solar P, et al. Multidrug resistance proteins in renal cell carcinoma. Folia Biol 2008;54:187–92.

39. Huang W, Huang C, Weng S, et al. Expression of the multidrug resistance protein MRP and the lung-resistance protein LRP in nasal NK/T cell lymphoma: further exploring the role of P53 and WT1 gene. Pathology 2009;41:127–32.

40. Zurita A, Diestra J, Condom E, et al. Lung resistance-related protein as a predictor of clinical outcome in advanced testicular germ-cell tumours. Cancer Res 2003;88:879–86.

41. Komdeur R, Klunder J, van der Graaf W, et al. Multidrug resistance proteins in rhabdomyosarcomas: comparison between children and adults. Cancer 2003;97:1999–2005.

42. Krishnakumar S, Mallikarjuna K, Desai N, et al. Multidrug resistant proteins: P-glycoprotein and lung resistance protein expression in retinoblastoma. Br J Opthalmol 2004;88:1521–6.

43. Uozaki H, Horiuchi H, Ishida T, et al. Overexpression of resistance-related proteins (metallothioneins, glutathione-S-transferase, heat shock protein 27,

and lung resistance-related protein) in osteosarcoma. Cancer 2000;79:2336–44.

44. Singhal S, Wiewrodt R, Malden L, et al. Gene expression profiling of malignant mesothelioma. Clin Cancer Res 2003;9:3080–97.

45. Schadendorf D, Makki A, Stahr C, et al. Membrane transport proteins associated with drug resistance expressed in human melanoma. Am J Pathol 1995; 147:1545–52.

46. Lara P, Lloret M, Clavo B, et al. Severe hypoxia induces chemo-resistance in clinical cervical tumors through MVP over-expression. Radiat Oncol 2009;4:29.

47. Raidl M, Berger W, Schulte-Hermann R, et al. Expression of the lung resistance-related protein in human and rat hepatocarcinogenesis. Am J Physiol Gastrointest Liver Physiol 2002;283:G1117–24.

48. van der Pol J, Blom D, Fiens M, et al. Multidrug resistance-related proteins in primary choroidal melanomas and in vitro cell lines. Invest Ophthalmol Vis Sci 1997;38:2523–30.

49. Meijer G, Schroeijers A, Flens M, et al. Increased expression of multidrug resistance related proteins Pgp, MRP1, and LRP/MVP occurs early in colorectal carcinogenesis. J Clin Pathol 1999;52:450–4.

50. Izquierdo M, Scheffer G, Flens M, et al. Broad distribution of the multidrug resistance-related vault lung resistance protein in normal human tissues and tumors. Am J Pathol 1996;148:877–87.

51. Berger W, Spiegl-Kreinecker S, Buchroithner J, et al. Overexpression of the human major vault protein in astrocytic brain tumor cells. Int J Cancer 2001;94:377–82.

52. Tews D, Nissen A, Kulgen C, et al. Drug resistance-associated factors in primary and secondary glioblastomas and their precursor tumors. J Neurooncol 2000;50:227–37.

53. Aronica E, Gorter J, van Vliet E, et al. Overexpression of the human major vault protein in gangliogliomas. Epilepsia 2003;44:1166–75.

54. Slesina M, Inman E, Rome L, et al. Nuclear localization of the major vault protein in U373 cells. Cell Tissue Res 2005;321:97–104.

55. Vasu S, Rome L. Dictyostelium vaults: disruption of the major proteins reveals growth and morphological defects and uncovers a new associated protein. J Biol Chem 1995;270:16588–94.

56. Kickhoefer V, Vasu S, Rome L. Vaults are the answer, what is the question? Trends Cell Biol 1999;6:174–8.

57. Scheffer G, Wingaard P, Flens M, et al. The drug resistance-related protein LRP is the human major vault protein. Nat Med 1995;1:578–82.

58. Slovak M, Ho J, Cole S, et al. The LRP gene encoding a major vault protein associated with drug resistance maps proximal to MRP on chromosome 16: evidence that chromosome breakage plays a key role in MRP or LRP gene amplification. Cancer Res 1995;55:4214–9.

59. van Zon A, Mossink M, Schoester M, et al. Structural domains of vault proteins: a role for the coiled coil domain in vault assembly. Biochem Biophys Res Commun 2002;291:535–41.

60. Stephen A, Raval-Fernandes S, Huynh T, et al. Assembly of vault-like particles in insect cells expressing only the major vault protein. J Biol Chem 2001;276:23217–20.

61. Kickhoefer V, Garcia Y, Mikyas Y, et al. Engineering of vault nanocapsules with enzymatic and fluorescent properties. Proc Natl Acad Sci U S A 2005;102:4348–52.

62. Mossink M, de Groot J, van Zon A, et al. Unimpaired dendritic cell functions in MVP/LRP knockout mice. Immunology 2003;110:58–65.

63. Schroeijers A, Reurs A, Scheffer G, et al. Up-regulation of drug resistance-related vaults during dendritic cell development. J Immunol 2002;168:1572–8.

64. Still I, Vince P, Cowell J. Identification of a novel gene (ADPRTL1) encoding a potential Poly(ADP-ribosyl) transferase protein. Genomics 1999;62:533–6.

65. Schreiber V, Dantzer F, Ame J, et al. Poly(ADP-ribose): novel functions for an old molecule. Nat Rev Mol Cell Biol 2006;7:517–28.

66. de Murcia G, Menissier de Murcia J. Poly(ADP-ribose) polymerase: a molecular nick-sensor. Trends Biochem Sci 1994;19:172–6.

67. D'Amours D, Desnoyers S, D'Silva I, et al. Poly(ADP-ribosyl)ation reactions in the regulation of nuclear functions. Biochem J 1999;342:249–68.

68. Smith S. The world according to PARP. Trends Biochem Sci 2001;26:174–9.

69. Shall S. Poly (ADP-ribosylation)—a common control process? Bioessays 2002;24:197–201.

70. Oliver F, Menissier de Murcia J, de Murcia G. Poly (ADP-ribose) polymerase in the cellular response to DNA damage, apoptosis, and disease. Am J Hum Genet 1999;64:1282–8.

71. Liu Y, Snow B, Kickhoefer V, et al. Vault poly(ADP-ribose) polymerase is associated with mammalian telomerase and is dispensable for telomerase function and vault structure in vivo. Mol Cell Biol 2004;24: 5314–23.

72. Raval-Fernandes S, Kickhoefer V, Kitchen C, et al. Increased susceptibility of vault poly (ADP-ribose) polymerase-deficient mice to carcinogen-induced tumorigenesis. Cancer Res 2005;65:8846–52.

73. Harrington L, McPhail T, Mar V, et al. A mammalian telomerase-associated protein. Science 1997;275: 973–7.

74. Nakayama J, Saito M, Nakamura H, et al. TLP1: a gene encoding a protein component of mammalian telomerase is a novel member of WD repeats family. Cell 1997;88:875–84.

75. Berger W, Steiner E, Grusch M, et al. Vaults and the major vault protein: novel roles in signal pathway regulation and immunity. Cell Mol Life Sci 2009;66:43–61.

76. Bateman A, Kickhoefer V. The TROVE module: a common element in telomerase, ro and vault ribonucleoproteins. BMC Bioinformatics 2003;4:49.

77. Poderycki M, Rome L, Harrington L, et al. The p80 homology region of TEP1 is sufficient for its association with the telomerase and vault RNAs, and the vault particle. Nucleic Acids Res 2005;33: 893–902.

78. van Zon A, Mossink M, Schoester M, et al. Multiple human vault RNAs: expression and association with the vault complex. J Biol Chem 2001;276: 37715–21.

79. Vilalta A, Kickhoefer V, Rome L, et al. The rat vault RNA gene contains a unique RNA polymerase III promoter composed of both external and internal elements that function syngergistically. J Biol Chem 1994;269:29752–9.

80. Stadler P, Chen J, Hackermüller J, et al. Evolution of vault RNAs. Mol Biol Evol 2009;26:1975–91.

81. Liu Y, Snow B, Hande M, et al. Telomerase-associated protein TEP1 is not essential for telomerase activity or telomere length maintenance in vivo. Mol Cell Biol 2000;20:8178–84.

82. Scheffer G, Pijenborg A, Smit E, et al. Multidrug resistance related molecules in human and murine lung. J Clin Pathol 2002;55:332–9.

83. Chugani D, Kedersha N, Rome L. Vault immunofluorescence in the brain: new insights regarding the origin of microglia. J Neurosci 1991;11:256–68.

84. Sasaki T, Hankins G, Helm G. Major vault protein/lung resistance-related protein (MVP/LRP) expression in nervous system tumors. Brain Tumor Pathol 2002; 19:59–62.

85. Komori N, Takemori N, Kim H, et al. Proteomics study of neuropathic and nonneuropathic dorsal root ganglia: altered protein regulation following segmental spinal nerve ligation injury. Physiol Genomics 2007;29:215–30.

86. Andersson U, Malmer B, Bergenheim A, et al. Heterogeneity in the expression of markers for drug resistance in brain tumors. Clin Neuropathol 2004;23:21–7.

87. Goldsmith L, Pupols M, Kickhoefer V, et al. Utilization of a protein "shuttle" to load vault nanocapsules with gold probes and proteins. ACS Nano 2009;3: 3175–83.

88. Ng B, Yu M, Gopal A, et al. Encapsulation of semiconducting polymers in vault protein cages. Nano Lett 2008;8:3503–9.

89. Esfandiary R, Kickhoefer V, Rome L, et al. Structural stability of vault particles. J Pharm Sci 2009;98: 1376–86.

90. Lai C, Wiethoffs C, Kickhoefer V, et al. Vault nanoparticles containing an adenovirus-derived membrane lytic protein facilitate toxin and gene transfer. ACS Nano 2009;3:691–9.

91. Kickhoefer V, Han M, Raval-Fernandes S, et al. Targeting vault nanoparticles to specific cell surface receptors. ACS Nano 2009;3:27–36.

92. Champion C, Kickhoefer V, Liu G, et al. A vault nanoparticle vaccine induces protective mucosal immunity. PLoS One 2009;4:e5409.

Clinical Trials with Immunotherapy for High-Grade Glioma

Jacob Ruzevick, BS, Christopher Jackson, BA, Jillian Phallen, BA, Michael Lim, MD*

KEYWORDS

- High-grade gliomas • Immunotherapy • Clinical trials • Vaccines

KEY POINTS

- Current strategies for immunotherapy against high-grade glioma include adoptive immunotherapy, active immunotherapy, and immunomodulation.
- Early clinical trials suggest that immunotherapy is safe and beneficial in a subset of patients.
- Major biologic challenges that must be overcome for immunotherapy to succeed include immune-editing, decreased antigen presentation by glioma cells, and decreased immune cell activation.
- The difficulty in predicting the success of immunotherapy trials as well as comparing the results across studies is the heterogeneous nature of immunotherapy trial design and reporting.

INTRODUCTION

High-grade gliomas (HGGs, World Health Organization [WHO] grade III and IV) make up most primary brain tumor diagnoses, with an incidence currently estimated at 14,000 new diagnoses per year.[1] These tumors are associated with high morbidity and mortality and a median survival of 2 to 5 years[2,3] for patients with anaplastic astrocytomas (WHO grade III) and 14.6 months[4] for patients with glioblastoma multiforme (GBM, WHO grade IV).

The current standard of care for patients with HGGs is summarized in **Table 1**, and includes maximal surgical resection followed by adjuvant chemotherapy and radiation therapy. In patients with anaplastic astrocytoma, a clear standard of care is lacking. The current treatment strategy typically includes maximal surgical resection in combination with adjuvant radiation with or without temozolomide (TMZ).[4–10] Advances in imaging, neuronavigation, and fluoroscopic guidance[11] have improved safety, decreased deficits associated with surgery, and allowed for more complete tumor resection, with more accurate surgical margins. Furthermore, medical treatment is often required to treat tumor-associated signs and symptoms, including seizures, edema, fatigue, and cognitive dysfunction.[12] These treatments carry their own set of side effects, which must be managed alongside side effects from radiation and chemotherapy.

Despite advances in surgical and medical management of HGGs, there is no current treatment that specifically targets tumor cells and spares normal brain parenchyma. Recently, immunotherapy has emerged as a promising treatment strategy against intracranial tumors. Although the brain has historically been considered immune-privileged, more recent evidence suggests that the immune system is capable of effecting vigorous responses in the central nervous system (CNS). Microglia are considered the first line of defense in the brain and possess the ability to phagocytose foreign cellular material and synthesize proinflammatory cytokines and chemokines.[13] Several

Department of Neurological Surgery, The Johns Hopkins University School of Medicine, Baltimore, MD, USA
* Corresponding author. Department of Neurosurgery, The Johns Hopkins University School of Medicine, Phipps 123, 600 North Wolfe Street, Baltimore, MD 21287.
E-mail address: mlim3@jhmi.edu

Neurosurg Clin N Am 23 (2012) 459–470
doi:10.1016/j.nec.2012.04.003
1042-3680/12/$ – see front matter © 2012 Elsevier Inc. All rights reserved.

Table 1	
Summary of standard treatments for HGGs	
Tumor	**Treatment Paradigm**
Anaplastic astrocytoma (WHO grade III)	Maximal surgical resection with the option of adjuvant radiation, TMZ, or combination radiation and TMZ
GBM (WHO grade IV)	Maximal surgical resection with adjuvant radiation therapy and TMZ or Gliadel (Eisai Inc, NC, USA) (implanted carmustine wafers)
Recurrent primary brain tumor	Resection of recurrent lesion, with adjuvant Gliadel placement, chemotherapy, or experimental treatments

groups have shown that lymphocytes and antigen-presenting cells (APCs), including macrophages and dendritic cells (DCs), are able to cross the blood-brain barrier and migrate to tumor within the brain parenchyma.[14–19] However, despite the ability of immune cells to traffic into intracranial lesions, the cells are generally unable to eradicate the primary tumor, in part because of the presence of an immunosuppressive tumor milieu. The release of immunosuppressive cytokines into the tumor microenvironment,[20,21] activation of immune checkpoints,[22,23] and an enriched population of CD4+CD25+FoxP3+ T regulatory (T_{reg}) cells[22] and T_H17 cells[24,25] are implicated in preventing an aggressive antitumor immune response.

Despite these challenges, immunotherapy has the potential to be advantageous over other chemotherapeutic strategies because of the potential for cellular level specificity and long-term surveillance. The potential of immunotherapy against cancers has recently been highlighted with the approval by the US Food and Drug Administration (FDA) of sipuleucel-T for treatment of castration-resistant prostate cancer[26] and ipilimumab for unresectable or metastatic melanoma.[27] There is no FDA-approved immunotherapy for HGGs, but the clinical evidence, as described later, suggests that immunotherapy may be a useful strategy to combat HGGs. This article reviews several strategies, including adoptive immunotherapy, active immunotherapy, and immunomodulation, that have been tested or are currently being tested in clinical trials as of August, 2011.

ADOPTIVE IMMUNOTHERAPY

Adoptive immunotherapy is a strategy in which immune cells are taken from the patient and activated ex vivo against tumor-specific antigens. The activated lymphocytes are then reintroduced into the patient, either directly into the tumor cavity or systemically.

Lymphokine-Activated Killer Cells

Lymphokine-activated killer (LAK) cells are peripheral lymphocytes that are cultured with interleukin 2 (IL-2) ex vivo. Once reintroduced, these cells possess cytotoxic abilities, but require activation against tumor cell antigens by host APCs. LAK cells have been studied in clinical trials and have been shown to be associated with varying levels of toxicity and antitumor activity.[28–33] In a study by Hayes and colleagues,[28] LAK cells were delivered via Ommaya reservoir 5 times every 2 weeks for 6 weeks, resulting in a median survival of 12.2 months compared with a median survival of 6.2 months in contemporary patients with recurrent GBM who were treated with surgery and chemotherapy. A similar trial in recurrent GBM showed a median survival of 9 months and a 1-year survival of 34%.[34] The most recent clinical trial in primary GBM, reported by Dillman and colleagues,[35] showed that introducing LAK cells into the tumor cavity in which patients who had undergone standard of care (radiation and TMZ) was safe and resulted in a median survival of 20.5 months with a 1-year survival rate of 75%. The use of corticosteroids was associated with lower total LAK count and worse survival. These trials are summarized in **Table 2**.

Cytotoxic T Cells

Other methods of adoptive immunotherapy for HGGs include infusion of cytotoxic T lymphocytes (CTL) that are isolated from a patient's own tissues, including peripheral blood mononuclear cells (PBMC),[36–38] tumor-infiltrating T lymphocytes (TILs),[18] draining lymph nodes, or PBMCs after vaccination with irradiated autologous tumor cells (ATCs).

Five studies were completed using CTLs isolated from PBMCs and TILs. Results from these 5 phase I/pilot studies showed that this strategy was safe and associated with only minor toxicities, including isolated side effects of hemorrhage and fever,[37] and transient cerebral edema in patients receiving TILs.[18] In each of these studies, the CTLs that were activated ex vivo were injected directly to the tumor cavity.

Table 2
Immunotherapy trials using LAK cells

Reference	Number of Patients	Trial Results
29	6	No PR or SD No toxicity
28	9	1 CR, 2 PR Median survival: 53 wk
32	9	Neurologic side effects in all patients 1 PR
33	20	Median survival: 63 wk (36–201) Use of steroids did not influence in vitro generation of LAK or autologous stimulated lymphocytes
46	19	4 PR Median survival after therapy: 30 wk
122	5	No survival benefit
123	9	1 CR, 2 PR, 4 stable disease Median survival: 18 mo
28	19	1 CR, 2 PR Median survival after therapy: 53 wk
45	9	2 PR Median survival: 78 wk
124	28	1 CR, 2 PR (GBM) Median survival: 53 wk (GBM)
34	40	Median survival: 17.5 mo
35	33	Median survival: 20.5 mo

Abbreviations: CR, complete response; OS, overall survival; PR, partial response; SD, stable disease.

Table 3
Immunotherapy trials using CTLs

Reference	Number of Patients	Trial Results
36	5	2 PR 1 patient's survival reported at 104 wk
125	4	3 PR
37	10	1 CR, 4 PR Median survival: 5 mo
38	5	3 SD
40	15	No PR Time to recurrence >8 mo (n = 7)
39	10	3 PR, 1 SD Survival >1 y (n = 4)
42	10	3 PR
41	9	3 PR Survival >4 y (n = 2)
43	19	1 CR, 7 PR Median survival: 12 mo
18	6	1 CR, 2 PR

Abbreviations: CR, complete response; OS, overall survival; PR, partial response; SD, stable disease.

Five other clinical trials studied the use of CTLs from draining lymph nodes[39] or PBMCs after injection of ATCs.[39–43] In these trials, all CTLs were injected intravenously. Similar to those studies that injected CTLs intracerebrally, the results from these studies showed acceptable safety with minimal toxicity. Isolated toxicities included delayed-type hypersensitivity (DTH) to the vaccine[43] and fever and myalgias lasting 24 hours.[42]

The clinical benefits of these studies have been generally promising. These trials are summarized in **Table 3**. Despite each being only a phase I or pilot study with primary outcomes of safety and toxicity, all but one[40] of these trials reported partial responses or stable disease. Despite this finding, Holladay and colleagues[40] reported a time to recurrence of approximately 8 months, with 1 patient experiencing recurrence of GBM after more than 40 weeks and 7 patients experiencing recurrence after 8 or more months.

In the 10 trials using LAK cells or CTLs, 2 variables consistently reported as significant were the total number of cells infused and the use of corticosteroids during treatment. In these trials, the number of CTLs injected ranged between 3×10^7 and 10×10^{10}, with between 1 and 13 injections. Because the total number of CTLs as well as the method of delivery differed between studies, Kronik and colleagues[44] sought to define the optimum dose using a mathematical model that incorporated data from in vitro and in vivo studies, interactions with CTLs and major histocompatibility complex (MHC) receptors, and the effect of transforming growth factor β (TGF-β) and interferon γ (IFN-γ) on the antitumor immune response. These investigators reported the optimum calculated dose of CTLs as 27×10^9 total CTLs. As a result, they concluded that many immunotherapy trials may not have been successful because the dose given to patients was often inadequate (sometimes 20-fold smaller than that predicted to be effective).

The use of corticosteroids to control peritumoral edema was another factor that varied between studies using LAKs or CTLs. Because of their immunosuppressive effect, corticosteroids were not used in 4 studies, suggesting that patients in these trials may have had a smaller tumor and potentially better outcomes compared with those patients who required steroid treatment.[29,34,35,45] Evidence for better survival when using LAK cells without the use of corticosteroids was reported by Dillman and colleagues[35] in their subset analyses. Other results point to the contrary, that corticosteroids did not have an effect on the number or functional activity of the infused effector cells.[31,33,46]

ACTIVE IMMUNOTHERAPY

Active immunotherapy involves administration of tumor antigens to prime the patient's endogenous immune system. Lysates of injected tumor antigens can be derived from irradiated tumor cells, nonspecific protein and mRNA lysates, and synthetic peptides. The delivery of these antigens is typically via vaccine, which often includes an immune adjuvant or the tumor antigen complexed to DCs, to increase the antitumor immune response. This strategy is considered advantageous because of the specificity afforded by directly injecting immunogenic tumor antigens and the long-term antitumor effect as a result of immunologic memory.

ATCs

ATCs have been studied in active immunotherapy strategies against HGG in 8 clinical trials and 2 case reports[47–54] for a total of 71 patients treated (**Table 4**). Of these studies, there was large heterogeneity in the number of cells infused, number of injections, and the use of immune adjuvants. The number of cells injected ranged from 10^6 to 10^{11} total cells per patient and they were given in 1 to 13 vaccinations. Only 2 of the 8 studies used immune adjuvants such as IL-2[48] and granulocyte-macrophage colony-stimulating factor (GM-CSF).[50] Although toxicities were minimal, 2 studies (n = 10 newly diagnosed GBM and n = 1 recurrent GBM), showed that no survival benefit was associated with treatment.[47,48]

Despite a large number of trials (n = 8), the available data do not show robust efficacy data despite most patients showing a strong immune response as assessed by ex vivo assays. Several studies reported a local skin reaction at the injection site.[48,50] Sobol and colleagues[47] reported an antitumor immune response mediated in part by CD8+ cytotoxic T cells, which were collected in the peripheral blood. Several groups reported significant increases of DTH reactions, numbers

Table 4
Immunotherapy trials using ATCs

Reference	Number of Patients	Trial Results
47	1	No survival benefit
48	11	Median survival: 46 wk
49	12	2 CR, 4 PR
50	1	Survival: 10 mo
51	23	Median progression-free survival: 40 wk Median survival: 100 wk
52	3	Prolonged recurrence-free survival
53	12	1 CR, 1 PR, 2 minor response, 1 SD Median survival: 10.7 mo
54	5	3 SD

Abbreviations: CR, complete response; OS, overall survival; PR, partial response; SD, stable disease.

of tumor-reactive memory T cells, and numbers of CD8(+) TILs in recurrent tumors. Despite the presence of increased antitumor immune activity, most studies were unable to show a survival benefit in patients.

DCs

Glioma cells are poor APCs because of downregulation of costimulatory molecules[55] and the release of immunoinhibitory cytokines.[56–58] DCs are professional APCs that phagocytose foreign antigens and present them in the context of MHC to activate innate and adaptive immune cells. DC therapy is based on the concept that GBM cells are poor stimulants of the host's immune system and thus require DCs, acting as APCs, to internalize GBM antigens and present them to activate antitumor immune cells.[59] Nineteen studies have been published using DCs, with a total of 323 patients studied.[60–79] The cellular material complexed with APCs included whole ATCs, tumor lysate, tumor peptides, including the epidermal growth factor vIII (EGFRvIII), or tumor mRNA.

DC vaccinations are typically prepared using GM-CSF and IL-4 as adjuvants, although several groups have reported stimulating DCs with other cytokines.[62,64,68,70,77,80] These vaccines are typically injected intradermally or intranodally. Nishioka and colleagues[81] reported delivering DCs that expressed IL-12 directly to the tumor cavity and found that these cells were able to traffic to draining lymph nodes and activate cytotoxic, antitumor immune cells. Phase I studies have reported that

DC vaccines are safe and associated with only grade I and II vaccine site responses.

Results of these studies are summarized in **Table 5**. In brief, immunologic, radiologic, and clinical benefits were seen in roughly 40% of patients. A peripheral immune response, as measured by ex vivo assays or DTH reactions, was present in more than half of patients. Clinically, 13 studies reported efficacy in terms of beneficial survival compared with historical controls. Two studies did not find a correlation between peripheral immune response and survival.[71,78]

A subset of these clinical trials used vaccines containing DCs that present the EGFRvIII tumor antigen. The EGFRvIII receptor is the most common variant of the EGF receptor and is present on 27% to 67% of GBMs,[82,83] with its expression indicating a negative prognosis.[84] Furthermore, its expression is limited to GBM cells and is not expressed in normal brain. The first clinical trial using DCs loaded with EGFRvIII antigen against HGG was the Vaccine for Intra-Cranial Tumors I (VICTOR I, n = 16 patients). This phase I study used mature DCs loaded with 500 μg of DCs that were pulsed with PEPvIII, a protein that spans the EGFRvIII fusion junction, and conjugated to keyhole limpet hemocyanin (KLH). Vaccines were given 2 weeks after the completion of radiation therapy. After vaccination, all patients showed ex vivo immune responses without any serious clinical side effects. The results of this study were promising, with 2 of the 3 patients with grade III glioma alive without evidence of tumor progression at 66.2 and 123.7 months after vaccination. In vaccinated patients with GBM, the median time to progression (TTP) was 46.9 weeks, with the median survival reported as 110.8 weeks.[85]

The follow-up phase II trial, A Complementary Trial of an Immunotherapy Vaccine Against Tumor-Specific EGFRvIII (ACTIVATE) used DCs loaded with PEPvIII. Similar to the phase I trial, after vaccination, ex vivo assays showed increased titers of anti-EGFRvIII and anti-KLH antibodies and an increase in CD8+, IFN-γ–expressing, EGFRvIII-specific T cells. Clinically, the median TTP was 64.5 weeks and median survival reported as 126.1 weeks.

Although the ACTIVATE study was ongoing, TMZ was initiated as standard of care, along with surgery and radiation. The ACTIVATE II trial was then initiated (n = 21 patients) to determine the efficacy of EGFRvIII vaccine (CDX-110) in combination with TMZ. In this trial, the CDX-110 vaccine was administered on day 21 of the 28-day TMZ cycle, which resulted in similar anti-EGFRvIII immune activity as seen in the previous trials.

IMMUNOMODULATION

One of the primary challenges in successful antitumor immune responses is the immunosuppressive milieu of the tumor microenvironment. The tumor microenvironment is a critical step in mediating antitumor immunity by the host immune system.

Cytokines

Of the multitude of immunosuppressive cytokines in the tumor microenvironment, a small number of cytokines have been targeted in clinical trials. TGF-β promotes immunosuppression in HGG by inhibiting T-cell activation and proliferation, blocking IL-2 production, suppressing activity of natural killer cells, and promoting T_{reg} activity.[86,87] Early phase I studies using trabedersen, a synthetic antisense phosphorothioate oligodeoxynucleotide that is complementary to the human TGFβ2 gene, showed that the drug was safe and associated with long-lasting remissions in some patients.[88] A phase IIb trial comparing trabedersen with standard chemotherapy in patients with recurrent HGG reported a median survival of 13.1 months with an 80-μM dose of trabedersen, 12.0 months with the 10-μM dose, and 11.0 months with standard chemotherapy. Overall survival at 12 months was not significantly different, although there was a trend toward increased survival in patients with grade III glioma receiving the 10-μM dose at 2 years.[89]

IL-2 is a proinflammatory cytokine that activates T cells and helps naive T cells differentiate along

Table 5
Immunotherapy trials using DCs

Reference	Number of Patients	Trial Results
62	8	6 SD
67	9	Median survival: 455 d
64	10	2 minor responses, 4 SD
66	10	Median survival: 133 wk
70	15	4 PR, 2 SD
71	12	Median survival: 23.4 wk
73	13	1 CR, 3 PR Survival >18 mo (n = 3)
74	34	Median survival: 642 d Time to progression: 167 d
76	12	Time to progression: 6.8 mo Median survival: 22.8 mo
Others:[61,63,65,68,69,72,75,77,80,126,127]		

Abbreviations: CR, complete response; OS, overall survival; PR, partial response; SD, stable disease.

the Th1 pathway.[90] Current trials using IL-2 are focused on local delivery because pharmacokinetic data show that high levels of systemically administered rIL-2 are needed to penetrate the CNS and are associated with prohibitive toxicities.[91] Early studies using IL-2 in combination with other immunotherapies including IFN-α[92] or LAK cells[32] reported high rates of neurologic side effects. When used in combination with IFN-α, patients experienced somnolence, headache, and increased peritumoral edema. When rIL-2 was used in combination with LAK cells, all patients had increases in cerebral edema. In another trial reported by Colombo and colleagues,[93] a total of 12 patients underwent gene therapy and received an intratumoral injection of retroviral IL-2 vector-producing cells (RVPCs). Results of this trial were promising in terms of safety because only grade I/II toxicities were noted. Biopsy samples after administration of the RVPCs showed an increase in Th1 cytokine levels. Progression-free survival and overall survival were reported as 47% and 58%, respectively, at 6 months and 14% and 25% at 1 year.

IFNs are secreted by immune cells in response to the presence of tumor cells and activate molecular pathways involved in coordinating an antitumor response against GBM. Three different IFNs have been tested in clinical trials; IFN-α, IFN-β, and IFN-γ.[94,95] Results of these studies are listed in **Table 6**.

Trials using IFN-α have produced mixed results in terms of both safety and efficacy. The first phase I study showed that treatment with IFN-α was safe and efficacious.[96] The follow-up phase II study of bis-chloroethyl-nitrosourea (BCNU) in combination with radiation and IFN-α resulted in a response rate of 29% in 35 patients with recurrent glioma. This phase II study also reported substantial constitutional side effects.[97] The phase III study of 214 patients with stable HGG involved randomization to BCNU or BCNU and IFN-α as a second course of treatment after they received surgery, radiation, and chemotherapy. Patients receiving IFN-α experienced fever, chills, myalgias, and neurocortical symptoms. Furthermore, there was no significant difference in TTP or overall survival.[98]

IFN-β has been tested in several trials, with mixed results. The first study evaluated escalating doses of IFN-β to 7 patients with recurrent glioma. The investigators reported that there was no radiographic response to the treatment, although stable disease was reported for 3 patients for a total of 8 to 26 weeks.[99] A phase I study in children with recurrent tumors (including glioma) tested a dose escalation of IFN-β, with the maximum tolerable dose reported as 500 mIU/m^2. Partial responses were seen in 4 patients (n = 2 high-grade astrocytoma, n = 2 brain stem glioma).[100] Fetell and colleagues[101] reported that a phase I study showed that infusion of

Table 6
Immunotherapy trials using immunomodulation

Reference	Number of Patients	Modulated Cytokine	Trial Results
88	24	TGF-β	3 CR, 7 SD Overall survival: 146.6 wk (anaplastic astrocytoma), 44 wk (GBM)
89	89	TGF-β	Median survival: 39.1 mo (10-μm dose) vs 35.2 mo (80-μm dose)
93	12	IL-2	4 minor response, 4 SD Progression-free survival at 6 mo (47%) and 12 mo (14%) Overall survival at 6 mo (58%) and 12 mo (25%)
96	15	IFN-α	Median survival: 44 mo
97	35	IFN-α	Median survival: 13.3 mo
98	275	IFN-α	No difference in TTP or overall survival
99	7	IFN-β	3 SD
100	21	IFN-β	4 PR
101	20	IFN-β	3 SD
94	28	IFN-γ	Median overall survival no different from historical controls
95	14	IFN-γ	No difference in survival from patients who did not receive IFN-γ
70	15	IL-12	4 SD, 1 mixed response

Abbreviations: CR, complete response; OS, overall survival; PR, partial response; SD, stable disease; TTP, time to progression.

IFN-β directly into the tumor cavity using Ommaya reservoir was well tolerated. Stable disease was reported in 3 patients, with the best response producing disease stability up to 539 days.

CHALLENGES
Challenges Presented by Tumor Biology

Three major challenges to immunotherapy presented by tumor biology include immune-editing, decreased antigen presentation by glioma cells, and decreased immune cell activation.

To eradicate a tumor, the immune system must be able to recognize a tumor-specific antigen, activate other immune cells, and then mount a substantial antitumor response. One major challenge presented to the immune system, and the use of immunotherapy as a treatment strategy, is the concept of immune-editing. Immune-editing consists of 3 phases: elimination, equilibrium, and escape. Elimination refers to the antitumor function of both the adaptive and innate immune system and is driven by the production of IFN-γ. Equilibrium is the period in which immune cells become latent to partially eradicated tumor. Escape is when the tumor escapes from immunosurveillance and becomes resistant to antitumor immune function, usually via genomic instability or downregulation of key antigens.[102] Immune-editing has been shown to exist in the treatment of HGG, especially in trials involving dendritic vaccines that target the EGFRvIII antigen. In the EGFRvIII vaccine trial reported by Sampson and colleagues,[76] 82% of patients with recurrent tumor had lost expression of EGFRvIII.

Another notable challenge is the presence of an immunosuppressive tumor microenvironment, causing decreased antigen recognition and depressed immune cell activation. Glioma cells show decreased HLA expression,[103] and in a recent study, Facoetti and colleagues[104] reported a loss of HLA-I expression in 50% of patients, with 80% of these patients showing a selective loss of HLA-A2. Macrophages and microglia also have a decreased potential for antigen presentation. In vitro data suggest monocytes lose phagocytic activity after exposure to glioma cells,[105] whereas in vivo data suggest that MHC class II activation is significantly depressed in microglia and macrophages isolated from glioma compared with normal brain.[106]

The other notable aspect of tumor-associated immunosuppression is depressed immune cell activation. CD4+ cells isolated from both tumor and peripheral blood show depressed function,[107,108] proliferative responses, and synthesis of IL-2 in patients with glioma.[109] Although increased CD8+ infiltrating lymphocytes have been shown in some studies to be associated with increased patient survival,[110–112] Hussain and Heimberger[15] reported that most tumor-infiltrating CD8+ cells are not activated.

The expression of immunosuppressive molecules and release of immunosuppressive cytokines are also associated with decreased immune cell activation. Increased expression of the surface molecules FAS, galectin-1, and B7-H1, which are all involved in regulating apoptosis, leading to subsequent decreases in tumor-infiltrating lymphocytes, have all been described.[113–116] Similarly, the release of cytokines such as IL-10,[117] prostaglandin E_2,[118,119] and TGF-β[120] are increased in the glioma microenvironment, leading to decreased immune cell activation.

Challenges Presented by Current Clinical Trials

Clinical trials for immunotherapy in HGG have mostly been small phase I or pilot studies in small cohorts of patients, leading to possible confounding prognostic variables. Although inclusion criteria usually require a histologic diagnosis of grade III/IV glioma, newer evidence suggests that a molecular classification of glioma may better subtype glioma tumors. This classification, reported by Verhaak and colleagues,[121] consists of classic, mesenchymal, proneural, and neural. Using a molecular diagnosis versus a histologic diagnosis as inclusion criteria for future clinical trials may lead to more uniform patient cohorts because differing responses to classic treatments are seen in patients with a molecular diagnosis. The investigators report a trend toward longer survival in the proneural subtype, despite poor responses to aggressive treatment protocols. Similarly, the same group report that the classic and mesenchymal subtypes showed a similar survival benefit; however, these tumors were susceptible to treatment.

Because of small patient cohorts typically seen in immunotherapy trials for HGG, dose escalation studies are rarely feasible, leading to a lack of a maximum tolerated dose. This heterogeneity in dose as well as the inability to reach a maximum tolerated dose may lead to results that may not reflect results seen at higher doses of vaccine.

SUMMARY

Despite several clinical trials evaluating immunotherapy as an adjuvant therapy for HGGs, robust efficacy for this treatment paradigm is lacking. Although nearly every clinical trial has reported induction of a peripheral immune response ex vivo, there was not a robust correlation between peripheral immune responses and patient survival.

One of the difficulties in predicting the success of immunotherapy trials as well as comparing the results across studies is the heterogeneous nature of immunotherapy trial design and reporting. Many intrinsic and extrinsic factors may influence trial results, including the use of other adjuvant agents that selectively deplete specific cell populations, patient selection, clinical trial design, and a wide variety of doses and methods of administration.

Despite these challenges, the cellular level specificity and surveillance against tumor cells are an appealing benefit to extending the survival of patients with HGG. Moving forward, well-designed clinical trials with standard doses and more homogenous patients will add stronger evidence for the use of immunotherapy as a standard adjuvant treatment of patients with HGG.

REFERENCES

1. Louis DN, Ohgaki H, Wiestler OD, et al. The 2007 WHO classification of tumors of the central nervous system. Lyon (France): IARC Press; 2007.
2. Scott CB, Scarantino C, Urtasun R, et al. Validation and predictive power of Radiation Therapy Oncology Group (RTOG) recursive partitioning analysis classes for malignant glioma patients: a report using RTOG 90-06. Int J Radiat Oncol Biol Phys 1998;40(1):51–5.
3. Davis FG, McCarthy BJ, Freels S, et al. The conditional probability of survival of patients with primary malignant brain tumors: surveillance, epidemiology, and end results (SEER) data. Cancer 1999; 85(2):485–91.
4. Stupp R, Mason WP, van den Bent MJ, et al. Radiotherapy plus concomitant and adjuvant temozolomide for glioblastoma. N Engl J Med 2005; 352(10):987–96.
5. Sathornsumetee S, Rich JN, Reardon DA. Diagnosis and treatment of high-grade astrocytoma. Neurol Clin 2007;25(4):1111–39, x.
6. Butowski NA, Sneed PK, Chang SM. Diagnosis and treatment of recurrent high-grade astrocytoma. J Clin Oncol 2006;24(8):1273–80.
7. Furnari FB, Fenton T, Bachoo RM, et al. Malignant astrocytic glioma: genetics, biology, and paths to treatment. Genes Dev 2007;21(21):2683–710.
8. Chi AS, Wen PY. Inhibiting kinases in malignant gliomas. Expert Opin Ther Targets 2007;11(4): 473–96.
9. Agarwal S, Sane R, Oberoi R, et al. Delivery of molecularly targeted therapy to malignant glioma, a disease of the whole brain. Expert Rev Mol Med 2011;13:e17.
10. Sathornsumetee S, Reardon DA, Desjardins A, et al. Molecularly targeted therapy for malignant glioma. Cancer 2007;110(1):13–24.
11. Stummer W, Pichlmeier U, Meinel T, et al. Fluorescence-guided surgery with 5-aminolevulinic acid for resection of malignant glioma: a randomised controlled multicentre phase III trial. Lancet Oncol 2006;7(5):392–401.
12. Wen PY, Schiff D, Kesari S, et al. Medical management of patients with brain tumors. J Neurooncol 2006;80(3):313–32.
13. Tambuyzer BR, Ponsaerts P, Nouwen EJ. Microglia: gatekeepers of central nervous system immunology. J Leukoc Biol 2009;85(3):352–70.
14. Yang I, Han SJ, Kaur G, et al. The role of microglia in central nervous system immunity and glioma immunology. J Clin Neurosci 2010;17(1):6–10.
15. Hussain SF, Heimberger AB. Immunotherapy for human glioma: innovative approaches and recent results. Expert Rev Anticancer Ther 2005;5(5): 777–90.
16. Serot JM, Foliguet B, Bene MC, et al. Ultrastructural and immunohistological evidence for dendritic-like cells within human choroid plexus epithelium. Neuroreport 1997;8(8):1995–8.
17. Calzascia T, Masson F, Di Berardino-Besson W, et al. Homing phenotypes of tumor-specific CD8 T cells are predetermined at the tumor site by crosspresenting APCs. Immunity 2005;22(2): 175–84.
18. Quattrocchi KB, Miller CH, Cush S, et al. Pilot study of local autologous tumor infiltrating lymphocytes for the treatment of recurrent malignant gliomas. J Neurooncol 1999;45(2):141–57.
19. Brabb T, von Dassow P, Ordonez N, et al. In situ tolerance within the central nervous system as a mechanism for preventing autoimmunity. J Exp Med 2000;192(6):871–80.
20. Platten M, Wick W, Weller M. Malignant glioma biology: role for TGF-beta in growth, motility, angiogenesis, and immune escape. Microsc Res Tech 2001;52(4):401–10.
21. Tada M, Suzuki K, Yamakawa Y, et al. Human glioblastoma cells produce 77 amino acid interleukin-8 (IL-8(77)). J Neurooncol 1993;16(1):25–34.
22. El Andaloussi A, Lesniak MS. An increase in CD4+CD25+FOXP3+ regulatory T cells in tumor-infiltrating lymphocytes of human glioblastoma multiforme. Neuro Oncol 2006;8(3):234–43.
23. Jacobs JF, Idema AJ, Bol KF, et al. Regulatory T cells and the PD-L1/PD-1 pathway mediate immune suppression in malignant human brain tumors. Neuro Oncol 2009;11(4):394–402.
24. Wainwright DA, Sengupta S, Han Y, et al. The presence of IL-17A and T helper 17 cells in experimental mouse brain tumors and human glioma. PLoS One 2010;5(10):e15390.
25. Langowski JL, Zhang X, Wu L, et al. IL-23 promotes tumour incidence and growth. Nature 2006; 442(7101):461–5.
26. Small EJ, Schellhammer PF, Higano CS, et al. Placebo-controlled phase III trial of immunologic

therapy with sipuleucel-T (APC8015) in patients with metastatic, asymptomatic hormone refractory prostate cancer. J Clin Oncol 2006;24(19):3089–94.

27. Cameron F, Whiteside G, Perry C. Ipilimumab: first global approval. Drugs 2011;71(8):1093–104.

28. Hayes RL, Koslow M, Hiesiger EM, et al. Improved long term survival after intracavitary interleukin-2 and lymphokine-activated killer cells for adults with recurrent malignant glioma. Cancer 1995; 76(5):840–52.

29. Jacobs SK, Wilson DJ, Kornblith PL, et al. Interleukin-2 or autologous lymphokine-activated killer cell treatment of malignant glioma: phase I trial. Cancer Res 1986;46(4 Pt 2):2101–4.

30. Yoshida S, Tanaka R, Takai N, et al. Local administration of autologous lymphokine-activated killer cells and recombinant interleukin 2 to patients with malignant brain tumors. Cancer Res 1988; 48(17):5011–6.

31. Merchant RE, Grant AJ, Merchant LH, et al. Adoptive immunotherapy for recurrent glioblastoma multiforme using lymphokine activated killer cells and recombinant interleukin-2. Cancer 1988;62(4): 665–71.

32. Barba D, Saris SC, Holder C, et al. Intratumoral LAK cell and interleukin-2 therapy of human gliomas. J Neurosurg 1989;70(2):175–82.

33. Lillehei KO, Mitchell DH, Johnson SD, et al. Long-term follow-up of patients with recurrent malignant gliomas treated with adjuvant adoptive immunotherapy. Neurosurgery 1991;28(1):16–23.

34. Dillman RO, Duma CM, Schiltz PM, et al. Intracavitary placement of autologous lymphokine-activated killer (LAK) cells after resection of recurrent glioblastoma. J Immunother 2004;27(5):398–404.

35. Dillman RO, Duma CM, Ellis RA, et al. Intralesional lymphokine-activated killer cells as adjuvant therapy for primary glioblastoma. J Immunother 2009;32(9):914–9.

36. Kitahara T, Watanabe O, Yamaura A, et al. Establishment of interleukin 2 dependent cytotoxic T lymphocyte cell line specific for autologous brain tumor and its intracranial administration for therapy of the tumor. J Neurooncol 1987;4(4):329–36.

37. Tsuboi K, Saijo K, Ishikawa E, et al. Effects of local injection of ex vivo expanded autologous tumor-specific T lymphocytes in cases with recurrent malignant gliomas. Clin Cancer Res 2003;9(9):3294–302.

38. Kruse CA, Cepeda L, Owens B, et al. Treatment of recurrent glioma with intracavitary alloreactive cytotoxic T lymphocytes and interleukin-2. Cancer Immunol Immunother 1997;45(2):77–87.

39. Plautz GE, Barnett GH, Miller DW, et al. Systemic T cell adoptive immunotherapy of malignant gliomas. J Neurosurg 1998;89(1):42–51.

40. Holladay FP, Heitz-Turner T, Bayer WL, et al. Autologous tumor cell vaccination combined with adoptive cellular immunotherapy in patients with grade III/IV astrocytoma. J Neurooncol 1996;27(2):179–89.

41. Wood GW, Holladay FP, Turner T, et al. A pilot study of autologous cancer cell vaccination and cellular immunotherapy using anti-CD3 stimulated lymphocytes in patients with recurrent grade III/IV astrocytoma. J Neurooncol 2000;48(2):113–20.

42. Plautz GE, Miller DW, Barnett GH, et al. T cell adoptive immunotherapy of newly diagnosed gliomas. Clin Cancer Res 2000;6(6):2209–18.

43. Sloan AE, Dansey R, Zamorano L, et al. Adoptive immunotherapy in patients with recurrent malignant glioma: preliminary results of using autologous whole-tumor vaccine plus granulocyte-macrophage colony-stimulating factor and adoptive transfer of anti-CD3-activated lymphocytes. Neurosurg Focus 2000;9(6):e9.

44. Kronik N, Kogan Y, Vainstein V, et al. Improving alloreactive CTL immunotherapy for malignant gliomas using a simulation model of their interactive dynamics. Cancer Immunol Immunother 2008;57(3):425–39.

45. Sankhla SK, Nadkarni JS, Bhagwati SN. Adoptive immunotherapy using lymphokine-activated killer (LAK) cells and interleukin-2 for recurrent malignant primary brain tumors. J Neurooncol 1996; 27(2):133–40.

46. Jeffes EW 3rd, Beamer YB, Jacques S, et al. Therapy of recurrent high grade gliomas with surgery, and autologous mitogen activated IL-2 stimulated killer (MAK) lymphocytes: I. Enhancement of MAK lytic activity and cytokine production by PHA and clinical use of PHA. J Neurooncol 1993;15(2):141–55.

47. Sobol RE, Fakhrai H, Shawler D, et al. Interleukin-2 gene therapy in a patient with glioblastoma. Gene Ther 1995;2(2):164–7.

48. Schneider T, Gerhards R, Kirches E, et al. Preliminary results of active specific immunization with modified tumor cell vaccine in glioblastoma multiforme. J Neurooncol 2001;53(1):39–46.

49. Andrews DW, Resnicoff M, Flanders AE, et al. Results of a pilot study involving the use of an antisense oligodeoxynucleotide directed against the insulin-like growth factor type I receptor in malignant astrocytomas. J Clin Oncol 2001;19(8):2189–200.

50. Okada H, Lieberman FS, Edington HD, et al. Autologous glioma cell vaccine admixed with interleukin-4 gene transfected fibroblasts in the treatment of recurrent glioblastoma: preliminary observations in a patient with a favorable response to therapy. J Neurooncol 2003;64(1–2):13–20.

51. Steiner HH, Bonsanto MM, Beckhove P, et al. Antitumor vaccination of patients with glioblastoma multiforme: a pilot study to assess feasibility, safety, and clinical benefit. J Clin Oncol 2004;22(21): 4272–81.

52. Parney IF, Chang LJ, Farr-Jones MA, et al. Technical hurdles in a pilot clinical trial of combined B7-2 and GM-CSF immunogene therapy for glioblastomas and melanomas. J Neurooncol 2006; 78(1):71–80.

53. Ishikawa E, Tsuboi K, Yamamoto T, et al. Clinical trial of autologous formalin-fixed tumor vaccine for glioblastoma multiforme patients. Cancer Sci 2007;98(8):1226–33.

54. Clavreul A, Piard N, Tanguy JY, et al. Autologous tumor cell vaccination plus infusion of GM-CSF by a programmable pump in the treatment of recurrent malignant gliomas. J Clin Neurosci 2010;17(7): 842–8.

55. Satoh J, Lee YB, Kim SU. T-cell costimulatory molecules B7-1 (CD80) and B7-2 (CD86) are expressed in human microglia but not in astrocytes in culture. Brain Res 1995;704(1):92–6.

56. Constam DB, Philipp J, Malipiero UV, et al. Differential expression of transforming growth factor-beta 1, -beta 2, and -beta 3 by glioblastoma cells, astrocytes, and microglia. J Immunol 1992;148(5): 1404–10.

57. Chen Q, Daniel V, Maher DW, et al. Production of IL-10 by melanoma cells: examination of its role in immunosuppression mediated by melanoma. Int J Cancer 1994;56(5):755–60.

58. Gabrilovich DI, Ishida T, Nadaf S, et al. Antibodies to vascular endothelial growth factor enhance the efficacy of cancer immunotherapy by improving endogenous dendritic cell function. Clin Cancer Res 1999;5(10):2963–70.

59. Constant S, Sant'Angelo D, Pasqualini T, et al. Peptide and protein antigens require distinct antigen-presenting cell subsets for the priming of CD4+ T cells. J Immunol 1995;154(10):4915–23.

60. Caruso DA, Orme LM, Neale AM, et al. Results of a phase 1 study utilizing monocyte-derived dendritic cells pulsed with tumor RNA in children and young adults with brain cancer. Neuro Oncol 2004;6(3):236–46.

61. De Vleeschouwer S, Van Calenbergh F, Demaerel P, et al. Transient local response and persistent tumor control in a child with recurrent malignant glioma: treatment with combination therapy including dendritic cell therapy. Case report. J Neurosurg 2004;100(Suppl Pediatrics 5):492–7.

62. Kikuchi T, Akasaki Y, Irie M, et al. Results of a phase I clinical trial of vaccination of glioma patients with fusions of dendritic and glioma cells. Cancer Immunol Immunother 2001;50(7): 337–44.

63. Liau LM, Black KL, Martin NA, et al. Treatment of a patient by vaccination with autologous dendritic cells pulsed with allogeneic major histocompatibility complex class I-matched tumor peptides. Case Report. Neurosurg Focus 2000;9(6):e8.

64. Yamanaka R, Abe T, Yajima N, et al. Vaccination of recurrent glioma patients with tumour lysate-pulsed dendritic cells elicits immune responses: results of a clinical phase I/II trial. Br J Cancer 2003;89(7): 1172–9.

65. Yamanaka R, Homma J, Yajima N, et al. Clinical evaluation of dendritic cell vaccination for patients with recurrent glioma: results of a clinical phase I/II trial. Clin Cancer Res 2005;11(11):4160–7.

66. Yu JS, Liu G, Ying H, et al. Vaccination with tumor lysate-pulsed dendritic cells elicits antigen-specific, cytotoxic T-cells in patients with malignant glioma. Cancer Res 2004;64(14):4973–9.

67. Yu JS, Wheeler CJ, Zeltzer PM, et al. Vaccination of malignant glioma patients with peptide-pulsed dendritic cells elicits systemic cytotoxicity and intracranial T-cell infiltration. Cancer Res 2001; 61(3):842–7.

68. Rutkowski S, De Vleeschouwer S, Kaempgen E, et al. Surgery and adjuvant dendritic cell-based tumour vaccination for patients with relapsed malignant glioma: a feasibility study. Br J Cancer 2004;91(9):1656–62.

69. Wheeler CJ, Das A, Liu G, et al. Clinical responsiveness of glioblastoma multiforme to chemotherapy after vaccination. Clin Cancer Res 2004; 10(16):5316–26.

70. Kikuchi T, Akasaki Y, Abe T, et al. Vaccination of glioma patients with fusions of dendritic and glioma cells and recombinant human interleukin 12. J Immunother 2004;27(6):452–9.

71. Liau LM, Prins RM, Kiertscher SM, et al. Dendritic cell vaccination in glioblastoma patients induces systemic and intracranial T-cell responses modulated by the local central nervous system tumor microenvironment. Clin Cancer Res 2005;11(15):5515–25.

72. Okada H, Lieberman FS, Walter KA, et al. Autologous glioma cell vaccine admixed with interleukin-4 gene transfected fibroblasts in the treatment of patients with malignant gliomas. J Transl Med 2007;5:67.

73. Walker DG, Laherty R, Tomlinson FH, et al. Results of a phase I dendritic cell vaccine trial for malignant astrocytoma: potential interaction with adjuvant chemotherapy. J Clin Neurosci 2008;15(2):114–21.

74. Wheeler CJ, Black KL, Liu G, et al. Vaccination elicits correlated immune and clinical responses in glioblastoma multiforme patients. Cancer Res 2008;68(14):5955–64.

75. De Vleeschouwer S, Fieuws S, Rutkowski S, et al. Postoperative adjuvant dendritic cell-based immunotherapy in patients with relapsed glioblastoma multiforme. Clin Cancer Res 2008;14(10):3098–104.

76. Sampson JH, Archer GE, Mitchell DA, et al. An epidermal growth factor receptor variant III-targeted vaccine is safe and immunogenic in patients with glioblastoma multiforme. Mol Cancer Ther 2009;8(10):2773–9.

77. Ardon H, De Vleeschouwer S, Van Calenbergh F, et al. Adjuvant dendritic cell-based tumour vaccination for children with malignant brain tumours. Pediatr Blood Cancer 2010;54(4):519–25.

78. Ardon H, Van Gool S, Lopes IS, et al. Integration of autologous dendritic cell-based immunotherapy in the primary treatment for patients with newly diagnosed glioblastoma multiforme: a pilot study. J Neurooncol 2010;99(2):261–72.

79. Fadul CE, Fisher JL, Hampton TH, et al. Immune response in patients with newly diagnosed glioblastoma multiforme treated with intranodal autologous tumor lysate-dendritic cell vaccination after radiation chemotherapy. J Immunother 2011;34(4):382–9.

80. Rosenberg SA, Yang JC, Restifo NP. Cancer immunotherapy: moving beyond current vaccines. Nat Med 2004;10(9):909–15.

81. Nishioka Y, Hirao M, Robbins PD, et al. Induction of systemic and therapeutic antitumor immunity using intratumoral injection of dendritic cells genetically modified to express interleukin 12. Cancer Res 1999;59(16):4035–41.

82. Humphrey PA, Wong AJ, Vogelstein B, et al. Anti-synthetic peptide antibody reacting at the fusion junction of deletion-mutant epidermal growth factor receptors in human glioblastoma. Proc Natl Acad Sci U S A 1990;87(11):4207–11.

83. Wong AJ, Ruppert JM, Bigner SH, et al. Structural alterations of the epidermal growth factor receptor gene in human gliomas. Proc Natl Acad Sci U S A 1992;89(7):2965–9.

84. Heimberger AB, Hlatky R, Suki D, et al. Prognostic effect of epidermal growth factor receptor and EGFRvIII in glioblastoma multiforme patients. Clin Cancer Res 2005;11(4):1462–6.

85. Sampson JH, Archer GE, Mitchell DA, et al. Tumor-specific immunotherapy targeting the EGFRvIII mutation in patients with malignant glioma. Semin Immunol 2008;20(5):267–75.

86. Wrann M, Bodmer S, de Martin R, et al. T cell suppressor factor from human glioblastoma cells is a 12.5-kd protein closely related to transforming growth factor-beta. EMBO J 1987;6(6):1633–6.

87. de Martin R, Haendler B, Hofer-Warbinek R, et al. Complementary DNA for human glioblastoma-derived T cell suppressor factor, a novel member of the transforming growth factor-beta gene family. EMBO J 1987;6(12):3673–7.

88. Hau P, Jachimczak P, Schlingensiepen R, et al. Inhibition of TGF-beta2 with AP 12009 in recurrent malignant gliomas: from preclinical to phase I/II studies. Oligonucleotides 2007;17(2):201–12.

89. Bogdahn U, Hau P, Stockhammer G, et al. Targeted therapy for high-grade glioma with the TGF-beta2 inhibitor trabedersen: results of a randomized and controlled phase IIb study. Neuro Oncol 2011; 13(1):132–42.

90. Gansbacher B, Zier K, Daniels B, et al. Interleukin 2 gene transfer into tumor cells abrogates tumorigenicity and induces protective immunity. J Exp Med 1990;172(4):1217–24.

91. Saris SC, Rosenberg SA, Friedman RB, et al. Penetration of recombinant interleukin-2 across the blood-cerebrospinal fluid barrier. J Neurosurg 1988;69(1):29–34.

92. Merchant RE, McVicar DW, Merchant LH, et al. Treatment of recurrent malignant glioma by repeated intracerebral injections of human recombinant interleukin-2 alone or in combination with systemic interferon-alpha. Results of a phase I clinical trial. J Neurooncol 1992;12(1):75–83.

93. Colombo F, Barzon L, Franchin E, et al. Combined HSV-TK/IL-2 gene therapy in patients with recurrent glioblastoma multiforme: biological and clinical results. Cancer Gene Ther 2005;12(10):835–48.

94. Wolff JE, Wagner S, Reinert C, et al. Maintenance treatment with interferon-gamma and low-dose cyclophosphamide for pediatric high-grade glioma. J Neurooncol 2006;79(3):315–21.

95. Farkkila M, Jaaskelainen J, Kallio M, et al. Randomised, controlled study of intratumoral recombinant gamma-interferon treatment in newly diagnosed glioblastoma. Br J Cancer 1994;70(1):138–41.

96. Rajkumar SV, Buckner JC, Schomberg PJ, et al. Phase I evaluation of radiation combined with recombinant interferon alpha-2a and BCNU for patients with high-grade glioma. Int J Radiat Oncol Biol Phys 1998;40(2):297–302.

97. Buckner JC, Brown LD, Kugler JW, et al. Phase II evaluation of recombinant interferon alpha and BCNU in recurrent glioma. J Neurosurg 1995;82(3):430–5.

98. Buckner JC, Schomberg PJ, McGinnis WL, et al. A phase III study of radiation therapy plus carmustine with or without recombinant interferon-alpha in the treatment of patients with newly diagnosed high-grade glioma. Cancer 2001;92(2):420–33.

99. Mahaley MS Jr, Dropcho EJ, Bertsch L, et al. Systemic beta-interferon therapy for recurrent gliomas: a brief report. J Neurosurg 1989;71(5 Pt 1):639–41.

100. Allen J, Packer R, Bleyer A, et al. Recombinant interferon beta: a phase I-II trial in children with recurrent brain tumors. J Clin Oncol 1991;9(5):783–8.

101. Fetell MR, Housepian EM, Oster MW, et al. Intratumor administration of beta-interferon in recurrent malignant gliomas. A phase I clinical and laboratory study. Cancer 1990;65(1):78–83.

102. Dunn GP, Old LJ, Schreiber RD. The immunobiology of cancer immunosurveillance and immunoediting. Immunity 2004;21(2):137–48.

103. Yang I, Kremen TJ, Giovannone AJ, et al. Modulation of major histocompatibility complex class I molecules and major histocompatibility complex-bound immunogenic peptides induced by interferon-alpha and interferon-gamma treatment of human

glioblastoma multiforme. J Neurosurg 2004;100(2): 310–9.

104. Facoetti A, Nano R, Zelini P, et al. Human leukocyte antigen and antigen processing machinery component defects in astrocytic tumors. Clin Cancer Res 2005;11(23):8304–11.

105. Parney IF, Waldron JS, Parsa AT. Flow cytometry and in vitro analysis of human glioma-associated macrophages. Laboratory investigation. J Neurosurg 2009;110(3):572–82.

106. Schartner JM, Hagar AR, Van Handel M, et al. Impaired capacity for upregulation of MHC class II in tumor-associated microglia. Glia 2005;51(4): 279–85.

107. Roszman TL, Brooks WH. Neural modulation of immune function. J Neuroimmunol 1985;10(1):59–69.

108. Roszman TL, Brooks WH, Steele C, et al. Pokeweed mitogen-induced immunoglobulin secretion by peripheral blood lymphocytes from patients with primary intracranial tumors. Characterization of T helper and B cell function. J Immunol 1985; 134(3):1545–50.

109. Elliott LH, Brooks WH, Roszman TL. Cytokinetic basis for the impaired activation of lymphocytes from patients with primary intracranial tumors. J Immunol 1984;132(3):1208–15.

110. Brooks WH, Markesbery WR, Gupta GD, et al. Relationship of lymphocyte invasion and survival of brain tumor patients. Ann Neurol 1978;4(3): 219–24.

111. Dunn GP, Dunn IF, Curry WT. Focus on TILs: prognostic significance of tumor infiltrating lymphocytes in human glioma. Cancer Immun 2007;7:12.

112. Palma L, Di Lorenzo N, Guidetti B. Lymphocytic infiltrates in primary glioblastomas and recidivous gliomas. Incidence, fate, and relevance to prognosis in 228 operated cases. J Neurosurg 1978; 49(6):854–61.

113. Yang BC, Lin HK, Hor WS, et al. Mediation of enhanced transcription of the IL-10 gene in T cells, upon contact with human glioma cells, by Fas signaling through a protein kinase A-independent pathway. J Immunol 2003;171(8):3947–54.

114. Parsa AT, Waldron JS, Panner A, et al. Loss of tumor suppressor PTEN function increases B7-H1 expression and immunoresistance in glioma. Nat Med 2007;13(1):84–8.

115. Ichinose M, Masuoka J, Shiraishi T, et al. Fas ligand expression and depletion of T-cell infiltration in astrocytic tumors. Brain Tumor Pathol 2001;18(1):37–42.

116. Rorive S, Belot N, Decaestecker C, et al. Galectin-1 is highly expressed in human gliomas with relevance for modulation of invasion of tumor astrocytes into the brain parenchyma. Glia 2001;33(3):241–55.

117. Nitta T, Hishii M, Sato K, et al. Selective expression of interleukin-10 gene within glioblastoma multiforme. Brain Res 1994;649(1–2):122–8.

118. Fontana A, Kristensen F, Dubs R, et al. Production of prostaglandin E and an interleukin-1 like factor by cultured astrocytes and C6 glioma cells. J Immunol 1982;129(6):2413–9.

119. Sawamura Y, Diserens AC, de Tribolet N. In vitro prostaglandin E2 production by glioblastoma cells and its effect on interleukin-2 activation of oncolytic lymphocytes. J Neurooncol 1990;9(2):125–30.

120. Couldwell WT, Yong VW, Dore-Duffy P, et al. Production of soluble autocrine inhibitory factors by human glioma cell lines. J Neurol Sci 1992;110(1–2):178–85.

121. Verhaak RG, Hoadley KA, Purdom E, et al. Integrated genomic analysis identifies clinically relevant subtypes of glioblastoma characterized by abnormalities in PDGFRA, IDH1, EGFR, and NF1. Cancer Cell 2010;17(1):98–110.

122. Blancher A, Roubinet F, Grancher AS, et al. Local immunotherapy of recurrent glioblastoma multiforme by intracerebral perfusion of interleukin-2 and LAK cells. Eur Cytokine Netw 1993;4(5): 331–41.

123. Boiardi A, Silvani A, Ruffini PA, et al. Loco-regional immunotherapy with recombinant interleukin-2 and adherent lymphokine-activated killer cells (A-LAK) in recurrent glioblastoma patients. Cancer Immunol Immunother 1994;39(3):193–7.

124. Hayes RL, Arbit E, Odaimi M, et al. Adoptive cellular immunotherapy for the treatment of malignant gliomas. Crit Rev Oncol Hematol 2001;39(1–2):31–42.

125. Tsurushima H, Liu SQ, Tuboi K, et al. Reduction of end-stage malignant glioma by injection with autologous cytotoxic T lymphocytes. Jpn J Cancer Res 1999;90(5):536–45.

126. Caruso DA, Orme LM, Amor GM, et al. Results of a phase I study utilizing monocyte-derived dendritic cells pulsed with tumor RNA in children with stage 4 neuroblastoma. Cancer 2005;103(6): 1280–91.

127. Wen PY, Macdonald DR, Reardon DA, et al. Updated response assessment criteria for high-grade gliomas: response assessment in neuro-oncology working group. J Clin Oncol 2010;28(11):1963–72.

IDH Mutations in Human Glioma

Won Kim, MD[a],*, Linda M. Liau, MD, PhD[b]

KEYWORDS

- IDH1 • IDH2 • Glioma • Isocitrate dehydrogenase • GBM • Brain tumor

KEY POINTS

- Isocitrate dehydrogenase-1 (IDH1) mutations are highly conserved to R132 within the enzyme's active site, suggesting that the mutation may have an oncogenic gain of function.
- IDH1 mutations are associated with other prognostically favorable alterations (TP53 mutations and 1p19q codeletions) and certain gene cluster profiles (proneural).
- IDH1 mutations are found across different molecular and histologic brain tumor subtypes, suggesting they are early genetic alterations in tumorigenesis.
- Novel IDH1 sequencing and staining techniques have allowed this marker to play an increasingly important role in the histologic determination of brain tumor specimens.

INTRODUCTION

The classification of human brain tumors by the World Health Organization (WHO) scale based on tumor histology remains the gold standard in the diagnosis and prognosis of glioma.[1] In addition to the traditional microscopic characteristics that subcategorize these tumor classes, mounting evidence has come to support distinct genetic aberrations associated with individual tumor sets within this grading scheme. For example, mutations in TP53 are commonly found in astrocytomas (50%–90%) and oligoastrocytomas (40%–50%) but are infrequent in oligodendrogliomas (5%–10%). On the other hand, 1p19q deletions are frequent in oligodendrogliomas (50%–70%) and less common to rare in oligoastrocytomas (30%–50%) and astrocytomas (0%–15%).[2–4] Although both TP53 mutations and 1p19q codeletions have been associated with improved prognosis, these mutations are mutually exclusive in gliomas, providing molecular evidence to support the histologic stratification of these tumors.

Recently, a sentinel paper by Parsons and colleagues[5] demonstrated the existence of a novel glioma-associated mutation in isocitrate dehydrogenase-1 (IDH1) in 12% of patients with glioblastoma (GBM) via high-throughput gene expression analysis of 20,661 protein coding genes. IDH1 is 1 of 3 metabolic enzymes (along with IDH2 and IDH3) that catalyze the oxidative decarboxylation of isocitrate to α-ketoglutarate (α-KG) while reducing $NADP^+$ to NADPH (NAD^+ to NADH in the case of IDH3).[6] Mutations in IDH1 were found to be associated with younger age, secondary GBMs (grade IV tumors that arise from biopsy-proven lower-grade predecessors), and increased overall survival (OS). Subsequently, a multitude of retrospective and prospective studies have emerged investigating the frequency, function, and prognostic utility of this mutation in human glioma.[7–36]

IDH1: FUNCTION

IDH1, -2, and -3 are enzymes involved in the citric acid cycle that catalyze the oxidative decarboxylation of isocitrate to α-ketoglutarate (α-KG) while reducing $NADP^+$ to NADPH (NAD^+ to NADH in the case of IDH3).[37] Although IDH1 is found within

No conflicts of interest to disclose.

[a] Department of Neurosurgery, University of California Los Angeles, Box 956901, Los Angeles, CA 90095-6901, USA; [b] Department of Neurosurgery, University of California Los Angeles Medical Center, 10833 Le Conte Avenue, CHS 74-145, Los Angeles, CA 90095-6901, USA
* Corresponding author.
E-mail address: wonkim@mednet.ucla.edu

Neurosurg Clin N Am 23 (2012) 471–480
doi:10.1016/j.nec.2012.04.009
1042-3680/12/$ – see front matter Published by Elsevier Inc.

the cytoplasm and peroxisomes, IDH2 and IDH3 are localized solely to the mitochondria.[38] The gene for IDH1 is located on 2q33.3 and is 1 of 5 IDH genes within the human genome.[39] Two of the 5 IDH genes produce homodimeric proteins (IDH1 and IDH2), whereas the remaining 3 IDH gene products constitute the subunits of the heterotetrameric protein IDH3 (2 IDH3α, IDH3β, and IDH3γ).[40] Human IDH1 contains 2 asymmetric active sites formed by small and large domains of each IDH1 molecule and transitions between an inactive open, an inactive semiopen, and a catalytically active closed conformation.[6,41] A critical structure in the enzymatic interaction with the substrate isocitrate is the arginine 132 (R132) found within the active site of IDH1 (arginine is conserved in the functionally analogous R172 of IDH2). This residue is unique among all others involved in the binding of isocitrate in that it forms 3 hydrogen bonds with the α- and β-carboxyl groups of the substrate, whereas other residues form no more than 2.[36] Moreover, it plays a critical role in facilitating the hinge movement between the open and closed conformations.[42,43] The R172 residue in IDH2 plays an identical role because it is the evolutionarily conserved homolog of R132 in IDH1.

Mutations in IDH1 and IDH2 are generally mutually exclusive, and there has only been one report of simultaneous IDH1 and IDH2 mutations to date.[34] Interestingly, apart from rare case reports, the mutations of IDH1 and IDH2 occur exclusively at these arginine residues (most commonly replaced by histidine, R132H in IDH1), which are highly conserved across species and malignancies that involve the mutation of isocitrate dehydrogenase.[44–46] The mutations are missense substitutions, with no evidence of inactivating nonsense deletions of base pairs. This slight modification in the active site of the enzyme disrupts the aforementioned hydrogen bonding of the critical R132 and results in a shift in the enzymatic equilibrium to favor the closed configuration and subsequently increased affinity for nicotinamide adenine dinucleotide phosphate (NADPH).[42] In addition, with the change in the active site conformation, there is a markedly reduced affinity for isocitrate. As a result of these changes, R132 mutations result in a greater than 80% reduction in activity compared with the wild-type (wt) enzyme.[36]

IDH1 MUTATIONS IN HUMAN GLIOMA

Following the first report that IDH1 mutations were found more frequently in secondary GBMs (sGBM) compared with primary GBMs (pGBM), other studies showed similar findings and elucidated other associations between IDH1 mutation status and WHO classification (**Table 1**). Indeed, IDH1 mutations are more frequently found in sGBMs, with reported frequencies ranging from 50% to 86% compared with pGBMs, which contain the mutation only 4% to 21% of the time.[8,9,18,21,24,25,28,31,34,35,47–50] sGBMs were frequently cited as being associated with younger patients; prognostically favorable genetic alterations, including 1p19q deletions and TP53 mutations; and an improved clinical course.[5,18,24,26,35] The association between IDH1 mutations and favorable overall prognosis was so striking that some groups argued that sGBMs lacking these characteristics may in fact be pGBMs that were underdiagnosed as anaplastic tumors on initial discovery; the molecular similarities with pGBMs of these IDH1 mutation-negative sGBMs and the fact that all said tumors were initially found as anaplastic gliomas supported this assertion.[24]

Table 1
Frequency of IDH1 mutations in various glial tumors based on results from direct sequencing

Tumor Type	Cases Studied	Mutations Detected	Frequency (%) (Range)
Diffuse astrocytoma[8,16,18,21,23,25,28,30,31,35,48,50–53,86]	887	669	75 (59–100)
Oligodendroglioma[8,16,18,23,28,35,47,48,51,53,86]	623	485	78 (67–93)
Oligoastrocytoma[8,16,18,23,28,35,47,48,51,53,86]	371	291	78 (50–100)
Anaplastic astrocytoma[8,9,16,18,21,23,25,28,30,31,34,35,48,50,51,53,86]	1084	674	62 (0–100)
Anaplastic oligodendroglioma[8,16,18,23,28,35,48,50,51,86]	721	482	67 (49–86)
Anaplastic oligoastrocytomas[8,16,18,21,28,32,34,35,48,50,86]	849	547	64 (63–100)
Secondary GBM[8,9,18,24,25,31,35,47,50,51]	134	96	72 (50–86)
Primary GBM[9,21,25,28,34,47–51,86]	1837	121	7 (4–21)
Pediatric GBM[8,27,35,51]	85	9	11 (0–16)

The reported rates of IDH1 mutation in low-grade gliomas (LGG) are comparable with those of sGBMs, ranging from 59% to 100% in diffuse astrocytomas, 67% to 93% in oligodendrogliomas, and 50% to 100% in oligoastrocytomas. WHO grade III tumors seem to share a similar rate of IDH1 mutations (0%–100% in anaplastic astrocytomas, 49%–86% in anaplastic oligodendrogliomas, and 63%–100% in anaplastic oligoastrocytomas); however, when calculated and compared across numerous series, they seem to have a lower overall frequency (see **Table 1**).[8,16,18,21,23,25,26,28,30,31,35,47,48,51–53] The ubiquitous nature of the mutation across histologic grades and traditionally dichotomized tumor groups (eg, oligodendroglial and astrocytic tumors) separated it from previously described genetic alterations and sparked great interest in elucidating its role in tumorigenesis and its value as a prognostic marker.

PUTATIVE ROLE OF IDH1 MUTATIONS IN GLIOMAGENESIS

It was initially thought that the loss of IDH1 enzymatic ability and subsequent decreased production of α-KG was a form of dominant negative activity and the driving force behind this mutation's oncogenic properties. Indeed, α-KG has critical ancillary roles aside from those of metabolism, as it is required by prolyl hydroxylases (PHD), enzymes that aid in the degradation of hypoxia induced factor-1α (HIF-1α). HIF-1α in turn serves as a key modulator of the transcription factor HIF-1, which is responsible for expressing genes implicated in tumor progression (eg, glucose metabolism, angiogenesis, and invasion) in response to low oxygen levels.[54] It seemed plausible that the loss of α-KG, resulting in the destabilization of PHDs and the accumulation of HIF-1α, could result in tumorigenesis as is seen in 2 other metabolic enzymes that have been found to serve as oncogenes: succinate dehydrogenase and fumarate hydratase.[55] Although initial work reported elevated levels of HIF-1α in IDH1 mutant tumors,[36] subsequent studies involving genome array, immunohistochemical, and fluorodeoxyglucose positron emission tomography analyses did not find significantly elevated levels of HIF-1α in IDH1 mutated gliomas.[23,31,56] Moreover, because the tumors associated with the loss of succinate dehydrogenase and fumarate hydratase are vascular because of the activated angiogenesis pathways, the lack of vascularity in IDH1-mutated LGG (tumors most frequently carrying the mutation) further argues against this as an underlying mechanism in their gliomagenesis.[57]

Other biochemical arguments against the role of reduced α-KG in gliomagenesis stem from the reasoning that a significant percentage of IDH1 molecules would need to exist as heterodimers in order for this mutation to exert dominant negative activity in vivo. A study by Jin and colleagues[58] demonstrated that although IDH1 R132 mutants have equal binding affinity for IDH1 wt proteins, IDH2 R172 mutants (which exhibit the same clinical and molecular profiles as IDH1 mutants) have little affinity for their IDH2-wt counterparts. This finding is supported by other studies that have shown that IDH1/2 containing glioma do not have significantly reduced levels of α-KG.[42,59]

Notwithstanding the controversial role of diminished oxidative decarboxylation of isocitrate to α-KG, IDH1/2 mutants do gain a neomorphic ability to convert α-KG to D-2-hydroxyglutarate (2-HG). This ability is likely secondary to the newly developed high affinity for NADPH by the R132/R172 mutant enzyme, which changes the equilibrium of the active site state to kinetically allow, and even favor, the conversion of α-KG to 2-HG.[42] Assays of 2-HG have shown increases in its concentration from 100- to 300-fold in glioma cells harboring IDH1 mutations.[42,59–61] Furthermore, the addition of 2-HG alone into glioma cells has been shown to decrease proliferation without inducing apoptosis as was found in IDH1 R132 mutant cells[61]; the addition of this metabolite also induced global metabolic changes in IDH1-wt glioma on metabolomic analysis, akin to those found in IDH1-R132H expressing cells.[62] The existence of a highly conserved mutation site without complete inactivation of the gene product, combined with data showing that the knockdown of IDH1-wt does not produce downstream changes shared by 2-HG–injected or IDH1-R132 mutant glioma, gives further credence to the idea that the isocitrate dehydrogenase gene serves as an oncogene with gain of function through its mutation.[6,57,62]

The notion that 2-HG may serve as an oncogenic metabolite in IDH1/2 mutated gliomas was appealing given the existence of congenital conditions, such as L-2HG aciduria whereby germ-line mutations of IDH result in the accumulation of the L-enantiomer of 2-HG, with some of these patients developing malignant brain tumors.[63,64] However, brain tumors are not found in the form of 2-HG aciduria that accumulates the D-enantiomer, although some suggest that because it is the more clinically severe form, these patients may not live long enough to develop intracranial neoplasms.[65,66] There is some evidence that the accumulation of 2-HG in cells may lead to epigenetic alterations because high levels of 2-HG have been shown to reduce the activity of histone demethylases and Translocated in liposarcoma, Ewing's sarcoma and TATA-binding protein-associated factor 15 (TET) 5-methylcyosine hydroxylases, which are 2 enzymes that have recently been implicated in the epigenetic control of gene transcription, although the exact mechanism is unclear.[60] Further studies are required to resolve the role of 2-HG in gliomagenesis.

IDH1 MUTATIONS AND OTHER GLIOMA-ASSOCIATED GENETIC CHARACTERISTICS

With mounting evidence that IDH1 mutations in glioma are associated with favorable molecular profiles and clinical outcomes, many studies began reporting on its association with other known significant genetic aberrations in human brain tumors. Traditionally, O^6-methylguanine-DNA methyltransferase (MGMT) promoter methylation, TP53 mutation, and deletions of 1p19q have been associated with improved outcomes in patients with glial tumors.[67-69] IDH1 mutations were found to be strongly associated with 1p19q codeletions in numerous studies,[18,22-24,28,32,70] although a few others did not find any significant relationship between the two.[8,14] Most of the published work to date regarding the association between these two genetic phenomena have indicated a high incidence of co-occurrence, with reported rates of 90% to 100% of IDH mutations in gliomas that have 1p19q deletions.[22,28] The correlation between TP53 and IDH1 mutations is not as robust[8,11,14,15,28]; however, the trend of evidence does suggest a high rate of simultaneous mutations in gliomas that have been studied to date.[10,19,23,24,31,35,48] MGMT promoter methylation was similarly found to be associated with IDH1 mutation in numerous studies,[10,15,28,29,31,32] although others did not find any significant relationship.[30,71,72]

The overwhelming presence of IDH1 mutations with 1p19q deletion and TP53 mutation, 2 events that have been classically dichotomized with distinct histologic and molecular groups, namely oligodendroglial and astrocytic tumors, alluded to an early genetic event that occurred before the differentiation of neural progenitor cells into these various tissue types. In the case of recurrent gliomas whereby multiple biopsies were taken, investigators were able to discern the presence of these genetic events in temporal sequence. In many cases, IDH1 mutations were found to be simultaneously present with TP53 mutations or 1p19q deletions, whereas in others, IDH1 mutations preceded them. In no case did TP53 mutations or 1p19q deletions precede the mutation of IDH1, indicating that this was indeed an early

event in the development of glioma.[25,35,70] Watanabe and colleagues[26] analyzed a series of glioma from patients with Li-Fraumeni syndrome, who on account of their disease have germ-line TP53 mutations, and found that 71% of their patients had an IDH1 mutation. Of note, 100% of these mutations were R132C substitutions, a rarer form of mutation (3.6%–4.6%) compared with R132H (~90%),[12] suggesting that this mutation may be the favored gliomagenic pathway in patients with preexisting mutations of TP53.[26] These findings indicate that although there seems to be a predilection for IDH1 mutations to be an early step in the formation of glioma, it is not the exclusive pathway in IDH1 mutation based gliomagenesis.

In addition to isolated changes in chromosome copy and gene mutations, some studies have investigated the relationship between IDH1 mutations and glioma genetics on a genome level. Recently, there has been mounting interest in chromosome methylation profiles of individual neoplasms. The cancer genome atlas project first identified DNA methylation, primary sequence, copy number, and gene expression changes characteristic of GBM tumors in 2008.[73] Noushmehr and colleagues[74] analyzed more than 200 gliomas for their glioma-CpG island methylator phenotype (G-CIMP) to ascertain if there was any relationship between IDH1 mutations and overall DNA methylation profiles. They found a tight association between G-CIMP with IDH1-mutation-containing tumors (18/23; 78%), whereas all 184 G-CIMP-negative tumors were IDH1-wt. They analyzed an additional 100 gliomas of all WHO grades and independently confirmed the strong relationship between IDH1-mutant tumors and G-CIMP (35/48; 72.9%). Similarly, Christensen and colleagues[10] clustered gliomas into separate groups based on their methylation status and found that only 2 distinct methylation classes had IDH1 or IDH2 mutants and that more than 98% of the tumors in these 2 classes possessed the mutation. Moreover, these methylation profiles were stable across the evolution of the tumor into more malignant grades, suggesting that these changes occurred early during gliomagenesis,[75] giving further credence to the idea that the mutation of IDH1 may have a role in the epigenetic modulation of gene expression.

Other cluster analyses based on overall gene expression have found that a high percentage of IDH1-mutants were associated with a proneural gene expression profile, a genetic gestalt that is commonly associated with younger age and improved prognosis compared with other expression constitutions (mesenchymal, neural, and classical).[74,76] Finally, recent reports have described the association between IDH1 mutation and internexin-α, a proneural gene encoding a neurofilament interacting protein that has previously been shown to be tightly related to 1p19q codeletions and a predictor of favorable outcomes in anaplastic oligoastrocytomas and anaplastic oligodendrogliomas.[77,78] Further studies will likely help add to the list of IDH1 mutation-associated genetic changes that interact in the oncogenesis of these unique tumors.

ROLE OF IDH1 MUTATION IN PROGNOSIS AND RESPONSE TO TREATMENT IN HUMAN GLIOMA

Since the publication of the first report on improved survival in patients with GBM with IDH1 mutations (45.6 vs 13.2 months in IDH1-mutations vs IDH1-wt respectively) by Parsons and colleagues,[5] numerous groups have been able to replicate similar findings.[12,18,22,24,28,31,32,34,35] In addition to improved OS, Sanson and colleagues[28] were able to demonstrate improved progression free survival (PFS) as well in their set of patients with GBM, with 55 months PFS in patients with IDH1 mutation versus 8.8 months PFS in those without it. The analysis was extended to anaplastic (WHO grade III) tumors because many groups were readily able to show an improved OS in grade III tumors that harbored the IDH mutation compared with those that did not in both univariate[18] and multivariate analyses.[22,28,32] In a prospective analysis, Wick and colleagues[34] found that grade III astrocytomas that possessed the IDH1 mutation were associated with greater PFS regardless of the treatment arm and conferred a stronger risk reduction than any other factor in multivariate analysis, including histology.

The evidence for LGG and the prognostic value of IDH1 mutations is slightly more controversial. Two independent groups found that IDH1 mutations in LGG were associated with significantly improved OS,[11,23] whereas others could not find any significant association.[18,70] Weller and colleagues[33] found improved PFS with IDH1 mutation in univariate and multivariate analyses but no significant improvement in OS in multivariate analysis.

It is still unclear if IDH1 mutational status is a prognostic indicator or a predictive measure of response to treatment. Houillier and colleagues[17] stratified a cohort of LGG into 3 groups based on prognostic factors based on the presence of 1p19q deletion, IDH1 mutation, or both together. They found that each of these factors was an independent predictor of improved clinical outcome in response to treatment with the chemotherapeutic agent temozolomide and that the group of patients with both mutations had the best treatment response (objective response in 80% with both mutations, 61% of IDH1-mutants without 1p19q deletion, 17% without either mutation). In a similar fashion, Hartman and colleagues[14] found that in their cohort of patients that received adjuvant therapies, IDH1 mutation status was the single most important predictor of PFS and OS; this was not seen in their cohort of patients that did not receive adjuvant therapy. These findings support the notion that IDH1 mutations may be an important predictor to treatment response. However, van de Bent and colleagues[32] reported that improved prognosis was found regardless of adjuvant therapy when investigating IDH1-mutant glioma in response to procarbazine (Matulane), lomustine (CCNU), and vincristine (Oncovin) chemotherapy. Future studies are necessary to better determine the prognostic versus predictive role of IDH1 status in human glioma.

DETECTION OF IDH1 MUTATIONS

There are 6 amino acid base pair substitutions at R132 of IDH1 that have been identified to date in human glioma: R132H (88.2%–92.7%), R132C (3.6%–4.6%), R132L (0.4%–4.3%), R132 G (0.6%–3.8%), R132S (0.8%–2.5%), and R132P (0.4%).[8,9,12,16,25,26,35] The identity of the amino acid does not seem to have any bearing on the function of the mutant enzyme as long as the arginine is replaced.[8] The R132C substitution has been found in greater frequency in astrocytomas[12,18] and gliomas associated with Li-Fraumeni syndrome, which were diffuse and anaplastic astrocytomas.[26] Recently Pusch and colleagues[44] identified 3 cases of R100Q substitutions within the IDH1 gene. In line with the preexisting dogma that it was the conformational alteration of the IDH1 protein that allowed neomorphic enzymatic activity, R100 is within the active site involved in binding isocitrate. Regardless of the location of the amino acid substituted, each of the identified IDH1 mutations seems to share the same molecular and clinical properties.

Given the increasing importance of IDH1 mutation status in glioma research, there has been considerable effort to develop novel ways to quickly and reliably detect this mutation in tissue specimens. Traditionally, and in most of the literature to date, IDH1 status was detected through traditional Sanger sequencing and polymerase chain reaction (PCR). Although this has the clear advantage of being able to detect non-R132H mutations, it is time consuming and requires there to be at least 20% mutant allele frequency within the tissue specimen for reliable detection.[51] Pyrosequencing is an alternative to traditional sequencing that allows for rapid high-throughput analysis of IDH1 mutations. This method has been recently used to detect IDH1 mutations in gliomas and demonstrated an advantage over classic Sanger sequencing in that it can detect mutated allele frequencies down to 5%.[71,79]

Derived cleaved amplified polymorphic sequence analysis is another alternative to DNA sequencing that uses mismatched primers for specific mutations, which, following PCR amplification, will create differing restriction endonuclease sites depending on the presence of the mutation.[80] The advantage of the technique is that it uses supplies commonly found in most laboratories, obviating expensive sequencing equipment. However, unlike sequencing, the method is limited in that it can only detect mutations being queried. Other PCR-based techniques include coamplification at lower temperature (COLD) PCR with high-resolution melting (HRM) and real-time PCR and post-PCR fluorescent melting curve analysis (FMCA). Through COLD PCR combined with HRM, Boisselier and colleagues[81] were able to detect mutant allele concentrations of 0.25% in a span of only 3 hours. However, because the technique requires the new mutation to have a T_m that is lower than IDH1-wt, it theoretically may not be able to detect R132 G mutations. Real-time PCR with post-PCR FMCA was shown by Horbinski and colleagues[82] to be more sensitive than Sanger sequencing with detection rates of as little as 10% mutant DNA and a processing time of 80 minutes.

A monoclonal antibody to detect IDH1-R132H mutations (mIDH1R132H) was developed with a reported sensitivity and specificity of 94% and 100%, respectively.[47,53] Other antibodies for R132H followed, including IMab-1[83] and DIA-H09,[15] with one report indicating that DIA-H09 was superior to IMab-1 in that it was generally crisper with better signal-to-noise ratio.[84] Proponents of immunohistochemistry-based antibody staining argue that the use of these antibodies to identify IDH1 mutations may even be superior to direct sequencing because there are reported cases in which these antibodies detect mutations missed by direct sequencing, likely because of poor tissue preservation of samples.[15,30] Their ability to detect even single IDH-mutant-containing tumor cells and distinguish them from non-neoplastic brain tissue or tissue contaminants, such as reactive gliosis, radiation necrosis, hemorrhage, and brain tumors with known absence of IDH-mutations (in addition to the technical simplicity of this method), make it a favorable alternative for clinical use.[53,85,86] However, because the antibodies are mutation specific, it can be expected that those designed to bind R132H will fail to detect IDH1 mutants approximately 10% of the time. Moreover, Ikota and colleagues[86] found that these antibodies may sometimes give false positives by staining antimitochondrial antibodies in the cytoplasm of certain cells, so microscopic interpretation should be done with caution to ensure that the antibody stains both the nucleus and the cytoplasm. Although there are other available antibodies to detect the less frequent mutations (eg, R132S),[87] current immunohistochemistry techniques may need to be complemented by other detection techniques to increase their sensitivity to 100%.[30]

IDH MUTATIONS IN OTHER BRAIN TUMORS

Multiple studies have reported the rate of IDH1 mutations in tumors other than glioma. In regard to central nervous system (CNS) tumors, IDH1 mutations do seem to favor glial tumors because the highest frequencies of mutations are found in astrocytic and oligodendroglial tumors of WHO grades II, III, and IV, as mentioned previously. Juvenile pilocytic astrocytomas do not seem to fall under the predilection of IDH1 mutations because there have been no reports of this gene mutation in this tumor type to date.[18,21,35] This finding suggests that despite their glial origin, these tumors arise from a distinct mechanism than other gliomas. Other CNS tumors that conspicuously lack IDH1 mutations include medulloblastomas,[8,18,35] dysembryoplastic neuroepithelial tumors,[18,51,53] schwannomas,[18] meningiomas,[51,53,86] pleomorphic xanthoastrocytomas,[8,35,51,71] subependymal giant cell astrocytomas,[8,35,51] and ependymomas.[8,18,25,35]

IDH1 mutations have been found with moderate frequency within gangliogliomas, and have been shown to confer a poorer prognosis in these patients. In a large-scale multi-institutional analysis of 98 gangliogliomas, Horbinski and colleagues[49] found that 8.2% (8/98) of the gangliogliomas harbored the R132H IDH1 mutation, and that these patients were older (46.1 vs 25.5 years of age), had greater risks of adverse outcomes (high-grade transformation or death), and shorter recurrence-free survival. On multivariate analysis, the presence of the IDH1 mutation was found to be the most powerful risk factor after age.

Pediatric gliomas have been reported to possess IDH mutations less frequently than their adult counterparts.[7,19] However, when analyzed across numerous studies, they seem to have a frequency comparable to primary GBM in adults (see **Table 1**).[8,27,35,51] Although they too are associated with older age,[88,89] they seem to have increased PFS and OS[27] when compared with patients possessing IDH-wt tumors. This finding was highlighted in a study by Pollack and colleagues[27] whereby 100% of their IDH mutations were in children aged older than 14 years (7/20, 35%), whereas none of their patients aged younger than 14 years were positive for the mutation. Given the paucity of studies, further reports will be needed before the exact frequency and prognostic value of IDH1 mutations in the pediatric population can be determined.

SUMMARY

The discovery of IDH1/2 mutations in gliomas was arguably one of the most significant breakthroughs in our understanding of the oncogenesis and classification of gliomas in the past decade. The presence of the mutation in both astrocytic and oligodendroglial tumor types suggests that it is an early event in the pathogenesis of brain tumors and has added novel insight in the way we view gliomas and their origins. Its value as a molecular prognosticator is becoming increasingly evident as more and more studies are published regarding its value in the clinical setting. Its ability to serve as a marker for improved clinical outcome over traditional measures, such as tumor grade and histopathology, has caused some to suggest it be added to the next addition of the WHO tumor classification scheme.[15] The use of IDH1 status to predict clinical outcome, aid diagnosis in histopathology, and illuminate the mechanisms underlying oncogenesis have been invaluable steps in glioma research to date. Future research will need to continue exploring these avenues to help further our understanding of this novel mutation and aid the development of novel therapies to target brain tumors that harbor it.

REFERENCES

1. Louis DN, Ohgaki H, Wiestler OD, et al. The 2007 WHO classification of tumours of the central nervous system. Acta Neuropathol 2007;114:97.
2. Ohgaki H, Kleihues P. Population-based studies on incidence, survival rates, and genetic alterations in astrocytic and oligodendroglial gliomas. J Neuropathol Exp Neurol 2005;64:479.
3. Okamoto Y, Di Patre PL, Burkhard C, et al. Population-based study on incidence, survival rates, and genetic alterations of low-grade diffuse astrocytomas and oligodendrogliomas. Acta Neuropathol 2004;108:49.
4. Figarella-Branger D, Colin C, Coulibaly B, et al. Histological and molecular classification of gliomas. Rev Neurol (Paris) 2008;164:505 [in French].
5. Parsons DW, Jones S, Zhang X, et al. An integrated genomic analysis of human glioblastoma multiforme. Science 2008;321:1807.
6. Reitman ZJ, Yan H. Isocitrate dehydrogenase 1 and 2 mutations in cancer: alterations at a crossroads of cellular metabolism. J Natl Cancer Inst 2010; 102:932.
7. Antonelli M, Buttarelli FR, Arcella A, et al. Prognostic significance of histological grading, p53 status, YKL-40 expression, and IDH1 mutations in pediatric high-grade gliomas. J Neurooncol 2010;99:209.
8. Balss J, Meyer J, Mueller W, et al. Analysis of the IDH1 codon 132 mutation in brain tumors. Acta Neuropathol 2008;116:597.
9. Bleeker FE, Lamba S, Leenstra S, et al. IDH1 mutations at residue p.R132 (IDH1(R132)) occur frequently in high-grade gliomas but not in other solid tumors. Hum Mutat 2009;30:7.
10. Christensen BC, Smith AA, Zheng S, et al. DNA methylation, isocitrate dehydrogenase mutation, and survival in glioma. J Natl Cancer Inst 2011; 103:143.
11. Dubbink HJ, Taal W, van Marion R, et al. IDH1 mutations in low-grade astrocytomas predict survival but not response to temozolomide. Neurology 2009;73: 1792.
12. Gravendeel LA, Kloosterhof NK, Bralten LB, et al. Segregation of non-p.R132H mutations in IDH1 in distinct molecular subtypes of glioma. Hum Mutat 2010;31:E1186.
13. Gravendeel LA, Kouwenhoven MC, Gevaert O, et al. Intrinsic gene expression profiles of gliomas are a better predictor of survival than histology. Cancer Res 2009;69:9065.
14. Hartmann C, Hentschel B, Tatagiba M, et al. Molecular markers in low-grade gliomas: predictive or prognostic? Clin Cancer Res 2011;17:4588.
15. Hartmann C, Hentschel B, Wick W, et al. Patients with IDH1 wild type anaplastic astrocytomas exhibit worse prognosis than IDH1-mutated glioblastomas, and IDH1 mutation status accounts for the unfavorable prognostic effect of higher age: implications for classification of gliomas. Acta Neuropathol 2010;120:707.
16. Hartmann C, Meyer J, Balss J, et al. Type and frequency of IDH1 and IDH2 mutations are related to astrocytic and oligodendroglial differentiation and age: a study of 1,010 diffuse gliomas. Acta Neuropathol 2009;118:469.
17. Houillier C, Wang X, Kaloshi G, et al. IDH1 or IDH2 mutations predict longer survival and response to temozolomide in low-grade gliomas. Neurology 2010; 75:1560.
18. Ichimura K, Pearson DM, Kocialkowski S, et al. IDH1 mutations are present in the majority of common

adult gliomas but rare in primary glioblastomas. Neuro Oncol 2009;11:341.

19. Jones DT, Mulholland SA, Pearson DM, et al. Adult grade II diffuse astrocytomas are genetically distinct from and more aggressive than their paediatric counterparts. Acta Neuropathol 2011; 121:753.

20. Kang MR, Kim MS, Oh JE, et al. Mutational analysis of IDH1 codon 132 in glioblastomas and other common cancers. Int J Cancer 2009;125:353.

21. Korshunov A, Meyer J, Capper D, et al. Combined molecular analysis of BRAF and IDH1 distinguishes pilocytic astrocytoma from diffuse astrocytoma. Acta Neuropathol 2009;118:401.

22. Labussiere M, Idbaih A, Wang XW, et al. All the 1p19q codeleted gliomas are mutated on IDH1 or IDH2. Neurology 2010;74:1886.

23. Metellus P, Coulibaly B, Colin C, et al. Absence of IDH mutation identifies a novel radiologic and molecular subtype of WHO grade II gliomas with dismal prognosis. Acta Neuropathol 2010;120:719.

24. Nobusawa S, Watanabe T, Kleihues P, et al. IDH1 mutations as molecular signature and predictive factor of secondary glioblastomas. Clin Cancer Res 2009;15:6002.

25. Watanabe T, Nobusawa S, Kleihues P, et al. IDH1 mutations are early events in the development of astrocytomas and oligodendrogliomas. Am J Pathol 2009;174:1149.

26. Watanabe T, Vital A, Nobusawa S, et al. Selective acquisition of IDH1 R132C mutations in astrocytomas associated with Li-Fraumeni syndrome. Acta Neuropathol 2009;117:653.

27. Pollack IF, Hamilton RL, Sobol RW, et al. IDH1 mutations are common in malignant gliomas arising in adolescents: a report from the Children's Oncology Group. Childs Nerv Syst 2011;27:87.

28. Sanson M, Marie Y, Paris S, et al. Isocitrate dehydrogenase 1 codon 132 mutation is an important prognostic biomarker in gliomas. J Clin Oncol 2009;27: 4150.

29. Taal W, Dubbink HJ, Zonnenberg CB, et al. First-line temozolomide chemotherapy in progressive low-grade astrocytomas after radiotherapy: molecular characteristics in relation to response. Neuro Oncol 2011;13:235.

30. Takano S, Tian W, Matsuda M, et al. Detection of IDH1 mutation in human gliomas: comparison of immunohistochemistry and sequencing. Brain Tumor Pathol 2011;28:115.

31. Toedt G, Barbus S, Wolter M, et al. Molecular signatures classify astrocytic gliomas by IDH1 mutation status. Int J Cancer 2011;128:1095.

32. van den Bent MJ, Dubbink HJ, Marie Y, et al. IDH1 and IDH2 mutations are prognostic but not predictive for outcome in anaplastic oligodendroglial tumors: a report of the European Organization for Research and Treatment of Cancer Brain Tumor Group. Clin Cancer Res 2010;16:1597.

33. Weller M, Felsberg J, Hartmann C, et al. Molecular predictors of progression-free and overall survival in patients with newly diagnosed glioblastoma: a prospective translational study of the German Glioma Network. J Clin Oncol 2009;27: 5743.

34. Wick W, Hartmann C, Engel C, et al. NOA-04 randomized phase III trial of sequential radiochemotherapy of anaplastic glioma with procarbazine, lomustine, and vincristine or temozolomide. J Clin Oncol 2009;27:5874.

35. Yan H, Parsons DW, Jin G, et al. IDH1 and IDH2 mutations in gliomas. N Engl J Med 2009;360:765.

36. Zhao S, Lin Y, Xu W, et al. Glioma-derived mutations in IDH1 dominantly inhibit IDH1 catalytic activity and induce HIF-1alpha. Science 2009;324:261.

37. Reitman ZJ, Olby NJ, Mariani CL, et al. IDH1 and IDH2 hotspot mutations are not found in canine glioma. Int J Cancer 2010;127:245.

38. Winkler BS, DeSantis N, Solomon F. Multiple NADPH-producing pathways control glutathione (GSH) content in retina. Exp Eye Res 1986;43:829.

39. Narahara K, Kimura S, Kikkawa K, et al. Probable assignment of soluble isocitrate dehydrogenase (IDH1) to 2q33.3. Hum Genet 1985;71:37.

40. Yen KE, Bittinger MA, Su SM, et al. Cancer-associated IDH mutations: biomarker and therapeutic opportunities. Oncogene 2010;29:6409.

41. Xu X, Zhao J, Xu Z, et al. Structures of human cytosolic NADP-dependent isocitrate dehydrogenase reveal a novel self-regulatory mechanism of activity. J Biol Chem 2004;279:33946.

42. Dang L, White DW, Gross S, et al. Cancer-associated IDH1 mutations produce 2-hydroxyglutarate. Nature 2010;465:966.

43. Kloosterhof NK, Bralten LB, Dubbink HJ, et al. Isocitrate dehydrogenase-1 mutations: a fundamentally new understanding of diffuse glioma? Lancet Oncol 2011;12:83.

44. Pusch S, Sahm F, Meyer J, et al. Glioma IDH1 mutation patterns off the beaten track. Neuropathol Appl Neurobiol 2011;37:428.

45. Ward PS, Patel J, Wise DR, et al. The common feature of leukemia-associated IDH1 and IDH2 mutations is a neomorphic enzyme activity converting alpha-ketoglutarate to 2-hydroxyglutarate. Cancer Cell 2010;17:225.

46. Dang L, Jin S, Su SM. IDH mutations in glioma and acute myeloid leukemia. Trends Mol Med 2010; 16:387.

47. Capper D, Weissert S, Balss J, et al. Characterization of R132H mutation-specific IDH1 antibody binding in brain tumors. Brain Pathol 2010;20:245.

48. Jha P, Suri V, Sharma V, et al. IDH1 mutations in gliomas: first series from a tertiary care centre in

India with comprehensive review of literature. Exp Mol Pathol 2011;91:385.

49. Horbinski C, Kofler J, Yeaney G, et al. Isocitrate dehydrogenase 1 analysis differentiates gangliogliomas from infiltrative gliomas. Brain Pathol 2011;21:564.

50. Sonoda Y, Kumabe T, Nakamura T, et al. Analysis of IDH1 and IDH2 mutations in Japanese glioma patients. Cancer Sci 2009;100:1996.

51. von Deimling A, Korshunov A, Hartmann C. The next generation of glioma biomarkers: MGMT methylation, BRAF fusions and IDH1 mutations. Brain Pathol 2011;21:74.

52. Camelo-Piragua S, Jansen M, Ganguly A, et al. A sensitive and specific diagnostic panel to distinguish diffuse astrocytoma from astrocytosis: chromosome 7 gain with mutant isocitrate dehydrogenase 1 and p53. J Neuropathol Exp Neurol 2011; 70:110.

53. Capper D, Reuss D, Schittenhelm J, et al. Mutation-specific IDH1 antibody differentiates oligodendrogliomas and oligoastrocytomas from other brain tumors with oligodendroglioma-like morphology. Acta Neuropathol 2011;121:241.

54. Semenza GL. Targeting HIF-1 for cancer therapy. Nat Rev Cancer 2003;3:721.

55. King A, Selak MA, Gottlieb E. Succinate dehydrogenase and fumarate hydratase: linking mitochondrial dysfunction and cancer. Oncogene 2006;25:4675.

56. Williams SC, Karajannis MA, Chiriboga L, et al. R132H-mutation of isocitrate dehydrogenase-1 is not sufficient for HIF-1alpha upregulation in adult glioma. Acta Neuropathol 2011;121:279.

57. Thompson CB. Metabolic enzymes as oncogenes or tumor suppressors. N Engl J Med 2009;360:813.

58. Jin G, Reitman ZJ, Spasojevic I, et al. 2-hydroxyglutarate production, but not dominant negative function, is conferred by glioma-derived NADP-dependent isocitrate dehydrogenase mutations. PLoS One 2011;6:e16812.

59. Seltzer MJ, Bennett BD, Joshi AD, et al. Inhibition of glutaminase preferentially slows growth of glioma cells with mutant IDH1. Cancer Res 2010; 70:8981.

60. Xu W, Yang H, Liu Y, et al. Oncometabolite 2-hydroxyglutarate is a competitive inhibitor of alpha-ketoglutarate-dependent dioxygenases. Cancer Cell 2011;19:17.

61. Bralten LB, Kloosterhof NK, Balvers R, et al. IDH1 R132H decreases proliferation of glioma cell lines in vitro and in vivo. Ann Neurol 2011;69:455.

62. Reitman ZJ, Jin G, Karoly ED, et al. Profiling the effects of isocitrate dehydrogenase 1 and 2 mutations on the cellular metabolome. Proc Natl Acad Sci U S A 2011;108:3270.

63. Moroni I, Bugiani M, D'Incerti L, et al. L-2-hydroxyglutaric aciduria and brain malignant tumors: a predisposing condition? Neurology 2004;62:1882.

64. Struys EA. D-2-Hydroxyglutaric aciduria: unravelling the biochemical pathway and the genetic defect. J Inherit Metab Dis 2006;29:21.

65. Struys EA, Salomons GS, Achouri Y, et al. Mutations in the D-2-hydroxyglutarate dehydrogenase gene cause D-2-hydroxyglutaric aciduria. Am J Hum Genet 2005;76:358.

66. Frezza C, Tennant DA, Gottlieb E. IDH1 mutations in gliomas: when an enzyme loses its grip. Cancer Cell 2010;17:7.

67. Nikiforova MN, Hamilton RL. Molecular diagnostics of gliomas. Arch Pathol Lab Med 2011;135:558.

68. Bourne TD, Schiff D. Update on molecular findings, management and outcome in low-grade gliomas. Nat Rev Neurol 2010;6:695.

69. Ducray F, El Hallani S, Idbaih A. Diagnostic and prognostic markers in gliomas. Curr Opin Oncol 2009;21:537.

70. Kim YH, Nobusawa S, Mittelbronn M, et al. Molecular classification of low-grade diffuse gliomas. Am J Pathol 2010;177:2708.

71. Felsberg J, Wolter M, Seul H, et al. Rapid and sensitive assessment of the IDH1 and IDH2 mutation status in cerebral gliomas based on DNA pyrosequencing. Acta Neuropathol 2010;119:501.

72. Jha P, Suri V, Jain A, et al. O6-methylguanine DNA methyltransferase gene promoter methylation status in gliomas and its correlation with other molecular alterations: first Indian report with review of challenges for use in customized treatment. Neurosurgery 2010;67:1681.

73. Cancer Genome Atlas Research Network. Comprehensive genomic characterization defines human glioblastoma genes and core pathways. Nature 2008;455:1061.

74. Noushmehr H, Weisenberger DJ, Diefes K, et al. Identification of a CpG island methylator phenotype that defines a distinct subgroup of glioma. Cancer Cell 2010;17:510.

75. Laffaire J, Everhard S, Idbaih A, et al. Methylation profiling identifies 2 groups of gliomas according to their tumorigenesis. Neuro Oncol 2011;13:84.

76. Verhaak RG, Hoadley KA, Purdom E, et al. Integrated genomic analysis identifies clinically relevant subtypes of glioblastoma characterized by abnormalities in PDGFRA, IDH1, EGFR, and NF1. Cancer Cell 2010;17:98.

77. Ducray F, Mokhtari K, Criniere E, et al. Diagnostic and prognostic value of alpha internexin expression in a series of 409 gliomas. Eur J Cancer 2011;47:802.

78. Mokhtari K, Ducray F, Kros JM, et al. Alpha-internexin expression predicts outcome in anaplastic oligodendroglial tumors and may positively impact the efficacy of chemotherapy: European organization for research and treatment of cancer trial 26951. Cancer 2011;117:3014.

79. Setty P, Hammes J, Rothamel T, et al. A pyrose-quencing-based assay for the rapid detection of IDH1 mutations in clinical samples. J Mol Diagn 2010;12:750.

80. Meyer J, Pusch S, Balss J, et al. PCR- and restriction endonuclease-based detection of IDH1 mutations. Brain Pathol 2010;20:298.

81. Boisselier B, Marie Y, Labussiere M, et al. COLD PCR HRM: a highly sensitive detection method for IDH1 mutations. Hum Mutat 2010;31:1360.

82. Horbinski C, Kelly L, Nikiforov YE, et al. Detection of IDH1 and IDH2 mutations by fluorescence melting curve analysis as a diagnostic tool for brain biopsies. J Mol Diagn 2010;12:487.

83. Kato Y, Jin G, Kuan CT, et al. A monoclonal antibody IMab-1 specifically recognizes IDH1R132H, the most common glioma-derived mutation. Biochem Biophys Res Commun 2009;390:547.

84. Preusser M, Wohrer A, Stary S, et al. Value and limitations of immunohistochemistry and gene sequencing for detection of the IDH1-R132H mutation in diffuse glioma biopsy specimens. J Neuropathol Exp Neurol 2011;70:715.

85. Gupta R, Webb-Myers R, Flanagan S, et al. Isocitrate dehydrogenase mutations in diffuse gliomas: clinical and aetiological implications. J Clin Pathol 2011;64:835.

86. Ikota H, Nobusawa S, Tanaka Y, et al. High-throughput immunohistochemical profiling of primary brain tumors and non-neoplastic systemic organs with a specific antibody against the mutant isocitrate dehydrogenase 1 R132H protein. Brain Tumor Pathol 2011;28:107.

87. Kaneko MK, Tian W, Takano S, et al. Establishment of a novel monoclonal antibody SMab-1 specific for IDH1-R132S mutation. Biochem Biophys Res Commun 2011;406:608.

88. De Carli E, Wang X, Puget S. IDH1 and IDH2 mutations in gliomas. N Engl J Med 2009;360:2248 [author reply: 2249].

89. Reitman ZJ, Parsons DW, Yan H. IDH1 and IDH2: not your typical oncogenes. Cancer Cell 2010;17:215.

Passive Immunotherapeutic Strategies for the Treatment of Malignant Gliomas

Daniel T. Nagasawa, MD[a], Christina Fong, BS[a],
Andrew Yew, MD[a], Marko Spasic, BA[a],
Heather M. Garcia, BS[a], Carol A. Kruse, PhD[a,b],
Isaac Yang, MD[a,b],*

KEYWORDS

- Malignant gliomas • Glioblastoma multiforme • Passive immunotherapy • Cellular therapy
- Brain tumors

KEY POINTS

- Glioblastoma multiforme has a proclivity for widespread invasion and destruction of healthy parenchyma, displaying a poor outcome despite aggressive conventional treatment.
- Immunotherapy offers the potential to selectively target tumor cells, thereby decreasing collateral damage to normal brain.
- Passive immunotherapy includes administration of monoclonal antibodies and the adoptive transfer of lymphocyte-activated killer cells or cytotoxic T lymphocytes.
- Although many clinical trials have demonstrated promising results, further prospective randomized studies will be necessary to validate the effects of various passive immunotherapeutic approaches.

Malignant gliomas are the most common primary intracranial tumor, with a proclivity for widespread invasion and rampant destruction of healthy parenchyma. This infiltrative process affords high-grade gliomas protection from traditional therapies and subjects the adjacent normal tissue to potential damage from nonspecific treatment modalities.[1,2] Immunotherapies involving antibodies or sensitized effector cells can offer selective targeting of protein-carbohydrate complexes on tumor cell surfaces that distinguish neoplastic from noncancerous cells.[1,3] Consequently, the treatment of malignant gliomas may be enhanced not only by increased specificity for tumor tissue but also from decreased toxicity to the host's healthy cells.[1] This review focuses on published findings from the use of passive immunotherapy for the treatment of high-grade gliomas, particularly glioblastoma multiforme (GBM).

PASSIVE IMMUNOTHERAPY

Passive immunotherapy can be broadly categorized into 2 treatment approaches: one that relies on the administration of antibodies that may

Daniel Nagasawa (first author) was partially supported by an American Brain Tumor Association Medical Student Summer Fellowship in Honor of Connie Finc. Carol Kruse (sixth author) was supported in part by NIH R01CA121258, R01CA125244, and R01CA154256. Isaac Yang (senior author) was partially supported by an Eli and Edythe Broad Center of Regenerative Medicine and Stem Cell Research UCLA Scholars in Translational Medicine Program Award, Visionary Fund Grant, and the Stein Oppenheimer Endowment Award.
a Department of Neurosurgery, University of California Los Angeles, 695 Charles East Young Drive South, Gonda 3357, Los Angeles, CA 90095-1761, USA; b Jonsson Comprehensive Cancer Center, University of California Los Angeles, 8-684 Factor Building, Box 951781, Los Angeles, CA 90095-1781, USA
* Corresponding author. UCLA Department of Neurosurgery, UCLA Jonsson Comprehensive Cancer Center, University of California, Los Angeles, David Geffen School of Medicine at UCLA, 695 Charles East Young Drive South, UCLA Gonda 3357, Los Angeles, CA 90095-1761.
E-mail address: iyang@mednet.ucla.edu

Neurosurg Clin N Am 23 (2012) 481–495
doi:10.1016/j.nec.2012.04.008
1042-3680/12/$ – see front matter © 2012 Elsevier Inc. All rights reserved.

further be coupled to a toxic counterpart molecule or one involving the adoptive transfer of an activated immune cell effector component to act against a neoplasm in the host. For cellular therapy, the most common types have included the adoptive transfer of nonspecifically activated lymphocyte-activated killer (LAK) cells or specifically sensitized cytotoxic T lymphocytes (CTLs).[4,5] In adoptive immunotherapy (AIT), patients' native immune cells are extracted and then activated ex vivo to increase antitumor activity. These cells are then reinfused back into the patients either intravenously or directly placed into the tumor resection cavity. Another technique of passive immunotherapy involves monoclonal antibodies (mAbs). Antibody-mediated immunotherapy uses mAbs to induce lymphocyte recruitment and complement system activation, thereby resulting in tumor cytotoxicity. In addition, radiolabeled antibodies may deliver localized radiation to the target-specific neoplastic tissue, with subsequent induction of cell death.

AIT: LAK CELLS

LAK cells are nonspecific effector cells that are derived from peripheral blood mononuclear cells (PBMC) and activated ex vivo with high-concentration interleukin 2 (IL-2) (T-cell growth factor) to induce antitumor properties.[6–10] IL-2 is an endogenously produced cytokine that aids in the host's natural immune system and is available in recombinant form to facilitate LAK cell generation.[8–17] The LAK cell's cytolytic properties against numerous tumor types have been demonstrated in various models, with the enhanced capability of destroying natural killer (NK) cell–resistant malignant gliomas and sparing of normal parenchyma.[8,18–26] Furthermore, it has been suggested that the use of IL-2/LAK cell immunotherapy may possess preventative properties against metastasis and recurrence of disease because intraventricular administration can induce a systemic response.[8] Yet, given the high toxicity of intravenous IL-2, local administration of this cytokine has been adopted for an increased therapeutic response and decreased morbidity.[8,27–29] In addition, LAK cells are unable to migrate to tumor sites, necessitating local therapeutic administration at the surgical resection cavity.[30] However, LAK AIT has remained limited, in part, by the need for leukapheresis to obtain significantly therapeutic numbers of LAK cells, a costly process that may inhibit its use for many patients with GBM.

Nevertheless, 12 trials[8,25,26,29,31–38] including 211 patients (170 GBM) have been reported using LAK cell AIT for the treatment of recurrent high-grade gliomas. Although historically disappointing, more recent findings have demonstrated improvement in median survival for patients with GBM compared with control groups.[25]

In most studies, patients were included at the time of relapse and received 1 to 15 injections, containing 10^6 to 10^{10} injected LAK cells. Adverse effects included neurologic toxicity, cerebral edema, aseptic meningitis, and hypereosinophlia.[7,39] However, the local presence of eosinophils has been positively correlated with long-term survival and may be an indicator of treatment response.[8]

Efficacy was typically reported based on radiological criteria, demonstrating 5 complete responses (CR), 13 partial responses (PR), and 6 stable diseases (SD) in a total of 118 patients.[36] Of the data exclusive to 88 GBM patients, the investigators reported 3 CR (3.4%), 8 PR (11.0%), and 6 SD (6.8%). However, these figures do not include the beneficial results observed in the two most recent studies that included 73 patients with GBM.[25,31] In the most promising of studies, Dillman and colleagues[25] reported results of their phase II clinical trial demonstrating a 20.5-month median survival and 75% 1-year survival rate in 40 patients with GBM treated with intralesional autologous LAK cells; this has been the only report thus far investigating patients with newly diagnosed GBM treated with LAK cells. In addition, patients who received higher doses of CD3+/CD16+/CD56+ (T-NK) cells were found to have an increased survival advantage compared with those with lower T-NK cell counts that presumably resulted from steroid use during the month before leukapheresis. Given these findings, the investigators conducted a 2-arm, randomized phase II trial using either intralesional LAK cells or carmustine (Gliadel) wafers, following standard treatment with surgical resection and radio- and chemotherapy with temozolomide. Results of this study are currently pending publication.

Additionally, 3 other trials have also demonstrated improved median survival for patients with GBM compared with control groups. In a study preceding this last one, Dillman and colleagues[31] reported findings of 31 patients with recurrent GBM tumors, surviving a median time of 17.5 months from the date of the original diagnosis, compared with 13.6 months for a control group. Hayes and colleagues[33] reported results of 19 total patients with recurrent malignant gliomas, demonstrating a median survival for 15 cases of GBM of 53 weeks after reoperation versus 25.5 weeks for patients treated with conventional therapy alone. In a subsequent report, Hayes and colleagues[8] presented results of 15 patients with recurrent GBM (28 total cases of recurrent malignant gliomas) improving median survival with similar findings as reported in their previous study.

However, findings from various other clinical trials using LAK cell immunotherapy have not indicated successful in vivo antitumor efficacy. In a study with 10 patients with recurrent malignant primary brain tumors (4 GBM), Sankhla and colleagues[32] reported no improvement in overall survival compared with patients receiving standard treatments, although partial and transient clinical responses were seen in 2 patients with grade II to III astrocytomas. Similarly, Jeffes and colleagues[36] failed to identify any significant relationship between clinical improvement and radiological response in 19 patients with recurrent gliomas, 14 of which had GBM. Merchant and colleagues. reported findings of 13 patients with recurrent GBM resulting in a median survival of less than 6 months and a 16% 60-day postoperative mortality.[25,38] Barba and colleagues[37] discussed findings for 9 patients in which 5 experienced significant toxicity and more than half were deceased within 4 months, with a 33% 60-day postoperative mortality. Similarly, Lillehei and colleagues[29] evaluated 11 patients with recurrent high-grade gliomas (9 GBM) and reported a median survival of less than 5 months following LAK cell therapy. Morbidity related to vascular leak syndrome caused by high-dose IL-2 was of considerable concern.

Given the findings that responders were noted more so in patients with lower-grade glioma and that there is now a precedent for treating patients with GBM earlier, additional prospective randomized trials will be necessary to fully elucidate the therapeutic potential of nonspecifically activated LAK cells in the management of patients with GBM.

AIT: CTL

Unlike LAK cells, AIT using CTL is advantageous because of its ability to migrate to target-specific antigens following administration. Furthermore, a T-cell subset has the capability to persist as memory cells, allowing for an extended period of antitumor response.[40] CTLs are most commonly generated by antigenic stimulation of PBMCs with autologous inactivated tumor cells (ATC).[39,41,42] This strong ex vivo priming of T cells overcomes the weak in vivo T-cell immune response to endogenous tumor-antigen stimulation.[43] Furthermore, CTLs can be expanded ex vivo to increase the numbers of effector T cells for adoptive transfer, compared with active immunotherapy relying on in situ or endogenous immune cell expansion.[44]

Various other methods of CTL generation have also been investigated, including the use of autologous HLA-displaying lymphocytes for allogeneic CTL stimulation.[43] In addition, CTL extraction from tumor-infiltrating lymphocytes (TIL) following IL-2 amplification, as well as lymphocyte collection from lymph nodes/PBMCs following stimulation with granulocyte-macrophage colony-stimulating factor and irradiated ATCs, have all been examined as sufficient means of collecting adequate quantities of T cells.[45–50] However, the lymphocytes obtained from these tumor-draining lymph nodes are pre-effector cells. As such, in vitro activation of the antitumor functions of these cells, in addition to the expansion of cells sensitized in situ, is required before their reinjection.[51]

To date, 4 phase I trials examining CTLs generated from PBMCs[39,41–43] and 1 pilot study using TILs[45] (**Fig. 1**) have been reported in the literature, investigating intracranial administration in a total of 30 patients with high-grade gliomas (19 GBM). A combined approach using strategies from both active and passive immunotherapy was examined in 3 phase I[46–48] and 2 pilot studies[49,50] in which CTLs of 62 patients (49 GBM) were extracted from lymph nodes or PBMCs after intradermal vaccination and reinjected either intravenously or by intracarotid infusion. In contrast to passive immunotherapy, active immunotherapeutic strategies attempt to sensitize the immune system using tumor-associated antigen vaccinations to activate endogenous tumor-specific T cells. Of these 10 total CTL immunotherapy clinical trials, patients received between 1 and 13 injections of CTL cells, ranging from 3×10^7 to 10×10^{10} cells,[7] and there were no grade III/IV adverse events.

Clinical trials using CTL AIT for the treatment of high-grade gliomas in a total of 92 patients (68 GBM) have resulted in 3 CR, 27 PR, and 16 SD.[49,52] However, of the data exclusively with 52 patients with GBM, the investigators reported 11 PR (21.2%) and 4 SD (7.7%). Although Sloan and colleagues[50] did not distinguish between tumor grades when reporting immunotherapeutic responses for their 19 patients (16 GBM), a favorable total of 1 CR (5.3%), 7 PR (36.8%), and 9 SD (47.4%) were documented for all of their patients.

Although a few studies demonstrated a survival benefit, many of these small phase I or I/II trials were not clinically designed or supported to effectively analyze survival outcomes against a control group.[7] Sloan and colleagues[50] reported an improved median survival of 12 months after tumor recurrence compared with 6 months for their historical controls. In addition, they demonstrated a correlation between increased survival with radiological response and a positive delayed-type hypersensitivity reaction. Likewise, Wood and colleagues[49] described a positive association between the concentration of CD8+ T cells in vaccine injections and clinical response. In their

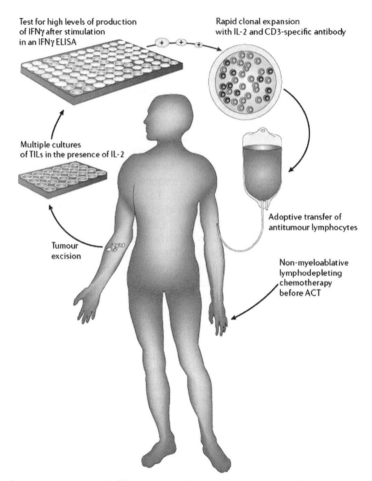

Fig. 1. A protocol for AIT using tumor-infiltrating lymphocytes in a patient with melanoma. A similar protocol may be used for patients with GBM, with adoptive transfer of CTLs directly into the tumor resection cavity. ACT, adoptive cell transfer; ELISA, enzyme-linked immunosorbent assay; IFN, interferon. (*From* Gattinoni L, Powell DJ Jr, Rosenberg SA, et al. Adoptive immunotherapy for cancer: building on success. Nat Rev Immunol 2006;6(5):383–93; This figure was reproduced with the kind permission of the Nature Publishing Group.)

study using autologous TIL, Quattrocchi and colleagues[45] suggested that the immunotherapeutic benefits of AIT may be patient-dependent because their case of complete response revealed a unique population of CD8+CD56+ cells. Kitahara and colleagues[41] found 1 of 4 patients with GBM to display a PR. Kruse and colleagues[43] found that 3 of 3 patients with World Health Organization grade III recurrent glioma demonstrated a long-term response, but no response was displayed by the 3 patients with GBM treated with intratumoral alloreactive CTL. The 12 patients with GBM treated by Holladay and colleagues[46] showed no responders; however, there was a significant relationship between adoptive T-cell immunotherapy and delayed recurrence of gliomas. Plautz and colleagues[47] reported on the limited efficacy of CTL immunotherapy; only 2 of 9 patients with

GBM demonstrated partial tumor regression. In a subsequent study, they identified only 1 of 6 patients with GBM to display a PR.[40] Similarly, Wood and colleagues[49] reported findings in 6 patients with recurrent GBM in which only 1 displayed partial transient decreased tumor growth.

Genetic Modulation of Adoptive T Cells

Ngo and colleagues suggested that the inability of AIT to produce more consistently promising results may be caused by functionally variable strengths of transferred cells and the proclivity of solid tumors to evade the human immune system by various techniques (**Fig. 2**).[53] Passive downregulation of major histocompatibility complex (MHC) or costimulatory molecules conceal tumors from T-cell targeting, whereas active expression of

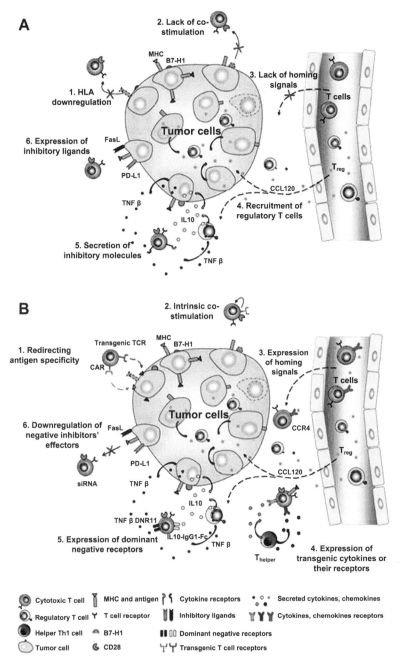

Fig. 2. Various mechanisms of (*A*) immune system evasion: (1) HLA down-regulation, (2) costimulation suppression, (3) homing signal suppression, (4) activation of Treg and Th2 subsets, (5) production of immunosuppressive cytokines, and (6) upregulation of inhibitory ligands; and (*B*) genetic modulations to counter the glioma microenvironment: (1) transgenic TCRs or CARs, (2) intrinsic costimulatory signals, (3) upregulation of homing signals, (4) production of transgenic cytokines, (5) dominant-negative receptors, and (6) depression of negative inhibition. CARs, chimeric antigen receptors; TCR, T-cell receptors; Th2, T helper type 2; Treg, T regulatory. (*From* Ngo MC, Rooney CM, Howard JM, et al. Ex vivo gene transfer for improved adoptive immunotherapy of cancer. Hum Mol Genet 2011;20(R1):R93–9. This figure was reproduced with the kind permission of Oxford University Press.)

inhibitory ligands and secretions allow for tumor escape from immune surveillance.[54] Furthermore, it may also be necessary to target brain tumor stem cells that display unique antigens.

Genetically modified CTLs may possess improved antitumor efficacy by their ability to counter the glioma's immunosuppressive microenvironment.[53] Specifically, augmentation with transgenic

T-cell receptors (TCRs) or chimeric antigen receptors (CARs) may facilitate increased quantities of tumor-specific T cells with a decreased reliance on tumor cell MHC expression. Morgan and colleagues[55] genetically engineered autologous T cells with a retroviral vector to display TCRs targeting the melanoma antigen recognized by T-cells (MART-1) melanoma antigen. Lymphocyte presence was detected up to a year following infusion, and tumor regression was documented in 4 of the 31 patients treated. However, because TCRs are limited in their function to MHC-matched tumors that have not yet evolved downregulation of their human leukocyte antigens (HLA), CARs may offer an alternative solution. These non–HLA-restricted synthetic receptors allow for targeted specificity without the disadvantage of dimerization with endogenous TCRs that may lead to loss of function in transgenic TCRs. CARs confer the added benefits of antigen recognition within a spectrum of posttranslational modifications,[56] with an increased binding affinity and a more stable immunologic synapse than those created by TCRs.[57] A phase I/II clinical trial investigating the effects of cytomegalovirus-specific CTLs expressing CARs targeting human epidermal growth factor receptor 2 (HER-2) in patients with GBM is currently underway, which may have the potential of destroying HER-2–positive CD133+ glioma cells.[58] However, concerns may arise from the potential binding to low-avidity off-target antigens[59] and adverse effects from supraphysiologic signaling activation induced by on-target cytokine expression.[53] Consequently, various safety mechanisms have been considered. For instance, suicide genes, such as the herpes simplex viral thymidine kinase gene or the inducible caspase 9 transgene (iCaspase9), are being incorporated to provide for their elimination should serious adverse reactions occur.[60,61]

Other genetic modifications to TCRs have also been postulated. Receptors specific for tumor-secreted chemokines may enhance T-cell homing to optimal tumor-specific sites.[53] Furthermore, T cells may be modified for transgenic expression of activating cytokines, such as IL-2 and IL-15. This action frees lymphocyte reliance on endogenous costimulatory factors for the activation and maintenance of functionality. In preclinical models, this technique applied in vivo has demonstrated increased antigen-specific T-cell expansion and enhanced antitumor activity.[62]

Dominant-negative receptors[63,64] and other genetic modifications[53] may also be used to enable T cells to overcome immunosuppressive factors present in the tumor microenvironment or immunosuppressive drug therapies. Transforming growth factor β (TGFβ) is one of the most potent inhibitory

cytokines and TGFβ2 is notably upregulated in patients with GBM.[65,66] In vitro studies and murine models of TGFβ-secreting Epstein-Barr virus–positive lymphoma have demonstrated T-cell resilience following the transgenic expression of dominant-negative TGFβ type II receptors.[67] A similar approach to circumvent the immunosuppressive effects of IL-10 is also being investigated.[68]

Despite the inconclusive results reported in the literature, adoptive transfer of CTL immunotherapy may be a promising treatment of GBM, necessitating further prospective trials to elucidate its potential effects. Studies that combine active immunotherapy with passive immunotherapy are also showing promise.[69] Furthermore, genetic modifications of CTLs may be a worthwhile approach to optimize the benefits of this technique for enhanced patient outcomes.

ANTIBODY-MEDIATED IMMUNOTHERAPY

Another passive immunotherapy strategy involves the use of monoclonal antibodies, which possess the capability of targeted tumor-antigen specificity with high binding affinity.[70] mAbs may be used either alone or coupled to radiation-emitting particles or toxins.[1] Yet, in order for mAbs immunotherapy to be effective, it has been suggested that GBM cells should display an epitope with a minimum of 10^5 surface markers per cell and maintain a low turnover time. Furthermore, the antigen should be glioma-associated to prevent damage to healthy brain parenchyma.[71]

Unlabeled Monoclonal Antibodies

The proposed mechanism of action for unlabeled mAbs involves the combination of several processes (**Fig. 3**). Although one of the major functions of this immunotherapeutic technique allows for the opsonization of glioma cells and induction of antibody-dependent cellular cytotoxicity (ADCC), mAb binding may also result in cross-linking or blocking of membrane receptors, with subsequent modulation of transmembrane molecular pathway signaling. Such activity may promote further cascades leading to decreased tumor growth and cellular apoptosis.[72–74] These concepts were supported by Bleeker and colleagues; they demonstrated anti–epidermal growth factor receptor (EGFR) mAb-induced cell death resulting from a combination of ADCC and a disruption of EGF signaling.[75]

In high-grade gliomas, EGFR is estimated to be overexpressed or mutated in 40% to 50% of all tumors.[1] EGFR activation is thought to induce cellular proliferation, motility, and increased tumor cell survival via downstream signaling related

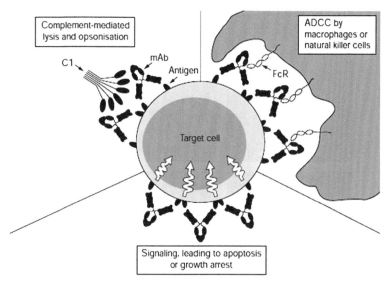

Fig. 3. Mechanisms of action for unlabeled monoclonal antibodies used in passive immunotherapy for the treatment of GBM. Antigen binding can induce subsequent C1 complement binding, activate antibody-dependent cellular cytotoxicity, or alter signaling pathways leading to reduced tumor growth or apoptosis. ADCC, antibody-dependent cellular cytotoxicity. (*From* Cragg MS, French RR, Glennie MJ. Signaling antibodies in cancer therapy. Cur Opin Immunol 1999;11(5):541–7; This figure was reproduced with the kind permission of Elsevier.)

to the PI3K/Akt, Ras/Raf/Mek/ERK, and PLC-gamma/PKC pathways.[76] Cetuximab is a mAb that has been demonstrated to inhibit the conformational changes necessary for EGFR to dimerize, thus preventing aberrant ligand-independent activation and signaling.[77] Confirmation of cetuximab's effects have been suggested by preclinical studies reporting GBM growth inhibition and increased apoptosis.[78,79] In a phase I/II trial with 17 patients with GBM, anti-EGFR mAb therapy demonstrated a median follow-up of 13 months. The investigators reported a 6-month progression-free survival (PFS) of 81%, whereas 87% of the patients were still alive at 1 year.[1] Neyns and colleagues[80] investigated the effects of cetuximab in 55 patients (**Fig. 4**) with recurrent GBM (28 with EGFR amplification and 27 without), noting evidence of some radiographic response (3 PR, 16 SD) but no overall improved outcome in survival. In a phase II trial combining cetuximab, bevacizumab (vascular endothelial growth factor [VEGF] inhibitor), and irinotecan (topoisomerase-1 inhibitor) for the treatment of 32 patients with recurrent GBM, available data for 27 patients demonstrated 1 CR (3.7%), 8 PR (30.0%), and 5 minor responses (18.5%, defined as 25%–50% regression and clinical improvement).[1]

Another promising antigen includes the EGFR variant III (EGFRvIII) protein.[81–84] EGFRvIII is restricted to only cancer cells and has been expressed in approximately 40% of all GBM cases. Furthermore, this EGFR mutation confers constitutively active signaling, resulting in increased tumor proliferation, invasion, and apoptotic resistance.[85,86] In animal models of brain tumors, the administration of anti-EGFRvIII mAbs have resulted in decreased tumor volume and increased survival.[85,87–90] Similarly, intratumoral administration of Y10 (mAb to an EGFRvIII murine homolog) for the treatment of EGFRvIII-expressing B16 melanoma increased the median survival by 286%.[91] Despite these promising preclinical results, there have not yet been any reports from clinical trials evaluating mAb for EGFRvIII targeting of GBM.[1] However, one phase I trial of 7 patients with various tumor types, including one anaplastic astrocytoma, showed the effects of a chimeric form of mAb 806 (ch806, one of the most tumor-specific EGFRvIII mAb), to demonstrate excellent target specificity, no evidence of normal tissue uptake, no significant toxicity, and stabilization of the patient's glioma.[92] Furthermore, an EGFRvIII-targeted dsFv-PE38K-DEL single fragment chain Pseudomonas exotoxin construct (MR1-1) is being used in a clinical trial for the treatment of patients with GBM.[85]

Other immunotherapeutic targets include the VEGF receptor. Literature suggests that glioma angiogenesis is the manifestation of definitive genetic mutations resulting in characteristic microvascular proliferation seen in GBM histopathology.[93,94] VEGF plays a role in endothelial cell survival, proliferation, invasion, and migration, which all

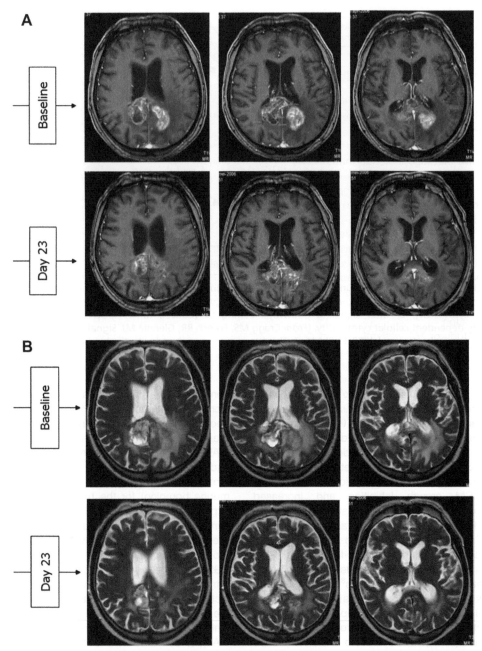

Fig. 4. (*A*) T1-weighted and (*B*) T2-weighted axial postcontrast magnetic resonance imaging of a patient with GBM at baseline and day 23 posttreatment with cetuximab. (*From* Neyns B, Sadones J, Joosens E, et al. Stratified phase II trial of cetuximab in patients with recurrent high-grade glioma. Ann Oncol 2009;20(9):1596–603. This figure was reproduced with the kind permission of Oxford University Press.)

participate in angiogenesis and tumor progression.[95] GBM have high levels of VEGF compared with other malignancies; high expression correlates with poor prognosis.[96,97] Accordingly, several studies have examined the therapeutic value of antiangiogenic mAbs, particularly bevacizumab, for GBM treatment.

In 2009, the Food and Drug Administration (FDA) approved bevacizumab for recurrent GBM based on its phase II demonstration of high treatment response rates and promising clinical improvements.[98] The first use of this therapy was by Dr Stark-Vance who treated 21 patients with recurrent GBM; this group documented a 43% response rate (1 CR, 8 PR).[99] Vredenburgh and colleagues[100] reported the administration of bevacizumab and irinotecan in 32 recurrent malignant gliomas (23 GBM) resulting in radiographic responses in 14 patients with GBM (61% of 23), with a 20-week median PFS and nearly doubled PFS at 6 months compared with control groups. However, overall survival was not significantly improved. These findings were reaffirmed in a retrospective review of 55 patients (33 GBM) that also included irinotecan.[101] However, Fine and colleagues[102] reported results from a phase II study of 79 patients with recurrent GBM treated with bevacizumab alone, establishing a 60% response rate, 30% PFS at 6 months, and a reduction in toxicity. Given the decreased adverse events and similar therapeutic effects of bevacizumab alone compared with other studies that have included the concurrent administration of irinotecan, the added benefits of this topoisomerase-1 inhibitor have been a point of investigation.

In a study of 167 patients with recurrent GBM assigned to either bevacizumab alone or in combination with irinotecan, response rates, PFS at 6 months, and median overall survival were 28% and 38%, 43% and 50%, and 9.2 months and 8.7 months, respectively.[103] However, despite these statistics, the median overall survival did not demonstrate clinically substantial improvements.[104–106] In a randomized trial by de Groot and colleagues,[99] they demonstrated an improvement in both the response rate and PFS with the addition of irinotecan, yet the median overall survival for both groups did not differ from historical controls. In a study evaluating bevacizumab alone, then in combination with irinotecan, Kreisl and colleagues[107] reported findings for 48 patients with recurrent GBM. Median PFS was 16 weeks, PFS at 6 months was 29%, and median overall survival was 31 weeks. Similar findings were reported in a recent study regarding outcomes in 225 patients with recurrent high-grade glioma (176 GBM) treated with bevacizumab alone or in combination with chemotherapy.[108] In summary, many investigations have evaluated the potential of chemotherapeutic agents in conjunction with bevacizumab, with most demonstrating clinical outcomes equivalent to those produced by anti-VEGF monotherapy.[100,103,109–112]

Although many previous studies have failed to identify an improvement in overall survival with the incorporation of bevacizumab to their treatment regimen, other trials have demonstrated more success.[95,100,103,107,110] Vredenburg and colleagues[96] later evaluated 75 patients with newly diagnosed GBM in a phase II trial for treatment with bevacizumab and irinotecan. Despite moderate toxicity in which 19 patients (25%) had to withdraw from the study early, results were promising. Compared with historical controls, this investigation demonstrated an improvement in median overall survival (21.2 months) and median PFS (14.2 months). These findings were similar to those of Lai and colleagues in which their phase II study of bevacizumab in patients with newly diagnosed GBM demonstrated an improved median overall survival of 19.6 months.[96,113] The experience of the University of California, Los Angeles group with bevacizumab has largely shown benefit radiographically, thus indicating that it may replace the need for high-dose steroids. In addition, a recent study of 14 recurrent high-grade gliomas (11 GBM) treated with bevacizumab and irinotecan within the Chinese population demonstrated an overall response detected within 9 patients with GBM (3 CR, 6PR), a median PFS of 6 months, a PFS at 6 months of 64%, and a median overall survival of 17 months.[114]

Since its inception, overall radiographic response and PFS following bevacizumab administration have achieved improvements up to fourfold greater than historical controls.[103,107,115–117] However, given the general lack of improvement to median overall survival, the true benefits of this antiangiogenic mAb remain controversial. Wong and colleagues[98] conducted a 15-study meta-analysis of 548 patients with recurrent GBM treated with bevacizumab. Their efforts demonstrated a 45% PFS at 6 months, 76% 6-month survival rate, and a 9.3-month overall survival, with no clear evidence of a dose-response benefit. Their 84% response rate included 6% CR, 49% PR, and 29% with SD. However, it has been suggested that radiological responses, on which demonstration of antitumor efficacy has been traditionally based, may represent the normalization of blood-brain-barrier function and resultant decreased contrast enhancement rather than valid glioma stability or regression. This concept has been supported by the findings of Norden and colleagues in which patients treated with bevacizumab demonstrated a lack of contrast enhancement, yet still displayed significant tumor dissemination.[101,104] This notion was the basis for which the European Medicines Agency denied approval for bevacizumab for recurrent GBM, stating that radiological response rates may not be the most appropriate measure of drug efficacy.[118] Furthermore, it has been postulated that the use of anti-VEGF treatment may induce a more invasive lesion with normal vessel cooption.[96,99] Given the continued controversy regarding the use of bevacizumab and its therapeutic benefits, further investigations will be necessary to establish the true value of this approach, with several phase III trials currently underway.[119] With the recent withdrawal of bevacizumab for breast cancer and the fast-tracked FDA approval of it for GBM, we may see withdrawal of this approval soon until better data become available to demonstrate its effects.

Radiolabeled Monoclonal Antibodies

Radiolabeled monoclonal antibodies confer added advantage over their unlabeled counterparts by providing delivered therapeutics. Similar to radiotherapy, treatment with radiolabeled mAbs uses radiation to induce cell death, with the enhanced benefit of an increased target specificity.

Emrich and colleagues[120] evaluated the use of ^{125}I-coupled mAbs against human A431 carcinoma cells, which have been demonstrated to display high concentrations of EGFR. In their phase II study of 180 patients of which 118 had a diagnosis of GBM, the overall median survival was 13.4 months for the patients with GBM, demonstrating a significant improvement in outcome. Furthermore, GBM patients less than 40 years old with a Karnofsky Performance Score greater than 70 had a median survival of 25.4 months. Casaco and colleagues[121] investigated the role of ^{188}Re (beta and gamma radionuclide) paired with nimotuzumab (anti-EGFR mAb) in 11 patients with recurrent malignant gliomas, 8 of which were GBM; there were 2 patients with CR (1 GBM), 1 with PR (1 GBM), and 2 with SD (1 GBM). However, no improvement in overall survival was reported, and 2 of 4 patients experienced severe adverse events, including hemorrhagic brain necrosis. Yet, in a recent study representing the largest series evaluating the use of radioimmunotherapy, Li and colleagues[122] reported findings of their phase II trial investigating ^{125}I-mAb 425 (anti-EGFR) for the treatment of newly diagnosed GBM in 192 patients. They demonstrated no National Cancer Institute common toxicities at grades 3/4 and an overall median survival of 15.7 months. Subgroup analysis determined that although those treated with ^{125}I-mAb 425 alone had an overall median survival of 14.5 months, those treated concurrently with temozolomide survived 20.2 months, indicating there may be no interference in the therapeutic effects of both agents when given simultaneously.

Another target of interest involves the extracellular matrix protein, tenascin-C, expressed in more than 90% of all GBM cases and implicated in glioma-associated angiogenesis.[71,123] Its function has been implicated in adhesion, migration, and proliferation, with increased expression being correlated with higher grades of tumor malignancy.[124–127] Riva and colleagues[128] reported findings for the treatment of 105 patients (58 GBM) with ^{131}I-labeled antitenascin mAbs (81C6). Their study identified a statistically significant improvement in survival (23 months) compared with controls, whereas others have demonstrated similar responses with increased stabilization of disease.[128–130] In another investigation of 21 patients with newly diagnosed malignant glioma (16 GBM) treated with 81C6, median overall survival was 91 weeks, with 87% of GBM patients alive at 1 year.[131,132] On later follow-up, the investigators found an average time to progression of 18 months and median overall survival of nearly 2 years.[1]

In a study by Zalutsky and colleagues,[133] 18 patients with recurrent high-grade gliomas (14 GBM) were treated with maximal surgical resection followed by ^{211}At (alpha-particle emitter) coupled with chimeric antitenascin mAbs. Alpha particles enable high-intensity radiation over short distances of 1 to 2 mm, thus targeting tumor cells at the resected margin. The investigators reported no grade 3/4 adverse reactions and a favorable 52-week median overall survival compared with 23 to 31 weeks observed for patients receiving conventional therapies.

Despite these promising results, there are still many obstacles that must be overcome before the treatment of GBM using monoclonal antibodies is optimized. One problem involves the host's immune system forming endogenous antibodies against the transferred mAbs. Furthermore, mAbs from passive immunotherapy may react with antigen-positive normal tissue causing collateral damage to healthy brain parenchyma. However, approaches that use intratumoral infusion of mAb may be capable of minimizing these potential complications.[71]

SUMMARY

The use of passive immunotherapeutic approaches for the treatment of GBM represents a promising adjuvant to current management strategies. However, given inconsistent findings between various studies, future prospective randomized trials will be necessary to validate the added benefits that the administration of LAK cells, CTLs, and mAbs may confer to this patient population.

REFERENCES

1. Mitra S, Li G, Harsh GR. Passive antibody-mediated immunotherapy for the treatment of malignant gliomas. Neurosurg Clin North Am 2010;21(1): 67–76.

2. Furnari FB, Fenton T, Bachoo RM, et al. Malignant astrocytic glioma: genetics, biology, and paths to treatment. Genes Dev 2007;21(21):2683–710.

3. Bolesta E, Kowalczyk A, Wierzbicki A, et al. DNA vaccine expressing the mimotope of GD2 ganglioside induces protective GD2 cross-reactive antibody responses. Cancer Res 2005;65(8):3410–8.

4. Herrlinger U, Weller M, Schabet M. New aspects of immunotherapy of leptomeningeal metastasis. J Neurooncol 1998;38(2–3):233–9.

5. Tjoa BA, Murphy GP. Progress in active specific immunotherapy of prostate cancer. Semin Surg Oncol 2000;18(1):80–7.

6. Quan WD Jr, Palackdharry CS. Common cancers–immunotherapy and multidisciplinary therapy: parts III and IV. Dis Mon 1997;43(11):745–808.

7. Vauleon E, Avril T, Collet B, et al. Overview of cellular immunotherapy for patients with glioblastoma. Clin Dev Immunol 2010;2010:689171.

8. Hayes RL, Arbit E, Odaimi M, et al. Adoptive cellular immunotherapy for the treatment of malignant gliomas. Crit Rev Oncol Hematol 2001; 39(1–2):31–42.

9. Lotze MT, Grimm EA, Mazumder A, et al. Lysis of fresh and cultured autologous tumor by human lymphocytes cultured in T-cell growth factor. Cancer Res 1981;41(11 Pt 1):4420–5.

10. Grimm EA, Mazumder A, Zhang HZ, et al. Lymphokine-activated killer cell phenomenon. Lysis of natural killer-resistant fresh solid tumor cells by interleukin 2-activated autologous human peripheral blood lymphocytes. J Exp Med 1982;155(6):1823–41.

11. Wang A, Lu SD, Mark DF. Site-specific mutagenesis of the human interleukin-2 gene: structure-function analysis of the cysteine residues. Science 1984;224(4656):1431–3.

12. Rosenberg SA, Lotze MT, Muul LM, et al. Observations on the systemic administration of autologous lymphokine-activated killer cells and recombinant interleukin-2 to patients with metastatic cancer. N Engl J Med 1985;313(23):1485–92.

13. Rosenberg SA, Lotze MT, Muul LM, et al. A progress report on the treatment of 157 patients with advanced cancer using lymphokine-activated killer cells and interleukin-2 or high-dose interleukin-2 alone. N Engl J Med 1987;316(15):889–97.

14. West WH, Tauer KW, Yannelli JR, et al. Constant-infusion recombinant interleukin-2 in adoptive immunotherapy of advanced cancer. N Engl J Med 1987;316(15):898–905.

15. Oldham RK. Cancer biotherapy: the first year. Cancer Biol Ther 1994;9(3):179–81.

16. Oldham RK, Blumenschein G, Schwartzberg L, et al. Combination biotherapy utilizing interleukin-2 and alpha interferon in patients with advanced cancer: a National Biotherapy Study Group trial. Mol Biother 1992;4(1):4–9.

17. Dillman RO, Church C, Oldham RK, et al. Inpatient continuous-infusion interleukin-2 in 788 patients with cancer. The National Biotherapy Study Group experience. Cancer 1993;71(7):2358–70.

18. Rosenstein M, Yron I, Kaufmann Y, et al. Lymphokine-activated killer cells: lysis of fresh syngeneic natural killer-resistant murine tumor cells by lymphocytes cultured in interleukin 2. Cancer Res 1984;44(5):1946–53.

19. Mule JJ, Shu S, Schwarz SL, et al. Adoptive immunotherapy of established pulmonary metastases with LAK cells and recombinant interleukin-2. Science 1984;225(4669):1487–9.

20. Mazumder A, Rosenberg SA. Successful immunotherapy of natural killer-resistant established pulmonary melanoma metastases by the intravenous adoptive transfer of syngeneic lymphocytes activated in vitro by interleukin 2. J Exp Med 1984; 159(2):495–507.

21. Ettinghausen SE, Lipford EH 3rd, Mule JJ, et al. Recombinant interleukin 2 stimulates in vivo proliferation of adoptively transferred lymphokine-activated killer (LAK) cells. J Immunol 1985; 135(5):3623–35.

22. Lafreniere R, Rosenberg SA. Successful immunotherapy of murine experimental hepatic metastases with lymphokine-activated killer cells and recombinant interleukin 2. Cancer Res 1985; 45(8):3735–41.

23. Kaaijk P, Troost D, Dast PK, et al. Cytolytic effects of autologous lymphokine-activated killer cells on organotypic multicellular spheroids of gliomas in vitro. Neuropathol Appl Neurobiol 1995;21(5):392–8.

24. George RE, Loudon WG, Moser RP, et al. In vitro cytolysis of primitive neuroectodermal tumors of the posterior fossa (medulloblastoma) by lymphokine-activated killer cells. J Neurosurg 1988;69(3):403–9.

25. Dillman RO, Duma CM, Ellis RA, et al. Intralesional lymphokine-activated killer cells as adjuvant therapy for primary glioblastoma. J Immunother 2009;32(9):914–9.

26. Jacobs SK, Wilson DJ, Kornblith PL, et al. Interleukin-2 or autologous lymphokine-activated killer cell treatment of malignant glioma: phase I trial. Cancer Res 1986;46(4 Pt 2):2101–4.

27. Papa MZ, Vetto JT, Ettinghausen SE, et al. Effect of corticosteroid on the antitumor activity of lymphokine-activated killer cells and interleukin 2 in mice. Cancer Res 1986;46(11):5618–23.

28. Mulvin DW, Kruse CA, Mitchell DH, et al. Lymphokine-activated killer cells with interleukin-2: dose toxicity and localization in isolated perfused rat lungs. Mol Biother 1990;2(1):38–43.

29. Lillehei KO, Mitchell DH, Johnson SD, et al. Long-term follow-up of patients with recurrent malignant gliomas treated with adjuvant adoptive immunotherapy. Neurosurgery 1991;28(1):16–23.

30. Hook GR, Greenwood MA, Barba D, et al. Morphology of interleukin-2-stimulated human peripheral blood mononuclear effector cells killing glioma-derived tumor cells in vitro. J Natl Cancer Inst 1988;80(3):171–7.

31. Dillman RO, Duma CM, Schiltz PM, et al. Intracavitary placement of autologous lymphokine-activated killer (LAK) cells after resection of recurrent glioblastoma. J Immunother 2004;27(5): 398–404.

32. Sankhla SK, Nadkarni JS, Bhagwati SN. Adoptive immunotherapy using lymphokine-activated killer (LAK) cells and interleukin-2 for recurrent malignant primary brain tumors. J Neurooncol 1996; 27(2):133–40.

33. Hayes RL, Koslow M, Hiesiger EM, et al. Improved long term survival after intracavitary interleukin-2 and lymphokine-activated killer cells for adults with recurrent malignant glioma. Cancer 1995; 76(5):840–52.

34. Boiardi A, Silvani A, Ruffini PA, et al. Loco-regional immunotherapy with recombinant interleukin-2 and adherent lymphokine-activated killer cells (A-LAK) in recurrent glioblastoma patients. Cancer Immunol Immunother 1994;39(3):193–7.

35. Blancher A, Roubinet F, Grancher AS, et al. Local immunotherapy of recurrent glioblastoma multiforme by intracerebral perfusion of interleukin-2 and LAK cells. Eur Cytokine Netw 1993;4(5):331–41.

36. Jeffes EW 3rd, Beamer YB, Jacques S, et al. Therapy of recurrent high grade gliomas with surgery, and autologous mitogen activated IL-2 stimulated killer (MAK) lymphocytes: I. Enhancement of MAK lytic activity and cytokine production by PHA and clinical use of PHA. J Neurooncol 1993;15(2):141–55.

37. Barba D, Saris SC, Holder C, et al. Intratumoral LAK cell and interleukin-2 therapy of human gliomas. J Neurosurg 1989;70(2):175–82.

38. Merchant RE, Grant AJ, Merchant LH, et al. Adoptive immunotherapy for recurrent glioblastoma multiforme using lymphokine activated killer cells and recombinant interleukin-2. Cancer 1988;62(4): 665–71.

39. Tsuboi K, Saijo K, Ishikawa E, et al. Effects of local injection of ex vivo expanded autologous tumor-specific T lymphocytes in cases with recurrent malignant gliomas. Clin Cancer Res 2003; 9(9):3294–302.

40. Plautz GE, Shu S. Adoptive immunotherapy of CNS malignancies. Cancer Chemother Biol Response Modif 2001;19:327–38.

41. Kitahara T, Watanabe O, Yamaura A, et al. Establishment of interleukin 2 dependent cytotoxic T lymphocyte cell line specific for autologous brain tumor and its intracranial administration for therapy of the tumor. J Neurooncol 1987;4(4):329–36.

42. Tsurushima H, Liu SQ, Tuboi K, et al. Reduction of end-stage malignant glioma by injection with autologous cytotoxic T lymphocytes. Jpn J Cancer Res 1999;90(5):536–45.

43. Kruse CA, Cepeda L, Owens B, et al. Treatment of recurrent glioma with intracavitary alloreactive cytotoxic T lymphocytes and interleukin-2. Cancer Immunol Immunother 1997;45(2):77–87.

44. Cheever MA, Chen W. Therapy with cultured T cells: principles revisited. Immunol Rev 1997;157: 177–94.

45. Quattrocchi KB, Miller CH, Cush S, et al. Pilot study of local autologous tumor infiltrating lymphocytes for the treatment of recurrent malignant gliomas. J Neurooncol 1999;45(2):141–57.

46. Holladay FP, Heitz-Turner T, Bayer WL, et al. Autologous tumor cell vaccination combined with adoptive cellular immunotherapy in patients with grade III/IV astrocytoma. J Neurooncol 1996;27(2): 179–89.

47. Plautz GE, Barnett GH, Miller DW, et al. Systemic T cell adoptive immunotherapy of malignant gliomas. J Neurosurg 1998;89(1):42–51.

48. Plautz GE, Miller DW, Barnett GH, et al. T cell adoptive immunotherapy of newly diagnosed gliomas. Clin Cancer Res 2000;6(6):2209–18.

49. Wood GW, Holladay FP, Turner T, et al. A pilot study of autologous cancer cell vaccination and cellular immunotherapy using anti-CD3 stimulated lymphocytes in patients with recurrent grade III/IV astrocytoma. J Neurooncol 2000;48(2):113–20.

50. Sloan AE, Dansey R, Zamorano L, et al. Adoptive immunotherapy in patients with recurrent malignant glioma: preliminary results of using autologous whole-tumor vaccine plus granulocyte-macrophage colony-stimulating factor and adoptive transfer of anti-CD3-activated lymphocytes. Neurosurg Focus 2000;9(6):e9.

51. Arca MJ, Mule JJ, Chang AE. Genetic approaches to adoptive cellular therapy of malignancy. Semin Oncol 1996;23(1):108–17.

52. Lokhorst HM, Liebowitz D. Adoptive T-cell therapy. Semin Hematol 1999;36(1 Suppl 3):26–9.

53. Ngo MC, Rooney CM, Howard JM, et al. Ex vivo gene transfer for improved adoptive immunotherapy of cancer. Hum Mol Genet 2011;20(R1):R93–9.

54. Gomez GG, Kruse CA. Mechanisms of malignant glioma immune resistance and sources of immunosuppression. Gene Ther Mol Biol 2006; 10(A):133–46.

55. Morgan RA, Dudley ME, Wunderlich JR, et al. Cancer regression in patients after transfer of genetically engineered lymphocytes. Science 2006;314(5796):126–9.

56. Sadelain M, Brentjens R, Riviere I. The promise and potential pitfalls of chimeric antigen receptors. Curr Opin Immunol 2009;21(2):215–23.

57. Beckman RA, Weiner LM, Davis HM. Antibody constructs in cancer therapy: protein engineering strategies to improve exposure in solid tumors. Cancer 2007;109(2):170–9.

58. Ahmed N, Salsman VS, Kew Y, et al. HER2-specific T cells target primary glioblastoma stem cells and induce regression of autologous experimental tumors. Clin Cancer Res 2010;16(2):474–85.

59. Heslop HE. Safer CARS. Mol Ther 2010;18(4): 661–2.

60. Bonini C, Brenner MK, Heslop HE, et al. Genetic modification of T cells. Biol Blood Marrow Transplant 2011;17(Suppl 1):S15–20.

61. Tey SK, Dotti G, Rooney CM, et al. Inducible caspase 9 suicide gene to improve the safety of allo-depleted T cells after haploidentical stem cell transplantation. Biol Blood Marrow Transplant 2007;13(8):913–24.

62. Quintarelli C, Vera JF, Savoldo B, et al. Co-expression of cytokine and suicide genes to enhance the activity and safety of tumor-specific cytotoxic T lymphocytes. Blood 2007;110(8):2793–802.

63. Bollard CM, Rossig C, Calonge MJ, et al. Adapting a transforming growth factor beta-related tumor protection strategy to enhance antitumor immunity. Blood 2002;99(9):3179–87.

64. Westwood JA, Kershaw MH. Genetic redirection of T cells for cancer therapy. J Leukoc Biol 2010;87(5): 791–803.

65. Olofsson A, Miyazono K, Kanzaki T, et al. Transforming growth factor-beta 1, -beta 2, and -beta 3 secreted by a human glioblastoma cell line. Identification of small and different forms of large latent complexes. J Biol Chem 1992;267(27):19482–8.

66. Kuppner MC, Hamou MF, Sawamura Y, et al. Inhibition of lymphocyte function by glioblastoma-derived transforming growth factor beta 2. J Neurosurg 1989;71(2):211–7.

67. Foster AE, Dotti G, Lu A, et al. Antitumor activity of EBV-specific T lymphocytes transduced with a dominant negative TGF-beta receptor. J Immunother 2008;31(5):500–5.

68. Weijtens ME, Willemsen RA, Valerio D, et al. Single chain Ig/gamma gene-redirected human T lymphocytes produce cytokines, specifically lyse tumor cells, and recycle lytic capacity. J Immunol 1996; 157(2):836–43.

69. Hickey MJ, Malone CC, Erickson KL, et al. Cellular and vaccine therapeutic approaches for gliomas. J Transl Med 2010;8:100.

70. Johnson LA, Sampson JH. Immunotherapy approaches for malignant glioma from 2007 to 2009. Curr Neurol Neurosci Rep 2010;10(4):259–66.

71. Wikstrand CJ, Cokgor I, Sampson JH, et al. Monoclonal antibody therapy of human gliomas: current status and future approaches. Cancer Metastasis Rev 1999;18(4):451–64.

72. Vitetta ES, Uhr JW. Monoclonal antibodies as agonists: an expanded role for their use in cancer therapy. Cancer Res 1994;54(20):5301–9.

73. Nadler LM, Stashenko P, Hardy R, et al. Serotherapy of a patient with a monoclonal antibody directed against a human lymphoma-associated antigen. Cancer Res 1980;40(9):3147–54.

74. Cragg MS, French RR, Glennie MJ. Signaling antibodies in cancer therapy. Curr Opin Immunol 1999; 11(5):541–7.

75. Bleeker WK, Lammerts van Bueren JJ, van Ojik HH, et al. Dual mode of action of a human anti-epidermal growth factor receptor monoclonal antibody for cancer therapy. J Immunol 2004;173(7):4699–707.

76. Ohno M, Natsume A, Ichiro Iwami K, et al. Retrovirally engineered T-cell-based immunotherapy targeting type III variant epidermal growth factor receptor, a glioma-associated antigen. Cancer Sci 2010;101(12):2518–24.

77. Ferguson KM. Active and inactive conformations of the epidermal growth factor receptor. Biochem Soc Trans 2004;32(Pt 5):742–5.

78. Eller JL, Longo SL, Hicklin DJ, et al. Activity of anti-epidermal growth factor receptor monoclonal antibody C225 against glioblastoma multiforme. Neurosurgery 2002;51(4):1005–13 [discussion: 1013–4].

79. Eller JL, Longo SL, Kyle MM, et al. Anti-epidermal growth factor receptor monoclonal antibody cetuximab augments radiation effects in glioblastoma multiforme in vitro and in vivo. Neurosurgery 2005;56(1):155–62 [discussion: 162].

80. Neyns B, Sadones J, Joosens E, et al. Stratified phase II trial of cetuximab in patients with recurrent high-grade glioma. Ann Oncol 2009;20(9):1596–603.

81. Bigner SH, Burger PC, Wong AJ, et al. Gene amplification in malignant human gliomas: clinical and histopathologic aspects. J Neuropathol Exp Neurol 1988;47(3):191–205.

82. Bigner SH, Humphrey PA, Wong AJ, et al. Characterization of the epidermal growth factor receptor in human glioma cell lines and xenografts. Cancer Res 1990;50(24):8017–22.

83. Humphrey PA, Gangarosa LM, Wong AJ, et al. Deletion-mutant epidermal growth factor receptor in human gliomas: effects of type II mutation on receptor function. Biochem Biophys Res Commun 1991;178(3):1413–20.

84. Humphrey PA, Wong AJ, Vogelstein B, et al. Amplification and expression of the epidermal growth factor receptor gene in human glioma xenografts. Cancer Res 1988;48(8):2231–8.

85. Zalutsky MR, Boskovitz A, Kuan CT, et al. Radioimmunotargeting of malignant glioma by monoclonal antibody D2C7 reactive against both wild-type and variant III mutant epidermal growth factor receptors. Nucl Med Biol 2012;39(1):23–34.

86. Lund-Johansen M, Bjerkvig R, Humphrey PA, et al. Effect of epidermal growth factor on glioma cell growth, migration, and invasion in vitro. Cancer Res 1990;50(18):6039–44.

87. Sampson JH, Crotty LE, Lee S, et al. Unarmed, tumor-specific monoclonal antibody effectively treats brain tumors. Proc Natl Acad Sci U S A 2000;97(13):7503–8.

88. Yang W, Barth RF, Wu G, et al. Development of a syngeneic rat brain tumor model expressing EGFRvIII and its use for molecular targeting studies with monoclonal antibody L8A4. Clin Cancer Res 2005;11(1):341–50.

89. Yang W, Barth RF, Wu G, et al. Molecular targeting and treatment of EGFRvIII-positive gliomas using boronated monoclonal antibody L8A4. Clin Cancer Res 2006;12(12):3792–802.

90. Perera RM, Narita Y, Furnari FB, et al. Treatment of human tumor xenografts with monoclonal antibody 806 in combination with a prototypical epidermal growth factor receptor-specific antibody generates enhanced antitumor activity. Clin Cancer Res 2005; 11(17):6390–9.

91. Mitchell DA, Fecci PE, Sampson JH. Immunotherapy of malignant brain tumors. Immunol Rev 2008;222:70–100.

92. Scott IU, Edwards AR, Beck RW, et al. A phase II randomized clinical trial of intravitreal bevacizumab for diabetic macular edema. Ophthalmology 2007;114(10):1860–7.

93. Birlik B, Canda S, Ozer E. Tumour vascularity is of prognostic significance in adult, but not paediatric astrocytomas. Neuropathol Appl Neurobiol 2006; 32(5):532–8.

94. Leon SP, Folkerth RD, Black PM. Microvessel density is a prognostic indicator for patients with astroglial brain tumors. Cancer 1996;77(2): 362–72.

95. Pope WB, Lai A, Nghiemphu P, et al. MRI in patients with high-grade gliomas treated with bevacizumab and chemotherapy. Neurology 2006; 66(8):1258–60.

96. Vredenburgh JJ, Desjardins A, Reardon DA, et al. The addition of bevacizumab to standard radiation therapy and temozolomide followed by bevacizumab, temozolomide, and irinotecan for newly diagnosed glioblastoma. Clin Cancer Res 2011;17(12): 4119–24.

97. Mendelsohn J, Baselga J. The EGF receptor family as targets for cancer therapy. Oncogene 2000; 19(56):6550–65.

98. Wong ET, Gautam S, Malchow C, et al. Bevacizumab for recurrent glioblastoma multiforme: a meta-analysis. J Natl Compr Canc Netw 2011;9(4):403–7.

99. de Groot JF, Yung WK. Bevacizumab and irinotecan in the treatment of recurrent malignant gliomas. Cancer J 2008;14(5):279–85.

100. Vredenburgh JJ, Desjardins A, Herndon JE 2nd, et al. Phase II trial of bevacizumab and irinotecan in recurrent malignant glioma. Clin Cancer Res 2007;13(4):1253–9.

101. Norden AD, Young GS, Setayesh K, et al. Bevacizumab for recurrent malignant gliomas: efficacy, toxicity, and patterns of recurrence. Neurology 2008;70(10):779–87.

102. Fine HA. Promising new therapies for malignant gliomas. Cancer J 2007;13(56):349–54.

103. Friedman HS, Prados MD, Wen PY, et al. Bevacizumab alone and in combination with irinotecan in recurrent glioblastoma. J Clin Oncol 2009;27(28): 4733–40.

104. Salmaggi A, Gaviani P, Botturi A, et al. Bevacizumab at recurrence in high-grade glioma. Neurol Sci 2011;32(Suppl 2):S251–3.

105. Addeo R, Caraglia M, De Santi MS, et al. A new schedule of fotemustine in temozolomide-pretreated patients with relapsing glioblastoma. J Neurooncol 2011;102(3):417–24.

106. Scoccianti S, Detti B, Sardaro A, et al. Second-line chemotherapy with fotemustine in temozolomide-pretreated patients with relapsing glioblastoma: a single institution experience. Anticancer Drugs 2008;19(6):613–20.

107. Kreisl TN, Kim L, Moore K, et al. Phase II trial of single-agent bevacizumab followed by bevacizumab plus irinotecan at tumor progression in recurrent glioblastoma. J Clin Oncol 2009;27(5):740–5.

108. Hofer S, Elandt K, Greil R, et al. Clinical outcome with bevacizumab in patients with recurrent high-grade glioma treated outside clinical trials. Acta Oncol 2011;50(5):630–5.

109. Reardon DA, Desjardins A, Peters KB, et al. Phase II study of carboplatin, irinotecan, and bevacizumab for bevacizumab naive, recurrent glioblastoma. J Neurooncol 2012;107(1):155–64.

110. Vredenburgh JJ, Desjardins A, Herndon JE 2nd, et al. Bevacizumab plus irinotecan in recurrent glioblastoma multiforme. J Clin Oncol 2007;25(30): 4722–9.

111. Reardon DA, Desjardins A, Vredenburgh JJ, et al. Metronomic chemotherapy with daily, oral etoposide plus bevacizumab for recurrent malignant glioma: a phase II study. Br J Cancer 2009; 101(12):1986–94.

112. Hasselbalch B, Lassen U, Hansen S, et al. Cetuximab, bevacizumab, and irinotecan for patients with primary glioblastoma and progression after radiation therapy and temozolomide: a phase II trial. Neuro Oncol 2010;12(5):508–16.

113. Lai A, Tran A, Nghiemphu PL, et al. Phase II study of bevacizumab plus temozolomide during and after radiation therapy for patients with newly diagnosed glioblastoma multiforme. J Clin Oncol 2011; 29(2):142–8.

114. Pu JK, Chan RT, Ng GK, et al. Using bevacizumab in the fight against malignant glioma: first results in Asian patients. Hong Kong Med J 2011;17(4): 274–9.

115. Lamborn KR, Chang SM, Prados MD. Prognostic factors for survival of patients with glioblastoma: recursive partitioning analysis. Neuro Oncol 2004; 6(3):227–35.

116. Wu W, Lamborn KR, Buckner JC, et al. Joint NCCTG and NABTC prognostic factors analysis for high-grade recurrent glioma. Neuro Oncol 2010;12(2):164–72.

117. Ballman KV, Buckner JC, Brown PD, et al. The relationship between six-month progression-free survival and 12-month overall survival end points for phase II trials in patients with glioblastoma multiforme. Neuro Oncol 2007;9(1):29–38.

118. Franceschi E, Brandes AA. Clinical end points in recurrent glioblastoma: are antiangiogenic agents friend or foe? Expert Rev Anticancer Ther 2011; 11(5):657–60.

119. Thompson EM, Frenkel EP, Neuwelt EA. The paradoxical effect of bevacizumab in the therapy of malignant gliomas. Neurology 2011;76(1):87–93.

120. Emrich JG, Brady LW, Quang TS, et al. Radioiodinated (I-125) monoclonal antibody 425 in the treatment of high grade glioma patients: ten-year synopsis of a novel treatment. Am J Clin Oncol 2002;25(6):541–6.

121. Casaco A, Lopez G, Garcia I, et al. Phase I single-dose study of intracavitary-administered nimotuzumab labeled with 188 Re in adult recurrent high-grade glioma. Cancer Biol Ther 2008;7(3):333–9.

122. Li L, Quang TS, Gracely EJ, et al. A phase II study of anti-epidermal growth factor receptor radioimmunotherapy in the treatment of glioblastoma multiforme. J Neurosurg 2010;113(2):192–8.

123. Zagzag D, Friedlander DR, Dosik J, et al. Tenascin-C expression by angiogenic vessels in human astrocytomas and by human brain endothelial cells in vitro. Cancer Res 1996;56(1):182–9.

124. Behrem S, Zarkovic K, Eskinja N, et al. Distribution pattern of tenascin-C in glioblastoma: correlation with angiogenesis and tumor cell proliferation. Pathol Oncol Res 2005;11(4):229–35.

125. Jallo GI, Friedlander DR, Kelly PJ, et al. Tenascin-C expression in the cyst wall and fluid of human brain tumors correlates with angiogenesis. Neurosurgery 1997;41(5):1052–9.

126. Leins A, Riva P, Lindstedt R, et al. Expression of tenascin-C in various human brain tumors and its relevance for survival in patients with astrocytoma. Cancer 2003;98(11):2430–9.

127. Sarkar S, Nuttall RK, Liu S, et al. Tenascin-C stimulates glioma cell invasion through matrix metalloproteinase-12. Cancer Res 2006;66(24):11771–80.

128. Riva P, Franceschi G, Arista A, et al. Local application of radiolabeled monoclonal antibodies in the treatment of high grade malignant gliomas: a six-year clinical experience. Cancer 1997;80(Suppl 12):2733–42.

129. Brown JM, Coates DM, Phillpotts RJ. Evaluation of monoclonal antibodies for generic detection of flaviviruses by ELISA. J Virol Methods 1996;62(2): 143–51.

130. Bigner DD, Brown MT, Friedman AH, et al. Iodine-131-labeled antitenascin monoclonal antibody 81C6 treatment of patients with recurrent malignant gliomas: phase I trial results. J Clin Oncol 1998; 16(6):2202–12.

131. Reardon DA, Akabani G, Coleman RE, et al. Salvage radioimmunotherapy with murine iodine-131-labeled antitenascin monoclonal antibody 81C6 for patients with recurrent primary and metastatic malignant brain tumors: phase II study results. J Clin Oncol 2006;24(1):115–22.

132. Reardon DA, Nabors LB, Stupp R, et al. Cilengitide: an integrin-targeting arginine-glycine-aspartic acid peptide with promising activity for glioblastoma multiforme. Expert Opin Investig Drugs 2008;17(8):1225–35.

133. Zalutsky MR, Reardon DA, Akabani G, et al. Clinical experience with alpha-particle emitting 211At: treatment of recurrent brain tumor patients with 211 At-labeled chimeric antitenascin monoclonal antibody 81C6. J Nucl Med 2008;49(1):30–8.

Use of Language Mapping to Aid in Resection of Gliomas in Eloquent Brain Regions

Matthew C. Garrett, MD, Nader Pouratian, MD, PhD,
Linda M. Liau, MD, PhD*

KEYWORDS

- Glioma • Brain tumor • Language mapping • fMRI • Electrical cortical stimulation

KEY POINTS

- Significant retrospective data exist to support the hypothesis that maximal safe resection benefits patients with glioma in terms of survival, accuracy of diagnosis, and response to chemotherapy.
- There are multiple modalities for preoperatively localizing eloquent language cortex and fibers, including anatomic landmarks, functional magnetic resonance imaging, and diffusion tensor imaging tractography.
- Considerable interpatient variation exists in the location of critical language areas. Thus, intraoperative cortical and subcortical electrostimulation mapping remains the gold standard.
- As our knowledge of human language function advances, our view of the brain will likely evolve from the identification of isolated areas of the cortex to a better understanding of integrated functioning circuits.

INTRODUCTION

It is thought that the cytoreduction of gliomas is a worthy goal and that adjuvant therapies (ie, radiation, chemotherapy, immunotherapy, and so forth) would be more effective with a smaller cell volume leading to delayed recurrence. However, studies looking at resection in high-grade gliomas have had mixed results.[1] Although there is a consensus that obtaining a histologic diagnosis and relieving compression and mass effect are worthwhile goals, the value of further microsurgical resection still remains controversial. This question becomes even more salient when considering a glioma located in eloquent areas, such as the language cortex. The risk of a postoperative language deficit in these surgeries has been reported to be as high as 26%.[2] Thus, the benefit of a gross total or near gross total resection needs to outweigh

these risks. Although there is some inconsistency in the literature regarding the impact of the extent of resection on outcomes, an increasing number of reports of both low-grade and high-grade gliomas suggest that extensive resection is beneficial.[1,3,4] As such, it is imperative to use all available strategies to obtain safe and extensive resections to ensure that any benefits of further resection outweigh the risks. The authors briefly review the literature regarding the value of the extent of resection. They proceed to the preoperative and intraoperative tools available to the neurosurgeon to distinguish eloquent from noneloquent language cortex and fibers, including the emerging roles of functional magnetic resonance imaging (fMRI) diffusion tensor imaging (DTI) tractography and direct cortical/subcortical stimulation in the surgical management of tumors in eloquent areas. Finally, the authors evaluate the postoperative course of these

UCLA Department of Neurosurgery, David Geffen School of Medicine at UCLA, 10833 Le Conte Avenue, Los Angeles, CA 90096-6901, USA
* Corresponding author. Department of Neurosurgery, UCLA Medical Center, 10833 Le Conte Avenue, CHS 74-145, Los Angeles, CA 90095-6901.
E-mail address: LLiau@mednet.ucla.edu

Neurosurg Clin N Am 23 (2012) 497–506
doi:10.1016/j.nec.2012.05.003
1042-3680/12/$ – see front matter © 2012 Elsevier Inc. All rights reserved.

patients and the effect of language deficits on their quality of life.

RATIONALE FOR EXTENSIVE RESECTION
High-Grade Gliomas

One of the earliest and most influential retrospective studies looking at the survival benefits of a gross total microsurgical resection for patients with glioblastomas was performed by Lacroix and colleagues[5] more than a decade ago. In this study, the investigators combined the results of 416 patients with newly diagnosed and recurrent glioblastomas and concluded that a 98% resection was associated with significantly improved survival. This finding has led to the all-or-none mentality that has existed over the last decade. This study, however, was designed to test whether complete or near complete resections had a survival advantage over biopsy and was not designed or powered to discover the threshold value whereby debulking had a survival advantage over biopsy. There were insufficient numbers of subtotal resections to perform this analysis.[1]

Since that time, there was an avalanche of case series attempting to quantify the benefit, if any, of subtotal resection. A recent review identified 28 studies between 1990 and 2007 that compared the outcome of patients with subtotal versus gross total resections.[1] Out of these studies, 16 demonstrated evidence that gross total resection was a significant predictor of overall survival or progression-free survival or both. Twelve studies, however, demonstrated no significant benefit based on extent of resection (EOR). The most quantitative study to date used compiled case series and Kaplan-Meier survival curve analyses, which suggested that a cutoff of 78% tumor resection provides a survival advantage.[4] However, all of these studies were nonrandomized and suffer from the same statistical confounder of selection bias. Despite some studies attempting to control for various tumor characteristics and baseline Karnofsky Performance Status (KPS), the fact remains that larger, more invasive, and difficult tumors in older patients with poor preoperative KPS scores are more likely to be subtotally resected, whereas younger patients with smaller tumors are more likely to get gross total resections.[6–8]

Low-Grade Gliomas

The evidence for extensive resection in low-grade gliomas (LGGs) is more persuasive than that for high-grade gliomas. LGGs differ significantly from their higher-grade counterparts in many important respects. A meta-analysis identified 10 studies investigating the benefit of resection in LGGs. Seven of the 10 studies found EOR to be a statistically significant predictor of survival. The survival benefit from gross total resection was approximately 30 months more than subtotal resection, with the average life expectancy increased from 61.1 to 90.5 months.[4,9] In regard to LGGs, although the question of when to observe versus intervene is still controversial, there exists consensus that once the tumor begins to show progression, the extent of resection does correlate with survival and all efforts should be made to obtain extensive resection. Besides the potential impact on survival, other compelling reasons exist for surgical resection, including the treatment of mass effect; potentially increasing the efficacy of adjuvant therapy; and, perhaps most importantly, increasing diagnostic accuracy.

Effect of Resection on Adjuvant Therapy

There is some indication in the literature that patients with extensive resection respond better to adjuvant therapy. There have been 2 prospective, randomized, phase 3 studies that have shown the efficacy of chemotherapy in patients with glioblastomas: one using carmustine (BCNU) wafers (Gliadel)[10] and one using temozolamide[11] in glioblastomas. In the case of BCNU wafers, the treatment was only significantly better than control in those patients who had a greater than 90% tumor resection. The increase in life expectancy was modest (14.8 vs 12. 6 months; $P = .01$) but significant. A similar trend was seen in the trial investigating the effectiveness of concurrent radiation and temozolomide following surgical resection.[11] Although this trial was not designed to examine the extent of resection and postoperative imaging was not mandated, patients were stratified into gross total resection (39%), partial resection (44%), and biopsy (16%). The survival advantage of radiation with concurrent temozolomide was greater in the gross total resection group (+4.1 months) than the partial resection group (+1.8 months) and was nonsignificant in the biopsy-only group (+1.5 months).

Diagnostic Accuracy

Finally, and perhaps most importantly, there is indisputable evidence that resection provides significantly superior diagnostic accuracy over stereotactic biopsy alone. Accurate diagnosis can be evasive when the histologic characteristics are heterogeneous. The grade of a glioma is defined by its most aggressive area, yet the tumor may still contain areas with less malignant features, which, if biopsied, may result in significant sampling and diagnostic error. Stereotactic biopsy series report a diagnostic yield of around 90%; however, a diagnosis made from such a biopsy cannot be confirmed unless the biopsy is followed by an extensive resection. In a series of 64 patients who had undergone stereotactic biopsy followed by a more extensive resection, Sawaya[2] found that the final diagnosis from resection was significantly different, leading to a change in therapy in 34 patients (53%). Further, as our ability to characterize gliomas on a genetic and molecular level increases, having more stored tumor may be vital to perform subsequent analyses and further personalized therapy.

Preventing Symptomatic Mass Effect

In patients who present with symptomatic mass effect, surgical resection is unequivocally indicated, even if the tumor involves eloquent areas. Prior studies have shown that gross total resections are associated with better patient neurologic performance scores than those observed after more limited resections.[12,13] Further, it is unusual for a large high-grade glioma with contrast enhancement to show a significant reduction in size after either radiation or chemotherapy, which, in some cases, requires the surgeon to perform a second surgery for symptomatic debulking.

PREOPERATIVE IMAGING FOR LANGUAGE MAPPING

Given the preponderance of evidence suggesting the importance of extensive resection, it behooves us to identify comprehensive strategies to safely resect gliomas without impairing eloquent function and quality of life. This point is particularly true when resecting tumors near or within canonical language areas. When planning surgery near perisylvian cortices in the dominant hemisphere, the localization of language cortices is of paramount importance in preventing postoperative deficits. The gold standard for locating essential language cortices has been electrical stimulation mapping (ESM). However, this technique is not without obstacles. Unlike intraoperative mapping of motor regions, patients must be awake and able to respond. This requirement leads to longer operative times, a higher chance of intraoperative seizures, and the potential for considerable patient distress. Moreover, awake intraoperative mapping is limited to those patients who have sufficient language ability and behavioral control to participate. Understandably, there is considerable interest in additional noninvasive modalities to identify patients in whom intraoperative awake mapping may be of low yield or not needed at all

as well as means to make intraoperative mapping safer and more efficient.

Anatomic Considerations

It has long been recognized that the human brain has a stereotypical pattern of gyri and sulci. As early as 1980, Kido and colleagues[14] described the relationship between the posterior end of the superior frontal sulcus and the precentral sulcus. Similarly in 1997, Yousry and colleagues[15] described the omega sign as a method to identify the hand portion of the precentral gyrus.

It was initially hoped that this link between structure and function would provide surgeons with much-needed guidance to distinguish an eloquent from a noneloquent cortex. However, with advances in neuro-functional imaging, we are finding more interpatient neuroanatomical variability even among typical patients. For example, the aforementioned omega sign can either represent a primary motor or premotor cortex.[16] Other groups have also reported variability in the functional organization of the primary sensorimotor cortices. For example, within the precentral gyrus, the stimulation of individual cortical sites has been shown to recruit both sensory and motor phenomenon; in other cases, stimulation has been shown to recruit motor movements in more than 1 motor group.[17–19]

The language cortices are even more variable. While performing cortical stimulation mapping on patients with gliomas undergoing resection, Quinones and colleagues[20] found more than 4 cm of variability in the localization of speech arrest when using classical anatomic landmarks. This finding may be because the cortical representation of speech is more complex than the motor cortex, with multiple essential and nonessential speech areas throughout the frontal, temporal, and parietal lobes. Fortunately, although the location of essential speech areas is variable among individuals, once it is found it is typically small and discrete.[21]

However, the difficulty still remains in predicting where the essential language areas will be in any individual patient. Although it is difficult to positively predict where vital areas will be, it is easier to define where they will not be. Ojemann and colleagues[22] reported that the posterior inferior frontal region is essential in 79% of patients, whereas the anterior middle temporal gyrus is essential in only 5% of patients. In perhaps the most extensive study of intraoperative mapping, Sanai and colleagues[23] tested 3281 cortical sites in 250 patients. In the 151 patients in whom the frontal lobe was tested, only 92 (60.9%) had essential areas of language that were identified on ESM. Further subdividing the frontal lobe squares revealed that even the most prevalent areas only yielded speech arrest in less than 25% of the stimulations.

The presence of an intracranial neoplasm seems to further compound this variability. Intracranial lesions can affect functional localization in 3 ways. First, developmental and vascular lesions may affect how the overlying cortex develops and which functions it assumes. Two studies have noted a greater preponderance of right-sided language lateralization in patients with cerebrovascular malformations.[24,25] Further, in patients with left temporal lobe epilepsy, earlier age of onset has been associated with a greater likelihood of right-sided or bilateral language lateralization.[26,27]

Second, intracranial pathologic conditions can lead to functional reassignment. Developmental lesions, destructive injuries, and malignancies acquired in adulthood can all lead the brain to compensate by reassigning neurologic functions to other areas of the cortex.[28] Lucas and colleagues compared language maps in patients with acquired pathologic conditions (gliomas, subarachnoid hemorrhage, and traumatic brain injury) with age-matched controls and found significant migration of language function to the nondamaged cortex in the pathologic group. The best evidence for this phenomenon is that, in stark contrast to ischemic stroke, LGGs rarely present with acute neurologic deficits. In fact, language mapping of patients with LGGs demonstrate multiple patterns of reorganization and compensation.[29] Robles and colleagues[30] reported on 2 patients in whom maps of eloquent language cortices changed between surgeries spaced by several years, allowing a multistage surgical approach for the resection of LGGs in eloquent cortices.

Third, the effect of intracranial disease on the accuracy of the imaging modality is unclear, possibly leading to disease-related imaging artifacts. It has long been suspected that fMRI cannot be used to map eloquent cortices adjacent to arteriovenous malformations (AVMs) because AVMs may alter the perfusion-dependent response that fMRI relies on or because AVMs cause susceptibility artifacts that can interfere with the detection of the blood oxygen level–dependent fMRI response. To investigate this claim, the authors' group specifically tested the accuracy and reliability of blood oxygen level–dependent fMRI mapping in patients with vascular malformations and found that fMRI is highly sensitive and specific for determining language localization in patients with vascular malformations, even directly adjacent to these lesions.[31] In the authors' practice

at the University of California, Los Angeles, it was found that relying on anatomic localization alone fails to identify up to 25% of the cases in which preoperative mapping (described later) suggested that awake intraoperative ESM mapping was necessary to achieve extensive resection.

fMRI

Recently, the use of fMRI has increased in prevalence. The use of the technology has expanded from simple language lateralization to specific language localization. fMRI works by detecting localized changes in blood flow and metabolism that is coupled to neuronal activity, such as during word language exercises. In contrast to ESM in which only essential cortices are identified, fMRI detects changes in all cortices (essential or not) that are activated during language tasks, resulting in an overly sensitive but nonspecific language map. A recent meta-analysis by Giussani and colleagues[32] identified 9 reports in the literature of case series in which patients with surgical lesions in the eloquent language cortex underwent preoperative fMRI followed by intraoperative electrocortical stimulation (ECS). Of the 9 studies cited, 5 of them computed a sensitivity and specificity of fMRI in comparison with ECS as a gold standard. The sensitivities ranged from 59% to 100% and the specificities ranged from 0% to 97%. The investigators stated that the varied methods and results used in these studies precluded any definitive conclusions about the utility of fMRI in preoperative planning. At this point, fMRI is not universally reliable and depends largely on the quality of the equipment and expert analysis and interpretation. Besides variability across institutions, the variability within a subject across cortices (frontal vs temporal vs parietal) is also not fully understood.

Despite its potential limitations, fMRI has been demonstrated at several institutions to be of value in identifying patients who require awake intraoperative language mapping and in identifying cortical regions that must be specifically interrogated intraoperatively for eloquence, thereby facilitating intraoperative awake mapping and making it more time efficient.

DTI Tractography

Gliomas often grow along white matter tracts in an infiltrative fashion. The method of DTI is a modification of diffusion-weighted imaging that is sensitive to the preferential diffusion of water along white matter fibers and can detect subtle changes in white matter structure and integrity.[33] Over the past 5 years, the authors have routinely integrated

DTI into the preoperative evaluation of patients harboring brain tumors (**Fig. 1**). This imaging modality can be used in a variety of capacities. For example, DTI can be used to differentiate normal white matter from edematous brain and nonenhancing tumor margins. More commonly, however, DTI has been used to evaluate the effect of intraparenchymal tumors on adjacent white matter tracts, including displacement, infiltration, and possible disruption by the tumor. Likewise, combined with functional imaging data (eg, fMRI), DTI has been used to identify the subcortical connections between essential eloquent cortices. This identification provides the surgeon with invaluable 3-dimensional information about spatial relationships of eloquent structures and their connectivity intraoperatively. It should be noted that DTI provides only anatomic and not functional information. Despite this limitation, the use of this technology can be useful in aiding the resection of tumors in the eloquent brain.[34,35] For instance, DTI, when combined with 3-dimensional intraoperative guidance, may be used to locate the pyramidal tracts in patients with insular gliomas or the arcuate fasciculus between the Broca area and Wernicke area.

INTRAOPERATIVE LANGUAGE TESTING AND ESM
ECS

Penfield introduced the method of direct cortical stimulation to assess motor function in the clinical setting in 1961.[36] Electric stimulation was delivered to the brain under local anesthesia to determine if there were any visible muscle contractions. Since that time, the awake craniotomy has become more sophisticated and allows the neurosurgeon to perform intraoperative electrical brain mapping with minimal risk (**Fig. 2**). Several studies have shown effective resection in eloquent areas previously thought to be inaccessible.[37–40] In a clinical case series by De Benedictis and colleagues,[36] the investigators reviewed the literature for 13 case series of patients with gliomas who underwent resection with intraoperative awake ECS mapping.[36] Of the 1460 patients reviewed, the severe permanent postoperative complication

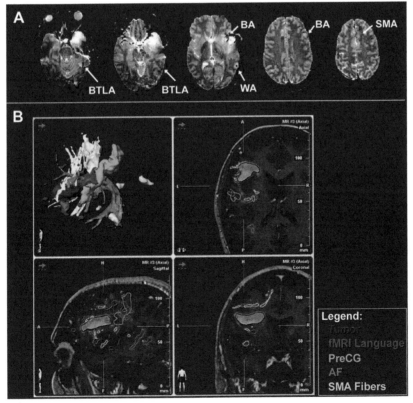

Fig. 1. fMRI and DTI tractography. (*A*) fMRI demonstrates areas of activation during language exercises. (*B*) Preoperative neuro-navigational imaging showing fMRI and DTI tractography fused to anatomic MRI to demonstrate important areas for intraoperative navigation. AF, arcuate fasciculus; BA, Broca area; BTLA, basal temporal language area; PreCG, precentral gyrus; SMA, supplementary motor area; WA, Wernicke area.

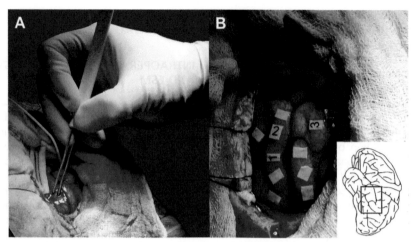

Fig. 2. ECS mapping. (*A*) Intraoperative photograph of ECS. (*B*) Results of intraoperative testing demonstrating essential (*letters*) and nonessential (*blank*) areas of cortex.

rate was 4.1% compared with a historical control of 19.0%.[41] Only 3 studies compared intraoperative mapping with traditional resection.

In the first of these studies, Reithmeier and colleagues[42] compared 42 patients who underwent ECS with 28 pair-matched controls who underwent resection between 1994 and 1997. The investigators noted a 14% incidence of postoperative deficit compared with a 29% incidence in the control group. In a study by Duffau and colleagues,[41] the investigators compared 100 patients with supratentorial LGGs undergoing traditional resection from 1985 to 1996 with 122 patients with similar tumors undergoing resection with intraoperative ECS mapping from 1996 to 2003 by the same surgical faculty. The investigators noted a 6% gross total resection rate and 17% severe permanent deficit rate in the control group compared with 25.4% and 6.5% in the awake intraoperative mapping group. In the third study, the investigators performed a re-resection using ECS on 9 patients who had undergone subtotal resections at another hospital for gliomas in the eloquent (defined as language or sensory motor) cortex. Five of the 9 patients were able to receive gross total resections. The investigators further noted that although only 6 of the 9 were able to work before surgery, all 9 were able to work after surgery.[43]

Negative Mapping

The first surgeries to use ECS mapping techniques were for epilepsy. These surgeries were typically done with large craniotomies to expose not only the region of surgical interest but also multiple other cortical sites involved in language production (positive sites). Until recently, it has been thought that such positive site controls must be established during language mapping before any other cortical area could be safely resected. Using this tactic, awake craniotomies traditionally identify positive language sites in 95% to 100% of the operative exposures.[23] However, the current trend is toward the identification of negative sites in which smaller tailored craniotomies often expose no positive functional language sites. Tumor resection is, therefore, directed by the localization of cortical regions that, when tested, contain no stimulation-induced language or motor function, which has led to less-extensive intraoperative mapping and a more time-efficient neurosurgical procedure.[44]

Direct Subcortical Stimulation

In addition to the identification of eloquent cortical brain areas, there is increased interest in using intraoperative direct subcortical stimulation (DSS) to functionally identify critical and eloquent white matter tracts that also must be preserved. DSS is similar to ECS in that it is performed intraoperatively with a awake patients; but instead of stimulating the cortex, the underlying white matter at the depths of the tumor resection cavity are interrogated. Because of the increased time required for the mapping of subcortical structures (relative to that required just for cortical mapping), subcortical mapping is often limited with respect to the number of tasks that can be performed before patients become too fatigued to cooperate. As an application of this concept, Lang and colleagues[45] used DSS on a series of insular gliomas but asserted that the technique did not give sufficient warning for the surgeon to alter his or her technique but rather served to inform the surgeon of damage that was already done. It should be noted that the surgeons stated that the "subcortical stimulation was used infrequently during tumor resection."[45] As such, critical damage may have occurred in between stimulations. Regardless of this experience, ECS associated with DSS is a potentially useful technique for preserving function and has been used by several surgeons to establish functional boundaries of tumors to guide maximal and safe resections to minimize both residual tumor and postoperative deficits.[46]

Neuropsychological Testing

As our technology of functional mapping improves, so does our understanding of the neuro-functional organization of the ability to understand and produce language. This, in turn, guides our clinical use of neuropsychological testing. By studying patients with strokes and traumatic brain injuries, it is clear that the language system can be separated into distinct subfunctions that can be selectively damaged or spared during surgical resections.

Surgeons and neuropsychologists have traditionally focused on naming exercises during intraoperative testing. However, the use of language requires numerous subcategories of function: semantics, pronunciation, inflection, prosody, connotation, sublexical procedures, reading, and writing. Further, each of these subcategories can have varying degrees of dysfunction. For these reasons, a thorough preoperative neuropsychiatric language evaluation is crucial before any surgical resection in eloquent brain areas.[47]

The first goal of neuropsychological testing is to provide a baseline for intraoperative and all postoperative evaluations. At a minimum, these evaluations should include sublexical processing, semantic and lexical knowledge, syntax, verbal short-term memory, and the ability to process auditory and visual stimuli as well as produce written and oral responses.

The second goal is to identify the most critical and feasible tasks for intraoperative testing. The list of tasks tested intraoperatively should include those that are both likely to be at risk during the surgery and functional at baseline. In regard to the former, when approaching a lesion in the superior temporal gyrus, a phoneme-discrimination task or a word picture with phonological foils will be appropriate considering the role played by this region in speech perception.[48] In other areas, simple picture naming may be sufficient or naming may need to be combined with comprehension, such as pairing an object with its intended action or naming an object both verbally and in written

form. Of note, the tested function need not be completely unimpaired. Making a preoperative deficit worse may be more devastating in some cases than causing a new postoperative deficit. Many language functions are not all-or-none phenomena but rather have different gradations of function. For example, a patient may have a mild lexical impairment for nouns (pure anomia). This type of deficit affects uncommonly used nouns more often that commonly used ones. Preoperatively, a list can be made of nouns that patients can name without error for use during the manipulation of suspected eloquent areas. Finally, the list of tasks must be defined and finite in length and performed in a reasonable amount of time so as to not excessively extend the operative time or cause patient fatigue.

Technical Considerations

The sensitivity and specificity of intraoperative language mapping also depends heavily on the neurosurgeon's skill. First and most simply, the intensity of the stimulation can affect the map produced. Low-intensity stimulation may be insufficient to affect the target, whereas high-intensity stimulation can excite neighboring areas, which leads to afterpotentials and false positives. Second, although most surgeons stimulate each area more than once, the number of stimulations differs among practitioners, as does the number and types of errors tolerated to define an essential language area. The electrical stimulation may produce an error at any of a variety of levels from simple dysarthria to true lexical semantic errors (tip-of-the-tongue states). Thus, the usefulness and benefit of intraoperative ECS and DSS mapping and, hence, the functional outcome of patients may vary depending on the experience of the surgeon with these techniques.

POSTOPERATIVE GOALS AND ASSESSMENT

The aim of any brain tumor treatment extends well beyond increasing survival. Palliation of symptoms and the maintenance/improvement of quality of life are important goals of any therapeutic intervention. Thus, the benefits of existing or new treatments need to be weighed against the side effects and possible impairment of patients' quality of life.

Aphasia and related language disabilities have wide-ranging impacts on the lives of those impaired and their families. These impacts can affect employment, social interactions, and familial roles regardless of how severe the linguistic impairment may be. Adults with aphasia and their relatives report numerous negative consequences of aphasia: changes in communication situations, changes in interpersonal relationships, difficulty controlling emotions, physical dependency, loss of autonomy, restricted activities, fewer social contacts, and recurring feelings of loneliness and despair.[49]

Surgeons tend to follow their patients throughout their inpatient course and for variable periods of time after discharge. As such, many surgeons may underestimate the potential for rehabilitation in the acute postoperative period. For many years, treatment of high-grade gliomas was considered palliative and neurologic rehabilitation was neglected. However, it is increasingly recognized that many patients who have undergone resection of gliomas in eloquent regions have significant functional impairment. Furthermore, these impairments can be responsive to rehabilitative physical, occupational, and speech therapy with corresponding improvements in functional status. Recently, studies have begun to compare the rehabilitative potential of patients with gliomas with those of patients who have had a stroke and found these two populations to be comparable in functional recovery.[50] Although many of these studies have used outcome tests that include language disturbances as a parameter, none have been sufficiently powered to look at language deficits specifically. Further outcome studies in the area of functional language recovery following glioma surgery are warranted.

Over the last several decades, neuroscientists and neurosurgeons have moved from a localizationist view of language in which language function was contained in discreet areas of neuronal cortex to an associationist view in which the visual and auditory linguistic information was processed in discreet cortical sites and then transported through subcortical white matter connections that are equally important.[51] As our white matter tractography imaging and DSS techniques improve and we are better able to map out and test functional connections, we may find that language follows a connectionist model, with multiple centers processing information in parallel. From Mesulam's large-scale neural network model of language in particular, it seems that there are 2 parallel pathways, the dorsal phonological stream and the ventral semantic stream, which converge to a common final tract allowing speech production.[52] Furthermore, the network is modulated by cortico-striato-pallido-thalamo-cortical loops. The next step to progress in the understanding of the brain connectivity might be a more accurate analysis of the interactions between the language circuit and the networks underlying the other cognitive functions, in particular the visuospatial component in which the role of the superior fronto-occipital fasciculus has been emphasized.[53]

The future neurosurgeon will need to be aware of how these different systems function in concert and identify which are peripherally involved with function versus essential to function. Additionally, neurosurgeons will need to understand and respect the role of subcortical structures and their associated connections because studies of stroke have taught us that lesions in the white matter can be significantly more damaging and debilitating than those found on the overlying cortex.[46]

SUMMARY

Although a clinical trial comparing biopsy with resection is not feasible, there exists sufficient retrospective uncontrolled evidence to conclude that a safe maximal resection will lead to the best outcome in most patients with glioma. A postoperative deficit in addition to an already debilitating disease can have serious and devastating consequences on a patient's quality of life. Identification and preservation of eloquent language regions in the brain are of critical importance to the neurosurgeon. As our understanding of the mechanisms of human speech and language expands, it is hoped that we will be better able to use current and future noninvasive imaging techniques to predict which areas of cortex and white matter are likely essential for speech production and language comprehension.

REFERENCES

1. Sanai N, Berger MS. Glioma extent of resection and its impact on patient outcome. Neurosurgery 2008; 62(4):753–64 [discussion: 264–6].
2. Sawaya R. Extent of resection in malignant gliomas: a critical summary. J Neurooncol 1999;42(3):303–5.
3. Sanai N, Berger MS. Extent of resection influences outcomes for patients with gliomas. Rev Neurol 2011;167(10):648–54.
4. Sanai N, Polley MY, McDermott MW, et al. An extent of resection threshold for newly diagnosed glioblastomas. J Neurosurg 2011;115(1):3–8.
5. Lacroix M, Abi-Said D, Fourney DR, et al. A multivariate analysis of 416 patients with glioblastoma multiforme: prognosis, extent of resection, and survival. J Neurosurg 2001;95(2):190–8.
6. Stummer W, van den Bent MJ, Westphal M. Cytoreductive surgery of glioblastoma as the key to successful adjuvant therapies: new arguments in an old discussion. Acta Neurochir 2011;153(6): 1211–8.
7. Albert FK, Forsting M, Sartor K, et al. Early postoperative magnetic resonance imaging after resection of malignant glioma: objective evaluation of residual

tumor and its influence on regrowth and prognosis. Neurosurgery 1994;34(1):45–60 [discussion: 60–1].

8. Stummer W, Reulen HJ, Meinel T, et al. Extent of resection and survival in glioblastoma multiforme: identification of and adjustment for bias. Neurosurgery 2008;62(3):564–76 [discussion: 564–76].

9. Sanai N, Polley MY, Berger MS. Insular glioma resection: assessment of patient morbidity, survival, and tumor progression. J Neurosurg 2010;112(1): 1–9.

10. Westphal M, Hilt DC, Bortey E, et al. A phase 3 trial of local chemotherapy with biodegradable carmustine (BCNU) wafers (Gliadel wafers) in patients with primary malignant glioma. Neuro Oncol 2003; 5(2):79–88.

11. Stupp R, Mason WP, van den Bent MJ, et al. Radiotherapy plus concomitant and adjuvant temozolomide for glioblastoma. N Engl J Med 2005;352(10): 987–96.

12. Ammirati M, Vick N, Liao YL, et al. Effect of the extent of surgical resection on survival and quality of life in patients with supratentorial glioblastomas and anaplastic astrocytomas. Neurosurgery 1987; 21(2):201–6.

13. Sawaya R, Hammoud M, Schoppa D, et al. Neurosurgical outcomes in a modern series of 400 craniotomies for treatment of parenchymal tumors. Neurosurgery 1998;42(5):1044–55 [discussion: 1055–6].

14. Kido DK, LeMay M, Levinson AW, et al. Computed tomographic localization of the precentral gyrus. Radiology 1980;135(2):373–7.

15. Yousry TA, Schmid UD, Alkadhi H, et al. Localization of the motor hand area to a knob on the precentral gyrus. A new landmark. Brain 1997;120(Pt 1): 141–57.

16. Shinoura N, Suzuki Y, Yamada R, et al. Precentral knob corresponds to the primary motor and premotor area. Can J Neurol Sci 2009;36(2):227–33.

17. Branco DM, Coelho TM, Branco BM, et al. Functional variability of the human cortical motor map: electrical stimulation findings in perirolandic epilepsy surgery. J Clin Neurophysiol 2003;20(1):17–25.

18. Farrell DF, Burbank N, Lettich E, et al. Individual variation in human motor-sensory (rolandic) cortex. J Clin Neurophysiol 2007;24(3):286–93.

19. Sanes JN, Donoghue JP, Thangaraj V, et al. Shared neural substrates controlling hand movements in human motor cortex. Science 1995;268(5218): 1775–7.

20. Quinones-Hinojosa A, Ojemann SG, Sanai N, et al. Preoperative correlation of intraoperative cortical mapping with magnetic resonance imaging landmarks to predict localization of the Broca area. J Neurosurg 2003;99(2):311–8.

21. Pouratian N, Bookheimer SY. The reliability of neuroanatomy as a predictor of eloquence: a review. Neurosurg Focus 2010;28(2):E3.

22. Ojemann G, Ojemann J, Lettich E, et al. Cortical language localization in left, dominant hemisphere. An electrical stimulation mapping investigation in 117 patients. J Neurosurg 1989;71(3):316–26.

23. Sanai N, Mirzadeh Z, Berger MS. Functional outcome after language mapping for glioma resection. N Engl J Med 2008;358(1):18–27.

24. Lehericy S, Biondi A, Sourour N, et al. Arteriovenous brain malformations: is functional MR imaging reliable for studying language reorganization in patients? Initial observations. Radiology 2002; 223(3):672–82.

25. Vikingstad EM, Cao Y, Thomas AJ, et al. Language hemispheric dominance in patients with congenital lesions of eloquent brain. Neurosurgery 2000; 47(3):562–70.

26. Brazdil M, Chlebus P, Mikl M, et al. Reorganization of language-related neuronal networks in patients with left temporal lobe epilepsy - an fMRI study. Eur J Neurol 2005;12(4):268–75.

27. Janszky J, Mertens M, Janszky I, et al. Left-sided interictal epileptic activity induces shift of language lateralization in temporal lobe epilepsy: an fMRI study. Epilepsia 2006;47(5):921–7.

28. Lucas TH 2nd, Drane DL, Dodrill CB, et al. Language reorganization in aphasics: an electrical stimulation mapping investigation. Neurosurgery 2008; 63(3):487–97 [discussion: 497].

29. Desmurget M, Bonnetblanc F, Duffau H. Contrasting acute and slow-growing lesions: a new door to brain plasticity. Brain 2007;130(Pt 4):898–914.

30. Robles SG, Gatignol P, Lehericy S, et al. Long-term brain plasticity allowing a multistage surgical approach to World Health Organization grade II gliomas in eloquent areas. J Neurosurg 2008;109(4): 615–24.

31. Pouratian N, Bookheimer SY, Rex DE, et al. Utility of preoperative functional magnetic resonance imaging for identifying language cortices in patients with vascular malformations. Neurosurg Focus 2002; 13(4):e4.

32. Giussani C, Roux FE, Ojemann J, et al. Is preoperative functional magnetic resonance imaging reliable for language areas mapping in brain tumor surgery? Review of language functional magnetic resonance imaging and direct cortical stimulation correlation studies. Neurosurgery 2010;66(1):113–20.

33. Le Bihan D. Looking into the functional architecture of the brain with diffusion MRI. Nat Rev Neurosci 2003;4(6):469–80.

34. Coenen VA, Krings T, Axer H, et al. Intraoperative three-dimensional visualization of the pyramidal tract in a neuronavigation system (PTV) reliably predicts true position of principal motor pathways. Surg Neurol 2003;60(5):381–90 [discussion: 390].

35. Holodny AI, Schwartz TH, Ollenschleger M, et al. Tumor involvement of the corticospinal tract: diffusion

magnetic resonance tractography with intraoperative correlation. J Neurosurg 2001;95(6):1082.

36. De Benedictis A, Moritz-Gasser S, Duffau H. Awake mapping optimizes the extent of resection for low-grade gliomas in eloquent areas. Neurosurgery 2010;66(6):1074–84 [discussion: 1084].

37. Bello L, Acerbi F, Giussani C, et al. Intraoperative language localization in multilingual patients with gliomas. Neurosurgery 2006;59(1):115–25 [discussion: 115–25].

38. Bello L, Gallucci M, Fava M, et al. Intraoperative subcortical language tract mapping guides surgical removal of gliomas involving speech areas. Neurosurgery 2007;60(1):67–80 [discussion: 80–2].

39. Chang EF, Potts MB, Keles GE, et al. Seizure characteristics and control following resection in 332 patients with low-grade gliomas. J Neurosurg 2008;108(2):227–35.

40. Duffau H. Intraoperative cortico-subcortical stimulations in surgery of low-grade gliomas. Expert Rev Neurother 2005;5(4):473–85.

41. Duffau H, Lopes M, Arthuis F, et al. Contribution of intraoperative electrical stimulations in surgery of low grade gliomas: a comparative study between two series without (1985-96) and with (1996-2003) functional mapping in the same institution. J Neurol Neurosurg Psychiatr 2005;76(6):845–51.

42. Reithmeier T, Krammer M, Gumprecht H, et al. Neuronavigation combined with electrophysiological monitoring for surgery of lesions in eloquent brain areas in 42 cases: a retrospective comparison of the neurological outcome and the quality of resection with a control group with similar lesions. Minim Invasive Neurosurg 2003;46(2):65–71.

43. Amorim RL, Almeida AN, Aguiar PH, et al. Cortical stimulation of language fields under local anesthesia: optimizing removal of brain lesions adjacent to speech areas. Arq Neuropsiquiatr 2008;66(3A):534–8.

44. Sanai N, Berger MS. Intraoperative stimulation techniques for functional pathway preservation and glioma resection. Neurosurg Focus 2010;28(2):E1.

45. Lang FF, Olansen NE, DeMonte F, et al. Surgical resection of intrinsic insular tumors: complication avoidance. J Neurosurg 2001;95(4):638–50.

46. Duffau H. New concepts in surgery of WHO grade II gliomas: functional brain mapping, connectionism and plasticity–a review. J Neurooncol 2006;79(1):77–115.

47. Pillon A, d'Honincthun P. The organization of the conceptual system: the case of the "object versus action" dimension. Cogn Neuropsychol 2011;27(7):587–613.

48. Hickok G, Poeppel D. The cortical organization of speech processing. Nat Rev Neurosci 2007;8(5):393–402.

49. Cruice M, Worrall L, Hickson L. Health-related quality of life in people with aphasia: implications for fluency disorders quality of life research. J Fluency Disord 2010;35(3):173–89.

50. Geler-Kulcu D, Gulsen G, Buyukbaba E, et al. Functional recovery of patients with brain tumor or acute stroke after rehabilitation: a comparative study. J Clin Neurosci 2009;16(1):74–8.

51. Geschwind N. The organization of language and the brain. Science 1970;170(961):940–4.

52. McClelland JL, Rogers TT. The parallel distributed processing approach to semantic cognition. Nat Rev Neurosci 2003;4(4):310–22.

53. Thiebaut de Schotten M, Urbanski M, Duffau H, et al. Direct evidence for a parietal-frontal pathway subserving spatial awareness in humans. Science 2005;309(5744):2226–8.

Quality of Life and Outcomes in Glioblastoma Management

Chaim B. Colen, MD, PhD[a],*, Elizabeth Allcut, MD[b]

KEYWORDS

- Glioblastoma • Health-related quality of life • Ethics

KEY POINTS

- Uniform evaluation of health-related quality of life (HRQOL) in patients with glioblastoma multiforme (GBM) is currently not in place.
- HRQOL can be altered by the patient's perception.
- Presurgical dialogue of the ultimate dismal outcome of GBM is very important.
- Discussion of postoperative QOL must be performed during the preoperative phase, to avoid misunderstandings and conserve patient expectations.
- Novel treatments for GBM should focus on improving survival while protecting HRQOL.
- Palliative services should be integrated into the overall multidisciplinary plan of treatment.

INTRODUCTION

Glioblastoma multiforme (GBM) is the most common primary brain tumor and unfortunately the most difficult tumor to effectively treat, despite the significant advances in recent research.[1,2] Because of this, unknowingly, many medical professionals might advocate for aggressive interventions that may adversely affect the quality of life (QOL) and outcome of these patients. Given the various neurologic deteriorations and psychopathological impairments that these patients tend to suffer during the course of this rapidly progressive disease, not all of these patients stand to benefit from certain of these therapies, at least from a QOL standpoint. In addition, there are few robust trials that have evaluated the QOL in patients with high-grade glioma.[3–6]

The goal of treatment for the cancer patient should go beyond increasing survival.[7] Rather, maintenance or improvement of the health-related QOL (HRQOL) must be a physician's prerogative when evaluating this goal. Hence, the benefits of the cancer treatment must be weighed against the adverse effects and potential psychopathological impairments. HRQOL, a multidimensional concept that includes self-reported measures of physical and mental health has become a tool to support clinical decision-making in patients with cancer that cannot be cured, such as GBM. Specifically, HRQOL evaluates physical, psychological, and social aspects of human functionality.[3,7]

Previously, the use of the Karnofsky Performance Status was a common method to evaluate QOL. However, this measure did not incorporate a multidimensional approach to cost, QOL, and return to work, all of which are gaining importance as outcome measures, especially because of the intense resource use that brain cancer treatment demands. Better technology and therapeutic

Disclosures: None.
Funding sources: None.
Conflict of Interest: None.
[a] Neurosurgical Oncology and Epilepsy Surgery, Department of Neurosurgery, Oakland Medical School, Beaumont Health System, 468 Cadieux Road, Grosse Pointe, Detroit, MI 48230, USA; [b] Wayne State University School of Medicine, Scott Hall, 540 East Canfield, Detroit, MI 48201, USA
* Corresponding author.
E-mail address: ccolen@colenpublishing.com

Neurosurg Clin N Am 23 (2012) 507–513
doi:10.1016/j.nec.2012.04.010

interventions have yielded a marginal increase in survival after surgery, radiation, and chemotherapy for GBM, and the attention is shifting toward evaluation of the QOL gained by these therapies during those additional weeks or months.[3,8]

Depending on tumor location, surgical intervention, and radiation therapy and chemotherapy administered, certain patients benefit from this marginal increase in survival, but may sustain a decline in their HRQOL. Other patients might do quite well after receiving treatment both clinically and from an HRQOL standpoint, which urges further research and clinical interventions.

The most commonly used metrics to evaluate HRQOL in patients with brain cancer are role participation, social functioning and global QOL, visual disorder, motor dysfunction, communication deficit, and drowsiness (**Box 1**).[9,10] Most papers agree that improvement in QOL is demonstrated by a 10-point positive change in HRQOL score from baseline.[11]

Divergent views of the HRQOL model exist, and there are several other formulations to evaluate physical and social functioning, and role participation that conceptualize disruptions caused by a disease to the community, family and work.[12] Because these formulations or metrics may vary by societal beliefs or norms, at least 1 paper has sought to establish equivalence of language and interpretation of the metric.[13] To add to this complexity, Herdman and colleagues[13] found 19 different types of equivalence, but these standards were not clearly defined, and the theoretical framework for equivalence lacked. Their literature review revealed vague or conflicting definitions to define HRQOL, particularly in the case of conceptual equivalence definitions of equivalence in the HRQOL literature. They concluded that conceptual equivalence definitions are cultural in nature, and there existed an urgent need to establish universalist standardized terminology within the HRQOL

field, which would require substantial changes to guidelines and more empiric work on the conceptualization of HRQOL in different cultures.

RADIOLOGICAL CONSIDERATIONS ON THE QUALITY OF LIFE AND OUTCOMES IN GBM

Radiological predictors of poor prognosis in GBM have been studied in multiple articles.[14–16] Intensity of enhancement of the tumor nodule and extent of peritumoral edema are commonly cited factors that portend a poorer prognosis (**Table 1**). Interestingly, location and tumor volume have not correlated as predictors of survival.[14]

Hobbs and colleagues[17] found that in GBM, the intensity of contrast enhancement on magnetic resonance imaging (MRI) correlated with differences in gene expression. The expression of certain genes has been used to determine the most appropriate individualized treatment. This intratumoral heterogeneity noted on MRI highlights the need for multidisciplinary multimodal treatment, to adequately address all aspects of the biology of GBMs and possibly extend the long-term HRQOL.[18] In summary, GBM patients with little or no necrosis and with less tumor nodule enhancement on preoperative MRI survive longer than patients with greater amounts of necrosis and greater degrees of tumor enhancement.

An increasing body of evidence demonstrates the utility of expression profiling in stratification of patients with GBM in terms of tumor classification and survival.[19]

SURGICAL CONSIDERATIONS ON THE QOL AND OUTCOMES IN GBM

Surgery in glioblastoma is mainstay treatment for both histopathological tissue diagnosis and tumor debulking.[20] Extent of tumor resection slightly increases survival, but this must be weighed against the removal of eloquent cortex, resection of which would decrease postoperative QOL. It is the opinion of the authors, that in cases where the malignant glial tumor invades eloquent cortex, a discussion of postoperative QOL must be performed during the preoperative phase, to avoid

---

Box 1
Common metrics used to evaluate quality of life in GBM

- Role participation
- Social functioning
- Global QOL
- Visual disorder
- Motor dysfunction
- Communication deficit
- Drowsiness

Table 1
Radiological predictors on the QOL

Poor Predictors	Good Predictors
Intense tumor enhancement	Low degree of tumor enhancement
Significant peritumoral edema	Little peritumoral edema

misunderstandings and conserve patient expectations. Many patients prefer to preserve functions like speech and movement, even at the expense of leaving behind significant amounts of tumor. Importantly, the continuum of open dialogue of specialists within a multidisciplinary team when caring for patients with GBM is key, since loss of communication among providers may result in delayed treatment. Interdisciplinary discussions are imperative, since aggressive early intervention retards tumor progression and leads to improved survival.[20] Surgery should be combined with chemotherapy and radiation, as both add survival benefit. Continuous communication of all parties involved with care of these patients is vital.

A presurgical consideration to preserve the QOL in patients with malignant glioma depends on 2 factors;

1. Location of the tumor
2. Aggressiveness of the tumor.

Tumors located within the left hemisphere, primary speech area, or primary motor areas are associated with decreased QOL. Preoperatively, patients with tumors located in the speech area of the brain may present with aphasia, or if in the motor area, with paresis, leading to the need for continuous dedicated care in the postoperative phase.

Rapidly progressive tumors are associated with a rapid decline of cognitive function. Early reoccurrence of tumors usually portends a poor prognosis, but pseudoprogression must be excluded.

Cognitive Impairments

Cognitive impairments that prevent return to work are more common than physical disability. It is unknown how many of the patients diagnosed with a GBM return to work for any period of time. Cognitive impairments are appraised through evaluation of role participation, social functioning, global QOL, communication deficit, and drowsiness. Cognitive impairments are greater when the tumor reoccurs, affects the left hemisphere, or is present in areas of the brain that facilitate comprehension.

Physical Disability

Presurgical consideration of potential postsurgical physical disability is central when trying to protect the QOL for these patients. This presurgical discussion of potential adverse outcomes in the postsurgical phase is crucial and creates improved patient expectations. Studies evaluating patient expectation scores to QOL are unknown, but based on the authors' experience, honest

discussion of postoperative expectation during the presurgical phase may improve postoperative role participation, social functioning, and global QOL scores.

According to Furlong and colleagues,[21] HRQOL is the value assigned to duration of life as modified by the impairments, functional states, perceptions, and social opportunities that are influenced by disease, injury, treatment, or policy.

However, since HRQOL can be altered by patient perception, presurgical dialogue of the ultimate dismal outcome of GBM is so important. For example, expectation of worsening weakness exists postsurgically, when the tumor invades the primary motor cortex and when preoperative weakness is present. Discussion of this fact can modify the patient's intrinsic perception of the weakness with improved HRQOL scores.

From another perspective, if a patient has a strong belief in the advancement of science despite shortcomings in current treatments, he or she may wish to become the subject of a clinical trial supporting scientific experimental technique that may or may not improve outcome or HRQOL. Thus, this calls for the incorporation of a universal HRQOL measurement tool into experimental studies, to begin to better understand outcomes of treatment from a patient's perspective. For example, a treatment that improves survival by 2 months, but causes the patient severe nausea and lethargy throughout the treatment period of 6 months, may not be seen and appraised favorably by the patient. On the other hand, without these trials, scientific advancement might not be made. Medicine thus becomes the science of balances, advancing scientific knowledge and novel treatments counterbalanced against potential patient suffering because of the experimental therapy.

RADIOTHERAPY CONSIDERATIONS ON THE QUALITY OF LIFE AND OUTCOMES IN GBM
Cognitive Impairments

Attention and psychopathological impairments are commonly associated with radiotherapy of the central nervous system (CNS). Most are dose-dependent and constitute limiting factors in the administration of treatments. Radiation-induced neurologic complications occur in 3 forms: acute, early delayed, or delayed (**Table 2**). Acute radiation necrosis is now uncommon, given improvements in accurate dose administration through advances in the design of safer radiation modalities.[22]

To preserve HRQOL, the clinician should be aware of 2 facts. First, patients harboring large GBMs, particularly with signs of increased intracranial pressure, should likely be treated with small

Table 2
Radiation-induced encephalopathy

Stages	Timing	Common Clinical Symptoms
Acute	Minutes to days	Increased intracranial pressure—headache, nausea, vomiting
Early delayed	2 wk to 4 mo	Prolonged drowsiness, somnolence syndrome
Late delayed	4 mo to 24 y	Dementia

doses per fraction (doses of 200 cGy per fraction or less appear to be better tolerated). Second, all patients undergoing brain irradiation should be protected with corticosteroids (8–16 mg of dexamethasone daily or more if increased intracranial pressure is symptomatic), preferably for at least 24 hours before the start of radiation therapy.[23]

The amelioration of the adverse effects of radiotherapy is fundamental in preserving long-term HRQOL. This also maintains patient satisfaction while undergoing further cancer treatment.

Physical Disability

Radiation of tumors affecting eloquent areas of the brain may adversely affect motor, speech, or sensory function over time. Precise stereotactic radiotherapy treatments, such as Gamma knife or Cyberknife demonstrate advantages over other radiotherapeutic modalities and assist in preservation of HRQOL.[24,25] However, such treatments are generally not recommended in large diffusely infiltrative GBMs. Because of its infiltrative characteristic, after surgical debulking, a margin of the surrounding brain should be included in the radiation treatment.[24] Effects of radiotherapy in GBM are usually seen in a semidelayed fashion (4–9 months), and it is paramount to bring up this issue during the initial radiotherapy discussions. It is known that informed patients have improved HRQOL scores despite the presence of significant disability.

CHEMOTHERAPEUTIC CONSIDERATIONS ON THE QOL AND OUTCOMES IN GBM
Cognitive Impairments

Aggressive chemotherapy may lead to cognitive impairment in 20% to 30% of cancer patients. These lasting effects, also known as chemotherapy-induced cognitive dysfunction," may result in decreased HRQOL, especially in the metric of social functioning.[26]

Through targeted chemotherapeutic approaches however, this metric can be improved. Literature suggests that there is benefit to the use of expression profiling in the stratification of patients, as well as the selection of targeted molecular and gene therapies used for successful treatment of malignancy. Although associated with less severe adverse effects than other chemotherapy agents, temozolomide should likely be used cautiously in cases where the tumor is unmethylated, since the tumor is not as responsive to this therapy. Temozolomide is an alkylating agent that adds methyl groups to DNA and is currently the standard of care for first-line chemotherapy for GBM. In a phase 3 study,[27] analysis of O^6-methylguanine–DNA methyltransferase (MGMT) promoter methylation status performed on a subset of tumor samples demonstrated a significant association between MGMT promoter methylation (which decreases protein expression) and improved patient outcome from treatment. Among the patients in the combined temozolomide and radiation therapy arm, those with MGMT promoter methylated tumors experienced a 2-year survival rate of 46% compared with 14% among patients with unmethylated tumors. Yet, MGMT tumor methylation might be a positive prognostic value that is intrinsic to these tumor subtypes, with a prognostic value that is independent from treatment with temozolamide. This is suggested by the fact that patients in this study who had methylated tumors but were treated with radiation alone also had improved survival.[27]

The use of systemic chemotherapy to treat GBM has been met with skepticism because of its limited efficacy and the significant adverse effects demonstrated in clinical trials. Nevertheless, based on findings in randomized trials of new agents, it has been suggested that further evaluation of the role of chemotherapy is warranted.

Temozolomide and Gliadel (carmustine wafers) are generally well tolerated due to their limited systemic toxicity. In addition, these agents appear particularly well suited for incorporation into multimodal treatment strategies.[18]

Although investigations of individual gene or protein alterations are important, because they can provide potentially important clinical markers of outcome or as therapeutic targets, a more powerful approach to stratify therapy while preserving HRQOL would be through the use of gene expression profiling using microarray-based platforms.[20]

This would allow the identification of novel molecular alterations associated with molecular subtypes of tumors or clinical outcome.

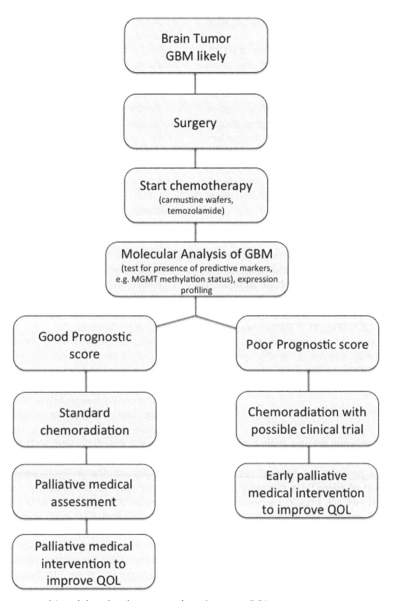

Fig. 1. Flow diagram: multimodal molecular approach to improve QOL.

Physical Disability

Toxic effects of chemotherapeutic agents on the CNS lead to impaired functionality. Central neurotoxicity ranges from acute toxicity such as aseptic meningitis, to delayed toxicities comprising cognitive deficits, hemiparesis, aphasia, and progressive dementia.

In one study,[28] the authors examined for evidence of cell death and cell division in the CNS. This study concluded the presence of chemotherapy-induced cognitive decline even in the absence of radiation. A second study suggested that neural progenitor cells are more vulnerable to DNA cross-linking agents in vitro than are many cancer cell lines. It is

becoming increasingly clear that not only CNS irradiation but also chemotherapy alone can cause severe neurotoxicity leading to cognitive decline.[29]

In summary, when discussing chemotherapy treatment, one must balance the need for survival with quality of life.

VALUE OF HOSPICE CARE

Malignant glioma is rapidly progressive despite treatment, and it behooves the physician to discuss this point together with the patient and his or her family. One study suggests that there exists limited provision of hospice care for supporting individuals in the palliative care stages of such an illness.[30]

Given the progressive illness trajectory of GBM, the complex symptoms experienced by such patients, and the requirement of extensive support, the options for palliative support should be discussed with the immediate family. Issues of those engaged in informal caregiving should be addressed, as this provides ease to the patient and to the family.[31] It is in the opinion of the authors that this topic might be raised by the physician providing immediate care to the patient, but should be formally addressed by a professional in the palliative medical services.

Baseline assessment of patients should be geared to identify 2 factors: first, the range of support services that both caregivers and patients require, and second, the uptake and response to these services. A multimodal molecular approach to GBM has been suggested, and the authors proposed a diagrammatical flow treatment paradigm to improve QOL (**Fig. 1**).[20] Each checkpoint should be documented throughout the illness trajectory. Following this or a similar protocol should improve HRQOL for the patient by relieving stressful tension in the family.[31]

SUMMARY

GBM is the most common primary brain tumor and the most difficult tumor to effectively treat, despite the significant advances in recent research. Uniform evaluation of HRQOL is currently not in place. A universal HRQOL should be adapted to cross-compare advances in clinical trials. Ultimately, excellent novel treatments for GBM should focus on improving survival while protecting HRQOL. Palliative services should be integrated into the overall multidisciplinary treatment plan.

ACKNOWLEDGMENTS

Dr Colen would like to acknowledge the invaluable editorial support of his mentor, Saroj Mathupala, PhD, and his wife, Roxanne E. Colen, PA-C.

REFERENCES

1. Colen CB, Shen Y, Ghoddoussi F, et al. Metabolic targeting of lactate efflux by malignant glioma inhibits invasiveness and induces necrosis: an in vivo study. Neoplasia 2011;13(7):620–32.
2. Colen CB, Seraji-Bozorgzad N, Marples B, et al. Metabolic remodeling of malignant gliomas for enhanced sensitization during radiotherapy: an in vitro study. Neurosurgery 2006;59(6):1313–23 [discussion: 1323–4].
3. Mauer M, Stupp R, Taphoorn MJ, et al. The prognostic value of health-related quality-of-life data in predicting survival in glioblastoma cancer patients: results from an international randomised phase III EORTC Brain Tumour and Radiation Oncology Groups, and NCIC Clinical Trials Group study. Br J Cancer 2007;97(3):302–7.
4. Garside R, Pitt M, Anderson R, et al. The effectiveness and cost-effectiveness of carmustine implants and temozolomide for the treatment of newly diagnosed high-grade glioma: a systematic review and economic evaluation. Health Technol Assess 2007;11(45):xi–xii, ix-221.
5. Bosma I, Reijneveld JC, Douw L, et al. Health-related quality of life of long-term high-grade glioma survivors. Neuro Oncol 2009;11(1):51–8.
6. Cheng JX, Zhang X, Liu BL. Health-related quality of life in patients with high-grade glioma. Neuro Oncol 2009;11(1):41–50.
7. Herdman M. The measurement of health related quality of life. Med Clin (Barc) 2000;114(Suppl):322–5 [in Spanish].
8. Osoba D, Brada M, Yung WK, et al. Health-related quality of life in patients treated with temozolomide versus procarbazine for recurrent glioblastoma multiforme. J Clin Oncol 2000;18(7):1481–91.
9. Torrance GW, Feeny DH, Furlong WJ, et al. Multiattribute utility function for a comprehensive health status classification system. Health Utilities Index Mark 2. Med Care 1996;34(7):702–22.
10. Yavas C, Zorlu F, Ozyigit G, et al. Health-related quality of life in high-grade glioma patients: a prospective single-center study. Support Care Cancer 2011. [Epub ahead of print].
11. Yavas C, Zorlu F, Ozyigit G, et al. Prospective assessment of health-related quality of life in patients with low-grade glioma: a single-center experience. Support Care Cancer 2011. [Epub ahead of print].
12. Taphoorn MJ, Sizoo EM, Bottomley A. Review on quality of life issues in patients with primary brain tumors. Oncologist 2010;15(6):618–26.
13. Herdman M, Fox-Rushby J, Badia X. A model of equivalence in the cultural adaptation of HRQoL instruments: the universalist approach. Qual Life Res 1998;7(4):323–35.
14. Hammoud MA, Sawaya R, Shi W, et al. Prognostic significance of preoperative MRI scans in glioblastoma multiforme. J Neurooncol 1996;27(1):65–73.
15. Oh J, Henry RG, Pirzkall A, et al. Survival analysis in patients with glioblastoma multiforme: predictive value of choline-to-N-acetylaspartate index, apparent diffusion coefficient, and relative cerebral blood volume. J Magn Reson Imaging 2004;19(5):546–54.
16. Li X, Jin H, Lu Y, et al. Identification of MRI and 1H MRSI parameters that may predict survival for

patients with malignant gliomas. NMR Biomed 2004; 17(1):10–20.

17. Hobbs SK, Shi G, Homer R, et al. Magnetic resonance image-guided proteomics of human glioblastoma multiforme. J Magn Reson Imaging 2003; 18(5):530–6.

18. Ashby LS, Ryken TC. Management of malignant glioma: steady progress with multimodal approaches. Neurosurg Focus 2006;20(4):E3.

19. Wiesner SM, Freese A, Ohlfest JR. Emerging concepts in glioma biology: implications for clinical protocols and rational treatment strategies. Neurosurg Focus 2005;19(4):E3.

20. Stupp R, Hegi ME, van den Bent MJ, et al. Changing paradigms—an update on the multidisciplinary management of malignant glioma. Oncologist 2006;11(2):165–80.

21. Furlong WJ, Feeny DH, Torrance GW, et al. The Health Utilities Index (HUI) system for assessing health-related quality of life in clinical studies. Ann Med 2001;33(5):375–84.

22. Kondziolka D, Flickinger JC, Bissonette DJ, et al. Survival benefit of stereotactic radiosurgery for patients with malignant glial neoplasms. Neurosurgery 1997;41(4):776–83 [discussion: 783–5].

23. Keime-Guibert F, Napolitano M, Delattre JY. Neurological complications of radiotherapy and chemotherapy. J Neurol 1998;245(11):695–708.

24. Crowley RW, Pouratian N, Sheehan JP. Gamma knife surgery for glioblastoma multiforme. Neurosurg Focus 2006;20(4):E17.

25. Combs SE, Widmer V, Thilmann C, et al. Stereotactic radiosurgery (SRS): treatment option for recurrent glioblastoma multiforme (GBM). Cancer 2005;104(10): 2168–73.

26. Nicholas MK. Glioblastoma multiforme: evidence-based approach to therapy. Expert Rev Anticancer Ther 2007;7(Suppl 12):S23–7.

27. Hegi ME, Diserens AC, Gorlia T, et al. MGMT gene silencing and benefit from temozolomide in glioblastoma. N Engl J Med 2005;352(10):997–1003.

28. Duffner PK, Cohen ME, Thomas PR, et al. The long-term effects of cranial irradiation on the central nervous system. Cancer 1985;56(Suppl 7):1841–6.

29. Dietrich J, Han R, Yang Y, et al. CNS progenitor cells and oligodendrocytes are targets of chemotherapeutic agents in vitro and in vivo. J Biol 2006; 5(7):22.

30. Faithfull S, Cook K, Lucas C. Palliative care of patients with a primary malignant brain tumour: case review of service use and support provided. Palliat Med 2005;19(7):545–50.

31. Arber A, Faithfull S, Plaskota M, et al. A study of patients with a primary malignant brain tumour and their carers: symptoms and access to services. Int J Palliat Nurs 2010;16(1):24–30.

High-Grade Gliomas in Children

Tene A. Cage, MD[a],*, Sabine Mueller, MD, PhD[b,c],
Daphne Haas-Kogan, MD[c,d], Nalin Gupta, MD, PhD[a,c]

KEYWORDS

- Glioblastoma multiforme • Anaplastic astrocytoma • Pediatric brain tumors • Radiation therapy
- Chemotherapy

KEY POINTS

- High-grade gliomas include anaplastic astrocytomas and glioblastomas. They account for 3% to 7% of primary brain tumors in children and peak in incidence during adolescence.
- Molecular mutations seen in pediatric glioblastoma multiforme and AAs include p53, PTEN, and LOH at 10q23. p53 and PTEN are associated with a poor prognosis.
- The goals of surgery include pathologic diagnosis and/or gross total resection. Longer progression-free survival is associated with a greater extent of resection.
- In children older than 3 years, chemotherapy plus radiation after surgery is the standard of care. In children younger than 3 years, radiation is associated with significant neurologic morbidity and should be used only when necessary.

INTRODUCTION

Gliomas are primary brain tumors derived from astrocytes and oligodendroglia and are historically separated into low- or high-grade categories according to the World Health Organization (WHO) classification system. Low-grade astrocytomas (WHO grade I and II) are approximately 40% of primary supratentorial tumors of childhood and are more common than high-grade astrocytomas (WHO grade III and IV).[1] Supratentorial high-grade gliomas (HGGs) are further divided into anaplastic astrocytomas (AAs, WHO grade III), anaplastic oligodendrogliomas (WHO grade III), mixed astrocytic tumors, and glioblastoma multiforme (GBM, WHO grade IV).[2] As expected, survival rates are poor and mortality is highest in patients with malignant astrocytomas.

EPIDEMIOLOGY

HGGs account for between 3% and 7% of newly diagnosed primary brain tumors in children.[3,4] GBM is the most common primary brain tumor in the adult population, but GBMs along with AAs account for only about 20% of pediatric supratentorial brain tumors.[1] In the pediatric population, malignant astrocytomas seem to affect boys and girls equally.[5] The incidence peaks during adolescence, although very young children can also develop malignant astrocytomas.[5]

At present, the only known risk factor associated with developing an HGG is prior radiation therapy.[6] Other rare risk factors include genetic syndromes such as Li-Fraumeni syndrome. This syndrome is characterized by 1 or more cancer occurrences in children, including HGGs.[7,8] Mutations of the p53

[a] Department of Neurological Surgery, University of California, San Francisco, 505 Parnassus Avenue, Room M779, San Francisco, CA 94143-0112, USA; [b] Department of Neurology, University of California, San Francisco, 505 Parnassus Avenue, Box 0114, San Francisco, CA 94143-0114, USA; [c] Department of Pediatrics, University of California, San Francisco, 505 Parnassus Avenue, M696, Box 0110, San Francisco, CA 94143, USA; [d] Department of Radiation Oncology, University of California, San Francisco, 505 Parnassus Avenue, San Francisco, CA 94143-0226, USA
* Corresponding author.
E-mail address: cageta@neurosurg.ucsf.edu

Neurosurg Clin N Am 23 (2012) 515–523
doi:10.1016/j.nec.2012.04.007
1042-3680/12/$ – see front matter © 2012 Published by Elsevier Inc.

tumor suppressor gene play a key role in tumorigenesis in these patients. Neurofibromatosis type 1 is an autosomal dominant genetic disorder caused by mutations of the neurofibromin gene. The clinical manifestations include cutaneous café au lait spots, neurofibromas in any organ system, optic gliomas, and intracranial HGGs.[9] Turcot syndrome, a disease of DNA mismatch repair characterized by adenomatous colorectal polyps and malignant neuroepithelial tumors, has been associated with HGGs in children.[10,11] Other diseases of constitutional mismatch repair deficiency, specifically expression of the MSH6 mismatch repair gene mutation has been linked to HGG development in children.[12] In addition, there have been case reports of GBM occurring in patients with Ollier disease and Maffucci syndrome, both diseases of cartilaginous dysplasia.[13] However, the significance of the occurrence of these malignancies in these syndromes is unknown.

PATHOLOGY
Histopathology

AAs are highly proliferative mitotically active tumors of glial origin with increased cellularity and cellular atypia. GBMs consist of active poorly differentiated astrocytes with high mitotic activity. These neoplasms are typically heterogeneous with areas of hypervascularity and necrosis. Often the necrotic areas are toward the center of the lesion and surrounded by dense hypervascular tissue. The peripheral zones of both AA and GBM are composed of less dense cellular layers that invade and infiltrate the surrounding brain tissue. Typically this invasion is along white matter tracts, including the anterior and posterior commissures, corpus callosum, fornix, and internal capsule. Infiltrating tumor cells are commonly found many centimeters from the original tumor location.

Molecular Features

The molecular profiles of pediatric and adult HGGs are distinct.[14] Mutations in the p53 tumor suppressor gene are characteristic features of pediatric GBMs and are associated with a poor prognosis. In a multi-institutional trial, the Children's Cancer Group (CCG) identified p53 mutations in 40.5% of pediatric HGGs.[15] This same p53 mutation is only seen in secondary adult GBMs. Secondary GBM refers to HGGs that have arisen from the progression of lower-grade gliomas. p53 overexpression in children is associated with a 5-year progression-free survival (PFS) rate of 17% in comparison with a PFS rate of 44% in patients with low p53 expression.[16,17]

Epidermal growth factor receptor (EGFR),[18] PTEN,[19] and the Ras pathway[20] are activated in most adult GBMs, although these alterations are only present in a subset of pediatric patients. EGFR amplification is rare (<10%) in children with GBMs than in adults with GBMs, although positive and elevated EGFR immunoreactivity is seen in 80% of pediatric tumors. The CCG trial reported that 24% of pediatric GBMs and AAs had PTEN deletions.[21] Although mutations in PTEN are rare in pediatric GBM than in GBM in adults, if present, a poorer prognosis can be expected. LOH at 10q23 is a common abnormality found in 80% of pediatric GBMs.

There are at least 2 molecular subtypes of pediatric GBM.[20] One has activation of the Ras/Akt and MAPK pathways and is associated with a poor clinical prognosis. The other subtype does not have Ras/Akt or MAPK pathway activation and has a much more favorable prognosis. In most adult GBMs, the Ras pathway is activated. In children with GBMs with Ras activation, high expression of CD133, nestin, dlx2, and MELK is also seen.

YB1, a protein involved in brain embryogenesis, is upregulated in 72% of pediatric GBMs.[20] This protein is unique to pediatric GBMs and, when localized to the nucleus, is associated with a poor prognosis. When expressed in the cytoplasm of Ras/Akt-negative GBMs, it was associated with a better outcome. A strong positive association between MIB-1 labeling, patient outcome, and histology has also been found. Mean labeling indices were 19.4 ± 2.66 for tumors classified as AA versus 32.1 ± 3.08 for those classified as GBM ($P = .0024$). The 5-year PFS was $33\% \pm 7\%$ in 43 patients whose tumors had MIB-1 indices of less than 18%, $22\% \pm 8\%$ in 27 patients whose tumors had indices between 18% and 36%, and $11\% \pm 6\%$ in 28 patients whose tumors had indices greater than 36% ($P = .003$), reflecting a significant inverse correlation between proliferative indices and PFS.[22]

Pediatric AAs are associated with both loss and gain of DNA copy number. The most common gains are on chromosome 5q (40%) and 1q (30%), whereas the most common losses are chromosomes 22q (50%) and 6q, 9q (40%).[23] Losses on 17p have also been reported. A shorter survival time is associated with a gain on the 1q arm.[23] PTEN mutation is rare (8%) in pediatric AA, but if present is associated with poor prognosis.[23] In addition, p53 mutations are present in 95% of pediatric AAs.[24]

Clinical Features

As with many brain tumors, the clinical presentation depends on the anatomic location of the tumor, associated effects on the surrounding brain, and the age of the patient. Constitutional symptoms such as fatigue, irritability, anorexia, loss of milestones, or failure to thrive can occur but are nonspecific in nature. Signs and symptoms of increased intracranial pressure, such as worsening headaches, nausea, and vomiting, are often seen with intracranial tumors regardless of their diagnosis or grade. Neurologic abnormalities related to tumor location may include hemiparesis; dysphasia; or, less commonly, worsening seizures related to tumor progression. Infants are a special population in whom signs and symptoms may be difficult to interpret. If the cranial sutures are still open, symptoms and signs of increased intracranial pressure may not be present; instead, the head circumference will increase, making room for the growing infiltrating tumor. A rapid increase in head circumference may be the first step in the diagnosis of a brain tumor in infants. The rate of tumor progression is related to tumor grade. Patients with HGGs have a hastening of functional decline and symptoms in comparison with those with lower-grade tumors.[25,26]

Diagnostic Imaging

HGGs can be identified on computed tomographic (CT) scans as an irregular isodense or hypodense lesion centered in the white matter. There may be heterogeneous enhancement of the lesion seen on postcontrast sequences. Although CT scans play an important diagnostic role in the early detection of brain tumors in children, magnetic resonance imaging (MRI) is the most sensitive imaging

tool and provides far more anatomic information. At a minimum, the following MRI sequences should be obtained: T1-weighted, precontrast and postcontrast administration, T2-weighted, and fluid-attenuated inversion recovery (FLAIR). Additional specialized magnetic resonance sequences include magnetic resonance spectroscopy (MRS), perfusion, diffusion-weighted imaging, and diffusion tensor imaging (DTI). Functional MRI (fMRI) can provide functional and structural information, which is particularly helpful for surgical planning.[27]

HGGs can have varying imaging features on MRI. They either can have an irregularly enhancing rim surrounding a necrotic core or can be poorly marginated with diffuse infiltration into white matter tracts such as the corpus callosum and anterior and posterior commissures. These tumors are usually solitary but can be multifocal. On precontrast T1-weighted sequences, these tumors are isointense or hypointense. After contrast administration, T1-weighted sequences typically show an irregular enhancing rim surrounding a nonenhancing area of central necrosis (**Fig. 1**). Hemorrhage is sometimes present within the tumor (**Fig. 2**). The enhancing portion typically represents mitotically active proliferating tumor cells. T2-weighted and FLAIR sequences usually show a heterogeneous mass with variable signal intensity surrounded by a broad zone of vasogenic edema. Infiltrating malignant tumor cells extend far beyond the area of enhancement. These aggressive tumors have elevated choline level, lactate level, and lipid peaks and decreased N-acetyl-aspartate peaks on MRS.[28] Because of the high proliferative index and elevated glucose metabolism

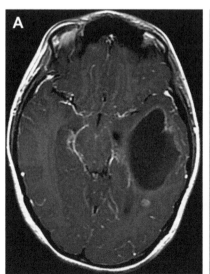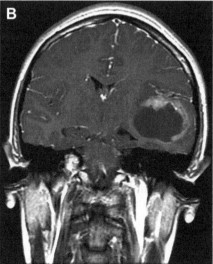

Fig. 1. A mainly cystic AA (WHO grade III) in a 6-year-old girl. On the postcontrast axial image (*A*), the tumor is mainly cystic in appearance. A rim of enhancement is better visualized on the coronal image (*B*).

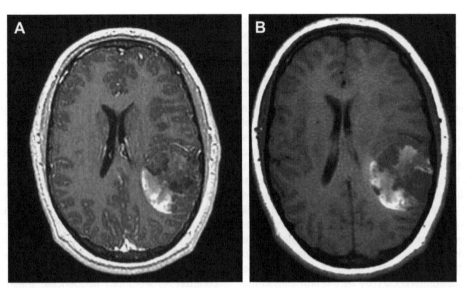

Fig. 2. A partially hemorrhagic GBM of the left parietal lobe in a 15-year-old boy. The precontrast image (*A*) shows areas of increased T1-weighted signal intensity consistent with hemorrhage. After gadolinium administration, there are irregular areas of enhancement within the tumor (*B*).

that characterizes HGGs, PET imaging reveals high fludeoxyglucose uptake in the lesion.

Gliomatosis cerebri is the most diffuse form of HGGs and is identified by tumor infiltration throughout multiple lobes and associated vasogenic edema. Imaging of the neuraxis is indicated when there is a concern for disseminated disease throughout the brain and spinal cord. The differential diagnosis based on imaging includes abscess, demyelination, or other primary malignant brain tumors of childhood, including primitive neuroectodermal tumors, ependymoma, or pleomorphic xanthoastrocytomas.

Following surgery, chemotherapy, and/or radiation therapy, patients should be monitored radiographically for tumor recurrence. Serial MRI with close clinical follow-up is required to detect early evidence of tumor progression.

TREATMENT
Surgery

The goals of surgery include obtaining tissue for pathologic diagnosis and achieving a gross total resection (GTR). Depending on tumor location, GTR must be balanced against the development of disabling neurologic deficits. Preoperative MRI sequences such as DTI or fMRI as well as intraoperative image guidance navigation can assist in safely achieving a greater extent of resection while preserving neurologic function for the patient. Because of the infiltrative nature and anatomic location of these tumors, GTR is often not possible. In circumstances in which the tumor is entirely deep in location with involvement of gray

matter nuclei, a limited biopsy may be the only safe option (**Fig. 3**). Once a diagnosis is obtained, adjuvant chemotherapy and/or radiation therapy can be planned.

If GTR cannot be achieved, debulking of the majority of the mass is beneficial. A longer PFS is associated with a greater extent of surgical resection.[29–31] In addition, by removing a portion of the mass, symptoms associated with mass effect can be partially or totally relieved. In the CCG 945 study, children with HGGs who underwent GTRs (defined as >90% resection) had a 5-year PFS rate of 35% (±7%) in comparison with 17% (±4%) in the group that underwent subtotal resection (STR) ($P = .006$).[32] Likewise, patients with AA who underwent GTRs had a 5-year PFS rate of 44% (±11%) in comparison with 22% (±6%) in those who underwent STRs ($P = .055$). Patients with GBM who underwent GTRs had a 5-year PFS rate of 26% (±9%) in comparison with 4% (±3%) in those who underwent STRs ($P = .046$).[32] In this same study, the 5-year event-free survival rate (event defined as relapse or death from any cause) for patients with oligoastrocytomas was 37.5% ± 17%.[33]

Radiation Therapy

Radiation therapy is the standard of care after surgical resection for children older than 3 years. The neurologic sequelae of radiation therapy include neurocognitive decline, secondary malignancy, endocrinopathy, and vasculopathy, depending on the location of the tumor and the required radiation treatment volume and dose.

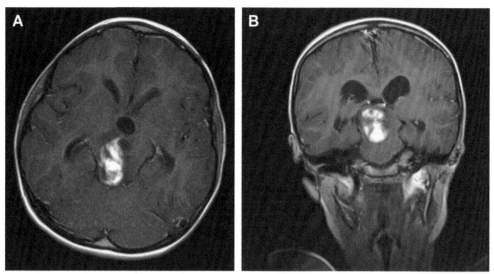

Fig. 3. A heterogeneous-appearing AA in the upper midbrain and thalamus. Lesion enhancement is observed following gadolinium administration in the axial (*A*) and coronal (*B*) images. This lesion was not amenable to GTR, and diagnosis was obtained by stereotactic biopsy.

Therefore, younger children, in particular those younger than 3 years, are often treated with chemotherapy after surgical resection to delay radiation therapy. For those patients older than 3 years, fractionated external beam radiation is the standard of care. Patients are treated with 54 to 60 Gy delivered in daily fractions of 1.8 to 2.0 Gy. Hyperfractionated radiotherapy, in which more than one fraction of radiation is administered daily, typically with a lower dose per fraction, has not proven to improve outcomes nor decrease associated side effects of radiation.[34,35]

Chemotherapy

Following surgical resection, chemotherapy is started usually in combination with radiation therapy, although it is often continued as maintenance therapy. For children younger than 3 years, chemotherapy can be administered as a primary therapy to delay radiation as long as possible. The effectiveness of adjuvant chemotherapy in addition to radiation therapy after surgical resection of HGGs in children is not well established, and most children with HGGs are treated on a clinical trial. The first randomized trial testing the efficacy of chemotherapy was conducted in the 1980s by the CCG. Children with HGGs were randomized after surgery to receive radiation therapy with or without chemotherapy with prednisone, lomustine, and vincristine. Children who received postradiation chemotherapy had better PFS (46%) than those who did not receive chemotherapy (26%).[36] This benefit was most apparent

in patients with GBM who had at least partial tumor resection. In a subsequent CCG study, patients were randomized to receive 1 of 2 chemotherapy regimens comparing an intensive "8-drugs-in-one-day" regimen with the standard regimen of prednisone, vincristine, and lomustine. No difference in 5-year PFS was seen between these regimens (33% vs 36%).[29] Based on these data, adding adjuvant chemotherapy to radiation seems to provide a small survival benefit.

Since these early studies, chemotherapy has been added to radiation therapy in different schedules, including a "sandwich" protocol (before and after radiation therapy), concomitant administration, and maintenance therapy. Single agents including etoposide, cyclophosphamide, irinotecan, platinum compounds, procarbazine, CCNU and vincristine, and topotecan have been studied in phase 2 trials with marginal effects on overall survival. Because concomitant temozolomide (TMZ) and radiation therapy for adult patients with GBM led to prolonged survival and is now considered the standard of care, several studies have tested the efficacy of this drug in pediatric patients.[37–40] Multiple other studies, including 2 large national Children's Oncology Group studies, had disappointing outcomes and failed to demonstrate a benefit of TMZ on long-term survival in pediatric patients with HGGs, including brainstem gliomas.[39,41–43] Ongoing trials are evaluating TMZ in combination with additional chemotherapeutic agents such as the PARP inhibitor ABT-888 or in combination with radiation and ABT-888 as upfront treatment of pediatric brainstem glioma.

High-dose myeloablative chemotherapy with autologous hematopoietic stem cell rescue (ASCR) has also been explored, and its role in the treatment of HGG remains unproved. The CCG 9922 study using thiotepa, BCNU, and etoposide followed by ASCR and focal radiation therapy resulted in a 2-year PFS rate of 46% (±14%).[44] This study was closed early after 5 of the 11 treated patients developed significant pulmonary complications. Another study using thiotepa in patients with newly diagnosed HGG showed a 4-year survival rate of 46%.[45] The most appropriate candidates for myeloablative therapy are those with complete or near-complete resection before myeloablative therapy.[46] The use of high-dose chemotherapy with ASCR may contribute to long-term disease control but at the expense of significant morbidity and mortality as a consequence of the regimens themselves. The associated side effects and resultant poor quality of life have led many investigators to question the benefit of high-dose chemotherapy with ASCR despite the potential for better disease control.

At present, a combination of surgery, radiation, and chemotherapy is the standard therapy for children with HGGs who are older than 3 years. The most effective chemotherapy regimen, however, is still under investigation.

OUTCOME

A diagnosis of HGG, either GBM or AA, carries a poor prognosis. In general, pediatric patients have a more favorable course than adults with the same diagnosis.[47] Histologic characteristics, amenability to surgical resection, and ability to tolerate adjuvant therapies all contribute to a patient's individual survival rate. Patients with grade IV tumors (GBM) have a worse prognosis than those with grade III tumors (AA).[29,48] Similarly, patients who undergo GTR have improved 5-year PFS in comparison with those who receive only STR or biopsy. In addition, patients who are able to tolerate radiation and chemotherapy after resection have an increased survival rate in comparison with those who do not undergo any adjuvant treatment.

Functional outcomes are influenced by location and extent of the tumor. For patients who have large tumors that involve the eloquent brain, preoperative deficits can be profound. Treatment side effects, particularly those associated with radiation therapy, to the developing neuraxis can translate into developmental comorbidities. Neuropsychological delay, endocrinopathies, vasculopathies, and cognitive delay/decline are not uncommon sequelae of radiation therapy.

Although prognosis is generally poor for patients with HGGs, secondary malignancies have been reported after undergoing radiation to the neuraxis and after exposure to chemotherapeutic agents (eg, alkylating agents and etoposide). Because of this, regular monitoring with serial MRI is crucial to follow up tumor progression.

FUTURE DIRECTIONS

Current studies and trials seek to identify new molecular targets for therapeutic intervention or attempt to uncover new drug combinations to limit treatment side effects while extending life expectancy. Significant progress in the last several years has greatly increased our understanding of the underlying molecular mechanisms that are involved in the tumorigenesis of pediatric HGGs. These findings are now being translated into targeted therapies and are entering early phase 1 clinical trials. For example, the PI3K/Akt/mTOR pathway as well as BRAF^{V600E} are promising new targets. An analysis of 74 pediatric HGGs revealed *EGFR* amplification in 4 of 43 pediatric GBMs (11%) and 2 of 11 pediatric AAs (14%). The constitutively active EGFRvIII mutant form was present in 6 of 35 (17%) cases.[49] *PDGFR* amplification is present in approximately 15% of pediatric HGGs, and gene expression pathway analysis revealed that RTK signaling is dysregulated in approximately 25% of pediatric HGGs.[49] These findings amongst others led to the development of a phase 1 trial with the new dual PI3K/mTOR inhibitor XL765 (Sanofi-Aventis) for treatment of recurrent pediatric HGGs. Further, Schiffman and colleagues[50] have reported a frequency of 25% (5/20) of BRAF^{V600E} mutations in pediatric HGGs, and a more recent analysis showed a frequency of 10% of BRAF^{V600E} mutations in an additional 60 pediatric HGGs.[51] At present, PLX4032, a specific inhibitor of BRAF^{V600E}, is being considered for a phase 1 clinical trial for children whose tumors carry this mutation. PLX4032 has already shown remarkable efficacy in patients with refractory metastatic melanoma with a reported response rate of 81% and only mild grade 2 toxicities.[52]

Receptor inhibitors, radiosensitization, and vaccine trials are techniques that are currently under further investigation as potential treatment strategies for these patients. Inhibitors of EGFR or platelet-derived growth factor receptor (PDGFR) are being tested in phase 1/2 trials with and without radiation as well as in combination with conventional chemotherapy.[53] Imatinib (PDGFR inhibitor) has been associated in a phase 1 trial with increased incidence of intracranial hemorrhage, especially in patients with brainstem glioma, which requires further investigation.[54] Results from a phase 2 trial (HIT-GMB-D) using high-dose methotrexate showed results superior to that in the control groups, and therefore this regimen is being tested as a phase 3 study.[55] Investigators are currently studying the increased effectiveness of chemotherapeutic agents used before radiation therapy as radiosensitizers.[56] Although vaccine trials have been used in adults with HGGs, there are less data for the pediatric population. Dendritic cell–based tumor vaccination trials in children with recurrent malignant brain tumors are underway.[57] Early results have shown that recurrent HGGs respond favorably to vaccination with a 6-month PFS of 42% and an overall survival of 21.2% at a median follow-up of 35.7 months after surgical resection and subsequent vaccination.

Laboratory investigations are setting the stage for further clinical therapies. For example, gefitinib, a GFR tyrosine kinase inhibitor, has been shown in the laboratory to alter EGFR phosphorylation.[58] Gene therapy using toxin-producing viral vector constructs to induce selective killing of rapidly proliferating tumor cells are also currently under investigation. Further analysis of the underlying molecular events leading to pediatric HGG will enhance clinicians' understanding and lead to improved targeted therapies.

SUMMARY

Pediatric HGGs include AAs, anaplastic oligodendrogliomas, and GBM. Pediatric patients present with a variety of clinical symptoms that vary greatly with age of the patient, making early diagnosis potentially more difficult than that in adults. MRI plays a critical role in the early detection of brain tumors in children, especially when clinical symptoms are nonspecific. Definitive diagnosis of HGG rests on gaining a tissue sample from surgical biopsy or resection. Although diagnosis is the main goal of surgery in these patients, debulking of the mass is critical both for symptomatic relief and to increase survival rates among patients. The standard of care in children includes surgical resection, radiation therapy (for children older than 3 years), and maintenance chemotherapy. Current clinical trials and laboratory studies are investigating new molecular targets, tumor cell sensitization to radiation and chemotherapy, and dendritic cell vaccinations.

REFERENCES

1. Pollack IF. Brain tumors in children. N Engl J Med 1994;331:1500.
2. Kleihues P, Louis DN, Scheithauer BW, et al. The WHO classification of tumors of the nervous system. J Neuropathol Exp Neurol 2002;61:215.
3. Tamber MS, Rutka JT. Pediatric supratentorial high-grade gliomas. Neurosurg Focus 2003;14:e1.
4. CBTRUS. 2009-2010 CBTRUS statistical report: primary brain and central nervous system tumors diagnosed in eighteen states in 2002-2006. Hinsdale (IL): Central Brain Tumor Registry of the United States; 2009.
5. Perkins S, Rubin J, Leonard J, et al. Glioblastoma in children: a single-institution experience. Int J Radiat Oncol Biol Phys 2011;80:1117.
6. Pettorini BL, Park YS, Caldarelli M, et al. Radiation-induced brain tumours after central nervous system irradiation in childhood: a review. Childs Nerv Syst 2008;24:793.
7. Li FP, Fraumeni JF Jr, Mulvihill JJ, et al. A cancer family syndrome in twenty-four kindreds. Cancer Res 1988;48:5358.
8. Varley JM, McGown G, Thorncroft M, et al. Germline mutations of TP53 in Li-Fraumeni families: an extended study of 39 families. Cancer Res 1997;57:3245.
9. Jouhilahti E, Peltonen S, Heape A, et al. The pathoetiology of neurofibromatosis 1. Am J Pathol 1932;178:2011.
10. Turcot J, Despres JP, St Pierre F. Malignant tumors of the central nervous system associated with familial polyposis of the colon: report of two cases. Dis Colon Rectum 1959;2:465.
11. Lusis E, Travers S, Jost S, et al. Glioblastomas with giant cell and sarcomatous features in patients with Turcot syndrome type 1: a clinicopathological study of 3 cases. Neurosurgery 2010;67:811.
12. Felsberg J, Thon N, Eigenbrod S, et al. Promoter methylation and expression of MGMT and the DNA mismatch repair genes MLH1, MSH2, MSH6 and PMS2 in paired primary and recurrent glioblastomas. Int J Cancer 2011;129:659.
13. Ranger A, Szymczak A, Hammond R, et al. Promoter methylation and expression of MGMT and the DNA mismatch repair genes MLH1, MSH2, MSH6 and PMS2 in paired primary and recurrent glioblastomas. J Neurosurg Pediatr 2009;4:363.
14. Pfister S, Witt O. Pediatric gliomas. Recent results. Cancer Res 2009;171:67.
15. Pollack IF, Hamilton RL, James CD, et al. Rarity of PTEN deletions and EGFR amplification in malignant gliomas of childhood: results from the Children's Cancer Group 945 cohort. J Neurosurg 2006;105:418.
16. Pollack IF, Finkelstein SD, Burnham J, et al. Age and TP53 mutation frequency in childhood malignant gliomas: results in a multi-institutional cohort. Cancer Res 2001;61:7404.
17. Pollack IF, Finkelstein SD, Woods J, et al. Expression of p53 and prognosis in children with malignant gliomas. N Engl J Med 2002;346:420.
18. Bredel M, Pollack IF, Hamilton RL, et al. Epidermal growth factor receptor expression and gene

amplification in high-grade non-brainstem gliomas of childhood. Clin Cancer Res 1999;5:1786.

19. Nakamura M, Shimada K, Ishida E, et al. Molecular pathogenesis of pediatric astrocytic tumors. Neuro Oncol 2007;9:113.

20. Faury D, Nantel A, Dunn S, et al. Molecular profiling identifies prognostic subgroups of pediatric glioblastoma and shows increased YB-1 expression in tumors. J Clin Oncol 2007;25:1196.

21. Liu W, James CD, Frederick L, et al. PTEN/MMAC1 mutations and EGFR amplification in glioblastomas. Cancer Res 1997;57:5254.

22. Pollack IF, Hamilton RL, Burnham J, et al. Impact of proliferation index on outcome in childhood malignant gliomas: results in a multi-institutional cohort. Neurosurgery 2002;50:1238.

23. Rickert C, Strater R, Kaatsch P, et al. Pediatric high-grade astrocytomas show chromosomal imbalances distinct from adult cases. Am J Pathol 2001;158:1525.

24. Sung T, Miller DH, Hayes RL, et al. Preferential inactivation of the p53 tumor suppressor pathway and lack of EGFR amplification distinguish de novo high grade pediatric astrocytomas from de novo adult astrocytomas. Brain Pathol 2000;10:249.

25. Mehta V, Chapman A, McNeely PD, et al. Latency between symptom onset and diagnosis of pediatric brain tumors: an Eastern Canadian geographic study. Neurosurgery 2002;51:365.

26. Duffner PK. Diagnosis of brain tumors in children. Expert Rev Neurother 2007;7:875.

27. Osborn A, Blaser S, Salzman K, et al. Diagnostic imaging brain. Salt Lake City (UT): Amirsys; 2007.

28. Steffen-Smith E, Shih J, Hipp S, et al. Proton magnetic resonance spectroscopy predicts survival in children with diffuse intrinsic pontine glioma. J Neurooncol 2011;105:365.

29. Finlay JL, Boyett JM, Yates AJ, et al. Randomized phase III trial in childhood high-grade astrocytoma comparing vincristine, lomustine, and prednisone with the eight-drugs-in-1-day regimen. Childrens Cancer Group. J Clin Oncol 1995;13:112.

30. Heideman RL, Kuttesch J Jr, Gajjar AJ, et al. Supratentorial malignant gliomas in childhood: a single institution perspective. Cancer 1997;80:497.

31. Wolff JE, Gnekow AK, Kortmann RD, et al. Preradiation chemotherapy for pediatric patients with high-grade glioma. Cancer 2002;94:264.

32. Wisoff JH, Boyett JM, Berger MS, et al. Current neurosurgical management and the impact of the extent of resection in the treatment of malignant gliomas of childhood: a report of the Children's Cancer Group trial no. CCG-945. J Neurosurg 1998;89:52.

33. Hyder D, Sung L, Pollack I, et al. Anaplastic mixed gliomas and anaplastic oligodendroglioma in children: results from the CCG 945 experience. J Neurooncol 2007;83:1.

34. Fulton DS, Urtasun RC, Scott-Brown I, et al. Increasing radiation dose intensity using hyperfractionation in patients with malignant glioma. Final report of a prospective phase I-II dose response study. J Neurooncol 1992;14:63.

35. Packer RJ, Boyett JM, Zimmerman RA, et al. Hyperfractionated radiation therapy (72 Gy) for children with brain stem gliomas. A Childrens Cancer Group Phase I/II Trial. Cancer 1993;72:1414.

36. Sposto R, Ertel IJ, Jenkin RD, et al. The effectiveness of chemotherapy for treatment of high grade astrocytoma in children: results of a randomized trial. A report from the Childrens Cancer Study Group. J Neurooncol 1989;7:165.

37. Stupp R, Dietrich PY, Ostermann Kraljevic S, et al. Promising survival for patients with newly diagnosed glioblastoma multiforme treated with concomitant radiation plus temozolomide followed by adjuvant temozolomide. J Clin Oncol 2002;20:1375.

38. Cohen BH, Zeltzer PM, Boyett JM, et al. Prognostic factors and treatment results for supratentorial primitive neuroectodermal tumors in children using radiation and chemotherapy: a Childrens Cancer Group randomized trial. J Clin Oncol 1995;13:1687.

39. Cohen K, Pollack I, Zhou T, et al. Temozolomide in the treatment of high-grade gliomas in children: a report from the Children's Oncology Group. Neuro Oncol 2011;13:317.

40. Cohen K, Heideman R, Zhou T, et al. Temozolomide in the treatment of children with newly diagnosed diffuse intrinsic pontine gliomas. Neuro Oncol 2011;13:410.

41. Nicholson HS, Kretschmar CS, Krailo M, et al. Phase 2 study of temozolomide in children and adolescents with recurrent central nervous system tumors: a report from the Children's Oncology Group. Cancer 2007;110:1542.

42. Lashford LS, Thiesse P, Jouvet A, et al. Temozolomide in malignant gliomas of childhood: a United Kingdom Children's Cancer Study Group and French Society for Pediatric Oncology Intergroup Study. J Clin Oncol 2002;20:4684.

43. Estlin EJ, Lashford L, Ablett S, et al. Phase I study of temozolomide in paediatric patients with advanced cancer. United Kingdom Children's Cancer Study Group. Br J Cancer 1998;78:652.

44. Grovas AC, Boyett JM, Lindsley K, et al. Regimen-related toxicity of myeloablative chemotherapy with BCNU, thiotepa, and etoposide followed by autologous stem cell rescue for children with newly diagnosed glioblastoma multiforme: report from the Children's Cancer Group. Med Pediatr Oncol 1999;33:83.

45. Massimino M, Gandola L, Luksch R, et al. Sequential chemotherapy, high-dose thiotepa, circulating

progenitor cell rescue, and radiotherapy for child-hood high-grade glioma. Neuro Oncol 2005;7:41.

46. Marachelian A, Butturini A, Finlay J. Myeloablative chemotherapy with autologous hematopoietic pro-genitor cell rescue for childhood central nervous system tumors. Bone Marrow Transplant 2008; 41:167.

47. Wolff J, Driever P, Erdlenbruch B, et al. Intensive chemotherapy improves survival in pediatric high-grade glioma after gross total resection: results of the HIT-GBM-C protocol. Cancer 2010;116:705.

48. Pollack I. Multidisciplinary management of child-hood brain tumors: a review of outcomes, recent advances, and challenges. J Neurosurg Pediatr 2011;8:135.

49. Bax D, Gaspar N, Little S, et al. EGFRvIII deletion mutations in pediatric high-grade glioma and response to targeted therapy in pediatric glioma cell lines. Clin Cancer Res 2009;15:5753.

50. Schiffman J, Hodgson J, VandenBerg S, et al. Onco-genic BRAF mutation with CDKN2A inactivation is characteristic of a subset of pediatric malignant astrocytomas. Cancer Res 2010;70:512.

51. Nicolaides T, Li H, Solomon D, et al. Targeted therapy for BRAFV600E malignant astrocytoma. Clin Cancer Res 2011;17:7595.

52. Flaherty K, Puzanov I, Kim K, et al. Inhibition of mutated, activated BRAF in metastatic melanoma. N Engl J Med 2010;363:809.

53. Gadji M, Crous A, Fortin D, et al. EGF receptor inhib-itors in the treatment of glioblastoma multiform: old clinical allies and newly emerging therapeutic concepts. Eur J Pharmacol 2009;625:23.

54. Pollack IF, Jakacki RI, Blaney SM, et al. Phase I trial of imatinib in children with newly diagnosed brainstem and recurrent malignant gliomas: a Pediatric Brain Tumor Consortium report. Neuro Oncol 2007;9:145.

55. Wolff J, Kortmann R, Wolff B, et al. High dose metho-trexate for pediatric high grade glioma: results of the HIT-GBM-D pilot study. J Neurooncol 2011;102:433.

56. van Vuurden D, Hulleman E, Meijer O, et al. PARP inhibition sensitizes childhood high grade glioma, medulloblastoma and ependymoma to radiation. Oncotarget 2011;2:984.

57. Ardon H, De Vleeschouwer S, Van Calenbergh F, et al. Adjuvant dendritic cell-based tumour vacci-nation for children with malignant brain tumours. Pediatr Blood Cancer 2010;54:519.

58. Hatziagapiou K, Braoudaki M, Karpusas M, et al. Evaluation of antitumor activity of gefitinib in pedi-atric glioblastoma and neuroblastoma cells. Clin Lab 2011;57:781.

Index

Note: Page numbers of article titles are in **boldface** type.

Printed and bound by CPI Group (UK) Ltd, Croydon, CR0 4YY

03/10/2024

01040359-0019